Motivational Interviewing in the Treatment of Psychological Problems

Edited by
HAL ARKOWITZ
HENNY A. WESTRA
WILLIAM R. MILLER
STEPHEN ROLLNICK

THE GUILFORD PRESS
New York   London

© 2008 The Guilford Press
A Division of Guilford Publications, Inc.
72 Spring Street, New York, NY 10012
www.guilford.com

Printed in the United States of America

This book is printed on acid-free paper.

Last digit is print number: 9   8   7   6   5   4   3   2   1

Library of Congress Cataloging-in-Publication Data

Motivational interviewing in the treatment of psychological problems / edited by Hal
Arkowitz ... [et al.].
    p. ; cm. — (Applications of motivational interviewing)
  Includes bibliographical references and index.
  ISBN-13: 978-1-59385-585-7 (hardcover : alk. paper)
  ISBN-10: 1-59385-585-0 (hardcover : alk. paper)
  1. Interviewing in psychiatry. I. Arkowitz, Hal, 1941– II. Series.
  [DNLM: 1. Nondirective Therapy—methods.   2. Interview, Psychological.
3. Mental Disorders—therapy.   4. Motivation. WM 420.5.N8 M918 2008]
  RC480.7.M68 2008
  616.89—dc22
                                                          2007015396

Motivational Interviewing in the Treatment of Psychological Problems

Edited by
HAL ARKOWITZ
HENNY A. WESTRA
WILLIAM R. MILLER
STEPHEN ROLLNICK

THE GUILFORD PRESS
New York   London

© 2008 The Guilford Press
A Division of Guilford Publications, Inc.
72 Spring Street, New York, NY 10012
www.guilford.com

Printed in the United States of America

This book is printed on acid-free paper.

Last digit is print number: 9 8 7 6 5 4 3 2 1

Library of Congress Cataloging-in-Publication Data

Motivational interviewing in the treatment of psychological problems / edited by Hal
Arkowitz ... [et al.].
    p. ; cm. — (Applications of motivational interviewing)
  Includes bibliographical references and index.
  ISBN-13: 978-1-59385-585-7 (hardcover : alk. paper)
  ISBN-10: 1-59385-585-0 (hardcover : alk. paper)
  1. Interviewing in psychiatry. I. Arkowitz, Hal, 1941– II. Series.
  [DNLM: 1. Nondirective Therapy—methods. 2. Interview, Psychological.
3. Mental Disorders—therapy. 4. Motivation. WM 420.5.N8 M918 2008]
  RC480.7.M68 2008
  616.89—dc22

                                   2007015396

About the Editors

Hal Arkowitz, PhD, is Associate Professor of Psychology at the University of Arizona. His main interests are in understanding how people change and why they don't. Dr. Arkowitz has published widely in the areas of anxiety, depression, psychotherapy, and psychotherapy integration. Most recently, he coauthored *Ambivalence in Psychotherapy: Facilitating Readiness to Change* (with David E. Engle; 2006, Guilford Press). Along with Scott O. Lilienfeld, Dr. Arkowitz is a co-columnist for the magazine *Scientific American Mind*. For 10 years, he served as Editor of the *Journal of Psychotherapy Integration*. Since receiving his doctorate, he has also maintained an active clinical practice and values the interplay between research and practice.

Henny A. Westra, PhD, is Associate Professor in the Department of Psychology and the Director of the Anxiety Research Clinic at York University in Toronto. Prior to this, she was the Clinical Director of the Anxiety and Affective Disorders Service at the London Health Sciences Centre. Dr. Westra has published over 30 peer-reviewed articles and book chapters, as well as given over 100 presentations and workshops, on the treatment of anxiety. She has received funding from the National Institute of Mental Health and the Canadian Institutes of Health Research for her research on motivational interviewing, expectations for change, and engagement with treatment.

William R. Miller, PhD, is Emeritus Distinguished Professor of Psychology and Psychiatry at the University of New Mexico. With over 400 publications, including 35 books, Dr. Miller introduced the concept of motivational interviewing in a 1983 article. He was named by the Institute for Scientific Information as one of the world's most cited scientists.

Stephen Rollnick, PhD, is a clinical psychologist and Professor of Health Care Communication in the Department of Primary Care and Public Health, Cardiff University, Wales, United Kingdom. He has published widely on motivational interviewing and health behavior change and has a special interest in challenging consultations in health and social care.

Contributors

Hal Arkowitz, PhD, Department of Psychology, University of Arizona, Tucson, Arizona

Brian L. Burke, PhD, Department of Psychology, Fort Lewis College, Durango, Colorado

Patrick W. Corrigan, PsyD, Institute of Psychology, Illinois Institute of Technology, Chicago, Illinois

Katherine M. Diskin, PhD, Addiction Centre, Foothills Medical Centre, Calgary, Alberta, Canada

David J. A. Dozois, PhD, Department of Psychology, University of Western Ontario, London, Ontario, Canada

Carl Åke Farbring, MA, National Prison and Probation Administration, Stockholm, Sweden

Nancy K. Grote, PhD, School of Social Work, University of Washington, Seattle, Washington

David Hodgins, PhD, Department of Psychology, University of Calgary, Calgary, Alberta, Canada

Wendy R. Johnson, MS, Department of Psychology, University of New Mexico, Albuquerque, New Mexico

Nicholas Maltby, PhD, Anxiety Disorders Center, The Institute of Living, Hartford, Connecticut

Steve Martino, PhD, Department of Psychiatry, Yale University School of Medicine, New Haven, Connecticut, and VA Connecticut Healthcare System, West Haven, Connecticut

Stanley G. McCracken, PhD, School of Social Service Administration, University of Chicago, Chicago, Illinois

William R. Miller, PhD, Department of Psychology, University of New Mexico, Albuquerque, New Mexico

Theresa B. Moyers, PhD, Center on Alcoholism, Substance Abuse, and Addictions, University of New Mexico, Albuquerque, New Mexico

Ronald T. Murphy, PhD, Department of Psychology, Francis Marion University, Florence, South Carolina

Stephen Rollnick, PhD, Department of General Practice, Cardiff University School of Medicine, Cardiff, United Kingdom

Ulrike Schmidt, MD, PhD, Section of Eating Disorders, Institute of Psychiatry, London, United Kingdom

Holly A. Swartz, MD, Department of Psychiatry, Western Psychiatric Institute and Clinic, University of Pittsburgh School of Medicine, Pittsburgh, Pennsylvania

David F. Tolin, PhD, Anxiety Disorders Center, The Institute of Living, Hartford, Connecticut, and Department of Psychiatry, University of Connecticut School of Medicine, Farmington, Connecticut

Janet Treasure, MD, PhD, Department of Academic Psychiatry, Kings College London, London, United Kingdom

Henny A. Westra, PhD, Department of Psychology, York University, Toronto, Ontario, Canada

Harry Zerler, MA, Hunterdon Medical Center, Flemington, New Jersey

Allan Zuckoff, PhD, Department of Psychiatry, Western Psychiatric Institute and Clinic, University of Pittsburgh School of Medicine, Pittsburgh, Pennsylvania

Preface

Motivational interviewing (MI) is an approach to helping people change that was originally developed by William R. Miller and Stephen Rollnick. It has had a tremendous impact on research and practice in the fields of substance abuse and health-related problems in the United States and many other countries.

There are several reasons for its appeal. First, it directly addresses a significant problem common to all therapies: resistance to change. In MI, resistance is seen as a result of ambivalence about change. Its primary goals are to help clients increase their intrinsic motivation and resolve ambivalence in order to facilitate behavior change. Second, it is flexible and can be used as a "stand-alone" approach, in combination with other therapies, or as an adjunct to other therapies. Third, there is a considerable body of research evidence supporting both the efficacy and effectiveness of MI with substance use and health-related problems. Fourth, research has demonstrated that MI is learnable, and achieves significant therapeutic effects in relatively few sessions.

Given all of these appealing features, it is rather surprising that MI has hardly been employed or studied outside of the fields of substance use and health-related problems. There have been some stirrings of interest in the field of psychotherapy. MI has been presented at several symposia and workshops at psychotherapy conferences, and we are aware of several grant applications in preparation or submitted that study MI with different clinical populations.

The time has come for clinical researchers and practitioners to seriously consider MI as a way to increase readiness to change and to enhance treatment outcomes with psychological problems. We hope that this book facilitates this goal. We invited researchers and practitioners who were already exploring MI for a variety of different clinical prob-

lems to contribute chapters describing their work. Each chapter describes the clinical problem and its usual treatments, how MI has been
used, any modifications that were necessary to tailor MI to the problem
and population, detailed clinical case histories, and a summary of relevant research.

This book represents a truly collaborative effort on the part of the
coeditors. Miller and Rollnick, the originators of MI, have done a great
deal of research and clinical work using MI with substance use disorders
and health-related problems. Arkowitz and Westra have done clinical work
and research extending the use of MI to depression and anxiety.

Clinical practitioners from a number of disciplines will find a
wealth of information in this book on clinical applications of MI, along
with numerous case histories and vignettes. Clinical researchers will
find in it a rich source of hypotheses to be tested regarding the efficacy,
effectiveness, and mechanisms of MI. Graduate students in clinical psychology, PsyD, counseling, rehabilitation, and social work programs
will also find this book of interest, as will psychiatry trainees.

One of us (HA) has taught a clinical-research practicum on MI to
clinical psychology graduate students at the University of Arizona for
several years. It has been very positively received by the students,
most of whom said they expected to incorporate it into their work.
Later contacts with those who took the practicum show that, for the
most part, they have. We hope other universities will offer courses
and practica on MI. If so, this book can serve as a text for such offer-
ings, or as supplementary readings in seminars and practica on other
forms of psychotherapy.

Contents

CHAPTER 1

Learning, Applying, and Extending Motivational Interviewing

Hal Arkowitz
William R. Miller

Since the first clinical description of motivational interviewing (MI; Miller, 1983), research and applications have mushroomed. First applied to problem drinking, MI has subsequently been used with a variety of other problems, including drug abuse, gambling, eating disorders, anxiety disorders, chronic disease management, and health-related behaviors. In this chapter, we present an overview of MI, including ways it has been used in clinical practice, outcome research, how it may work, and how clinicians learn it.

MOTIVATION IN CLINICAL PRACTICE AND RESEARCH

For decades, the concept of motivation has played a significant role in research on learning (e.g., Cofer & Apley, 1964; Sorrentino & Higgins, 1996), but it has had surprisingly little impact in the field of psychotherapy. Over two decades ago, Miller (1985) reviewed research relating motivational variables and interventions to treatment entry, compliance, and outcome. His review highlighted the importance of motivational variables in treatment, anticipating the further development of MI (Miller & Rollnick, 1991, 2002).

1

The concept of motivation is particularly useful when psychotherapy clients seem "stuck." The view of most traditional psychotherapy approaches is that "stuckness" represents resistance to change. However, the term "resistance" has a pejorative connotation, implying willful (albeit often unconscious) stubbornness. In addition, each school of psychotherapy has a different view of what constitutes resistance and how to work with it. Using the term "motivation" not only is more respectful, but also it directs therapists toward a more integrated understanding of why clients *do* change and toward ways of facilitating change (Engle & Arkowitz, 2006).

MI works from the assumption that many clients who seek therapy are ambivalent about change and that motivation may ebb and flow during the course of therapy. Therapists therefore should be attuned to such variations, working with them rather than against them.

A central goal of MI is to increase intrinsic motivation to change— that which arises from personal goals and values rather than from such external sources as others' attempts to persuade, cajole, or coerce the person to change. In fact, external pressure to change can create a paradoxical *decrease* in the desire to change. Brehm and Brehm (1981) proposed that an aversive state of reactance arises when people perceive a threat to their personal freedoms. One way that this aversive state can be reduced is by behaving oppositionally when directed to change. Such reactance is less likely to occur when the therapist is supportive rather than directive (Miller, Benefield, & Tonigan, 1993; Patterson & Chamberlin, 1994), making change more likely.

The importance of intrinsic motivation was highlighted in a study by Lepper, Greene, and Nisbett (1973). They observed young children in the classroom to determine which activities the children engaged in on their own without apparent external prompting or incentives. The assumption was that these activities were intrinsically motivated. In a second phase of the study, the experimenters praised each child for engaging in that activity. Contrary to the usual prediction that such reinforcement should increase those behaviors, the investigators found that the preferred behaviors *decreased* when praised. Their interpretation was that external praise undermined intrinsic motivation, since it may have seemed to the children that they were now engaging in the behaviors to please the adult rather than themselves. This in turn may have diminished their interest in engaging in the behaviors. In addition, studies have found that changes attributed to oneself are more likely to endure (cf. Davison, Tsujimoto, & Glaros, 1973; Davison & Valins, 1969) than are those attributed to external sources (e.g., therapist or medication).

MI and the Stages of Change

There is some similarity between MI and the transtheoretical model of Prochaska and his associates (e.g., Prochaska & Norcross, 2004), although they were developed independently. Both assume that people approach change with varying levels of readiness. The transtheoretical model suggests that different stages of change are associated with different degrees of readiness to change, specifically proposing five stages through which people pass: precontemplation, contemplation, preparation, action, and maintenance. There is oscillation rather than smooth progression through these stages. For example, people in the action stage may revert to contemplation for a period of time and from there may either further regress to precontemplation or again move ahead to action. The model describes certain processes of change that are most often used at each stage of change. For example, consciousness raising is commonly used in the precontemplation or contemplation stages, whereas contingency management is used more often in the later action and maintenance stages. Prochaska and Prochaska (1991) suggest that if there is a mismatch between processes and stages (e.g., contingency management in the precontemplation stage), movement through the stages will be impeded and the person will appear resistant or noncompliant.

Ambivalence is regarded as normal both in MI and in the transtheoretical model where it is characteristic of the contemplation stage. People for whom the cons of change outweigh the pros will appear relatively unmotivated to change. When the pros outweigh the cons, the person will be more motivated to change. Casting the issue as ambivalence rather than resistance leads to an examination of each side of the ambivalence and their dynamic relationship to each other. Reasons for not changing are regarded as valid and are considered in the change equation. MI is designed to enhance motivation by resolving ambivalence in the direction of change.

WHAT IS MI?

Miller and Rollnick defined MI as "a client-centered directive method for enhancing intrinsic motivation to change by exploring and resolving ambivalence" (2002, p. 25). It is strongly rooted in the client-centered therapy of Carl Rogers (1951, 1959) in its emphasis on understanding the client's internal frame of reference and present concerns, and in discrepancies between behaviors and values. In both MI and client-centered therapy, the therapist provides the conditions for growth and change by communicating attitudes of accurate empathy and unconditional positive regard.

MI can be thought of as client-centered therapy with a twist. Unlike client-centered therapy, MI has specific goals: to reduce ambivalence about change and to increase intrinsic motivation to change. In this sense, MI is both client-centered and directive. The MI therapist creates an atmosphere in which the client rather than the therapist becomes the main advocate for change as well as the primary agent of change.

The MI spirit, consisting of collaboration, evocation, and autonomy, is central to MI. Without it, one can use MI methods, but it would not be MI. But MI is not defined by the MI spirit alone. In addition to the MI spirit, MI consists of specific principles (express empathy, develop discrepancy, roll with resistance, and support self-efficacy) and methods, the most important of which is to elicit and differentially reinforce change and commitment talk to help resolve ambivalence, increase motivation to change, and promote behavior change.

In their review of outcome research on MI, Burke, Arkowitz, and Menchola (2003) made the rather surprising observation that none of the studies in the literature at the time used a "pure" MI approach. Virtually all published studies had modified the basic MI approach in some ways. Many combined MI with other treatments such as cognitive-behavioral therapies. In the most common adaptation, the client (usually with alcohol or drug problems) is given feedback based on individual results from standardized assessment measures (Miller, Sovereign, & Krege, 1988), a combination now known as motivational enhancement therapy (MET; Miller, Zweben, DiClemente, & Rychtarik, 1992). This feedback, which concerns the client's level of severity on target symptoms as compared to norms, is delivered in a motivational interviewing style. Such feedback is not an integral part of MI (although it might still be very helpful), and less is known about the effects of MI itself without feedback.

Principles and Strategies of MI

Miller and Rollnick (2002) described four basic principles of MI along with specific clinical strategies that are derived from them.

Principle 1: Express Empathy

An empathic therapist strives to experience the world from the client's perspective without judgment or criticism. In doing so, the client's thoughts, feelings, and actions make a great deal more sense. For example, one of us (Hal Arkowitz) worked with a man with uncontrolled life-threatening hypertension. Although in his early 50s and quite aware that he was at high risk for stroke or heart attack, he did not take his medications regularly, nor did he follow his doctor's diet and exercise recommendations. His doctor and his family, seeing his condition from an external frame of reference, couldn't make sense of his actions and kept trying to persuade him to live more healthily. However, when seen from the client's perspective, his actions were more comprehensible. The client reported that his job was "OK," his family was "OK," and his life was "OK." These statements were made in a tone of voice distinctly lacking in energy and enthusiasm. However, when discussing his favorite foods (none of which was healthy for him), he became animated. Eating those foods provided him with the pleasure and zest for life that was lacking in other areas. When the therapist inquired about his medication noncompliance, the client immediately described his elderly parents, who analyzed every morsel of food that they put in their mouths and carefully counted out their pills daily to be sure to take them correctly. The client said: "I don't want to live my life that way; I'd rather go out having a good time than live like them." Seen from his perspective, his behavior made perfect sense.

Empathy involves a nonjudgmental attitude in which the therapist tries to see the world from the client's perspective. It doesn't mean that the therapist condones the behaviors, but neither does it mean that the therapist is disapproving or critical of the choices people make. What it does imply is that the behaviors are more comprehensible when understood from the client's perspective.

Principle 2: Develop Discrepancy

Motivation is a function of the discrepancy between the client's present behaviors and values. Awareness of these discrepancies can increase motivation to change. For example, a drug-dependent person who strongly values being a good parent will experience discomfort when he or she becomes more aware of the discrepancy between drug use and his or her commitment to quality parenting. This discomfort can enhance motivation to change. The MI therapist reflects discrepancies between behaviors and values to the client in order to accomplish this. In MI, the therapist pays particular attention to the client's arguments for change, compared to his or her arguments for not changing. The therapist differentially elicits and explores the client's own arguments for change as a path out of ambivalence.

Principle 3: Roll with Resistance

In MI, resistance to change is viewed as a normal and expected part of the change process and a valuable source of information about the client's experience rather than an obstacle to be overcome. Ambivalence illuminates the client's hopes, desires, and fears. Clients may see the advantages of changing and also have concerns about changing that may include fear of failure, fear of the demands and responsibilities they believe will occur if they do change, or apprehension that change will confront them with the unknown and unpredictable.

In MI, the therapist strives to understand and respect both sides of the ambivalence from the client's perspective. When arguments against change arise, they are met with empathy and acceptance. It can be a profound experience for clients to talk about the *advantages* of having the problem and to find the therapist listening and responding compassionately without becoming an advocate for change. Rolling with resistance tends to defuse rather than amplify it.

Principle 4: Support Self-Efficacy

In MI, the therapist supports the client's self-efficacy, the belief that he or she can carry out the necessary actions and succeed in changing. People often have the knowledge and resources to make desired changes once they have decided to do so. If not, the therapist acts as a consultant or guide, suggesting possible ways to proceed. However, in MI, the client remains the final arbiter of the change process.

Basic Skills of MI

Miller and Rollnick (2002) have described a number of foundational skills that are consistent with the principles discussed above. They divided MI into two phases. In the first, the client is ambivalent about change, and motivation may be insufficient to accomplish change. Accordingly, the goals in this phase are to resolve ambivalence and build intrinsic motivation to change. The second phase begins with the client showing signs of readiness to change, such as increased talk about change, questions about change, and envisioning of a future that includes the desired changes. In this phase, the focus shifts to strengthening the commitment to change and helping the client develop and implement a change plan.

Several of the MI skills come directly from Rogers's (1951) client-centered therapy include *asking open-ended questions, listening reflec-*

tively, affirming, and *summarizing.* However, one method—*eliciting change talk*—is intentionally directive and specific to MI.

Ask Open-Ended Questions

In MI, the client should do most of the talking, and open-ended questions are used to achieve this goal. Through the use of selective open-ended questions and reflections, the therapist focuses the client on those areas that seem important for working with ambivalence and change.

Listen Reflectively

Reflective listening is probably the single most important skill in MI. Miller and Rollnick suggested that "The essence of a reflective listening response is that it makes a guess as to what the speaker means" (2002, p. 69). People don't always clearly express what they mean. They may not verbalize their true meanings because of fears, concerns, lack of awareness of what they mean, or simply not being able to find the proper words to convey their experience. Reflective listening helps them verbalize their meanings and make them more explicit. Table 1.1 illustrates various levels of reflection.

Many therapists learn about reflective listening as part of their early training in basic interviewing skills. It is easy to underestimate the difficulty of skillful empathic reflection. High-quality reflective listening is a core MI skill for increasing motivation and commitment to change. A majority of the MI therapist's utterances are reflective guesses about the client's meaning. Our experience in teaching MI to novices as well as experienced professionals is that it is initially quite difficult for them to rely primarily on empathic reflection without also relating in ways that impose an external frame of reference.

Affirm

In order to encourage and support the client during the change process, the MI therapist frequently affirms the client in the form of statements of appreciation or understanding. Some simple examples of affirmations are "It took courage to do that" or "That's a really good idea."

Summarize

Summaries play an important role throughout MI sessions. Not only do they show that the therapist has been listening, but also they link mate-

TABLE 1.1. Levels of Reflection in Motivational Interviewing

Client statement

"Even though nothing has happened, I've been feeling more depressed lately."

	Definition	Example of response
Repeat	Repeating an element of what the speaker said.	*"You've been more depressed lately."*
Rephrase	Staying close to what the speaker has said with some rephrasing and synonyms	*"So your sadness is getting worse and you don't know why."*
Paraphrase	Inferring or guessing at the meaning of what the speaker has said and reflecting this back	*"You would like to understand why your mood changes like that."*
Reflect feeling	Emphasizing the emotional dimension through feeling statements and metaphors	*"It's scary not to be able to understand your depressed feelings."*

rial together and can help emphasize certain points. Summaries are particularly used to collect and reinforce "change talk," the client's own statements of motivations for change.

Elicit Change Talk

While the four methods discussed above are basic to MI, they don't necessarily provide the client with a way out of their ambivalence. One could simply go around in circles by asking, reflecting, affirming, and summarizing. In the fifth method, eliciting change talk, the therapist intentionally elicits change talk without becoming an advocate for change. Change talk consists of statements reflecting desire, perceived ability, need, readiness, reasons, or commitment to change. Amrhein, Miller, Yahne, Palmer, and Fulcher (2003) found that statements reflecting commitment to change were the strongest predictors of outcome in therapy for drug use. The MI therapist asks open questions to elicit change talk, explores and reflects what the client offers, and provides summaries that collect change-talk themes.

Working with Ambivalence

All of the strategies discussed above are used to work with ambivalence. Two-sided reflections may be used to highlight the client's dilemma, such as: "So, part of you feels like you really want to end the relationship, and another part feels unsure whether that's the right thing for you to do." Periodic summaries are helpful to collect and reinforce change talk.

When the therapist senses that the client may be leaning toward a resolution of the ambivalence, an open question such as "What are you thinking you'll do at this point?" might be used. The client may respond with some openness to action or may signal that they don't know if they're ready to do anything yet. In the latter case, the therapist returns to Phase 1 strategies for working with ambivalence until it's appropriate to test the waters again.

Phase 2 MI: Commitment and Action

This phase of MI involves developing a change plan and strengthening the client's commitment to it. Miller and Rollnick (2002) discuss signs of readiness that suggest that the client is entering Phase 2. These include:

- Decreased resistance to change.
- Decreased discussion about the problem and a feeling of waiting for the next step.
- A sense of resolution in which the client may seem more relaxed and unburdened about the problem.
- Increased change talk.
- Increased questions about change.
- Greater envisioning a future that includes the changes.
- Experimenting with possible change actions between sessions.

We should note that people will often vacillate in their degree of motivation and ambivalence. As Mahoney (1991) has suggested, change is best described as an oscillating process.

Furthermore, change is seldom unidimensional. Most people who seek therapy have more than one problem or are weighing change at various levels. For example, depression is often accompanied by relationship problems and substance abuse. There may be different degrees of motivation for change in these different problem areas. In addition, Arkowitz and Burke (Chapter 6, this volume) and Zuckoff, Swartz, and Grote (Chapter 5, this volume) distinguish between motivation to change the overall problem (e.g., anxiety) and motivation to engage in the actions necessary to accomplish the change (e.g., exposure). A person highly motivated to decrease distress may nevertheless be unwilling to pursue a particular strategy for doing so. There may be ambivalence about one or both of these.

The MI style encourages a change plan that comes primarily from the client rather than the therapist. The therapist may encourage the client to think about change with questions like "How do you think you can make that happen?" At times, clients may be motivated to change but may not know what they need to do in order to accomplish the change (e.g., to reduce panic attacks). At such times, the therapist's expertise is a useful and necessary part of therapy. The issue isn't whether or not advice and suggestions are offered but *how and when* they are offered. In MI, this input is given by a therapist who takes the role of guide or change consultant. A guide doesn't decide when or where you should go, but instead helps you get to where you want to go. If the client wishes, the therapist may make suggestions about how to proceed, but does so tentatively and with the attitude that the client will choose those options that fit best at that point. For example, a therapist might say the following to a client who appears ready to change but doesn't know how to do it: "I have some thoughts about approaches that have been helpful for other people with a similar problem. Would you be interested in hearing them?" In this way, the therapist conveys respect for clients' ability to choose what's best for them, while being ready to provide input to facilitate change.

Varieties of MI in Clinical Practice

MI can be used as a "stand-alone" treatment like other therapeutic approaches. Even relatively brief exposure to stand-alone MI (one to four sessions) can lead to significant change (Hettema, Miller, & Steele, 2005). For example, in a major comparative outcome study on the treatment of alcohol dependence (Project Match Research Group, 1997), clients receiving 4 sessions of motivational enhancement therapy fared as well on measures of percentage of days abstinent and drinks per drinking day during the 1-year posttreatment period as those receiving 12 sessions of cognitive-behavioral or 12-step treatments. Since MI specifically focuses on motivation, it also has the potential to act as a catalyst to other therapeutic approaches. In fact, it has been used in conjunction with other therapies as a pretreatment, adjunct, or else combined and integrated with other therapies.

MI has been used successfully as a pretreatment to enhance motivation in subsequent treatment. Meta-analyses of MI have found larger effect sizes (Burke et al., 2003) and longer-lasting results (Hettema et al., 2005) for MI as a pretreatment than when used as a stand-alone.

Furthermore, Connors, Walitzer, and Dermen (2002) found that an MI pretreatment was more effective in enhancing the effects of cognitive-behavior therapy for alcoholism than a role induction pretreatment originally developed by Jerome Frank (1974) and his associates. The role induction interviewer discussed the rationale of the therapy with the client and the expectations of the client and therapist in the therapy process. MI pretreatments have also improved treatment outcomes in more directive inpatient (Brown & Miller, 1993) and outpatient (Bien, Miller, & Boroughs, 1993) programs. It may be that, once there is sufficient intrinsic motivation to change, people can make use of a directive program because they are less resistant to change.

Arkowitz and Westra (2005) have discussed another use of MI in clinical practice. It involves shifting to MI during the course of another treatment in order to better address emergent ambivalence and resistance. MI may be integrated into another therapy by having the therapist use MI at any point in the sessions when low motivation or ambivalence is encountered. In addition, the therapist can shift into MI style (often sharing with the client that they are doing so) for a series of sessions specifically focused on working on ambivalence. Since MI removes the pressure for change, it might liberate individuals to explore the factors inhibiting change. The multisite COMBINE study similarly tested a combination of cognitive-behavior therapy for alcohol dependence with the overall clinical style of MI (Miller, 2004), finding it to be more effective than placebo and comparable to naltrexonepharmacotherapy within the context of medical monitoring (Anton et al., 2006).

Relationship of MI to Other Psychotherapies

As discussed earlier, MI is more of a way of being with people than it is another "school" of therapy. Yet, as in other types of psychotherapy, the goal is to facilitate therapeutic change. In this section, we will compare and contrast MI with other psychotherapies and briefly discuss how MI can be used in conjunction with these other therapies.

While MI is strongly rooted in Carl Rogers's client-centered therapy, it also shares similarities with other therapeutic approaches. MI and psychoanalytic therapies view ambivalence and resistance as providing meaningful information that can be used productively in therapy. However, they differ sharply in the types of information that they consider important and how they work with ambivalence. In psychoanalytic theories, ambivalence is usually thought of as conflict, usually unconscious, between parts of the personality. In a psychodynamic view, ambivalence provides information about repressed conflicts that are carried over from the past as well as threats to a stable self-image, pathogenic beliefs, fear of change, and secondary gain. By contrast, MI is very much in the here and now, without a priori views about why resistance and ambivalence occur. Ambivalence and resistance are not seen as pathological. In MI, what is important is to understand the client's perspective on the pros or cons of changing.

In cognitive-behavioral therapy (CBT), resistance and ambivalence are not given any special status. Nonetheless, some behavior therapists (e.g., Patterson & Forgatch, 1985) and cognitive-behavioral therapists (e.g., Leahy, 2002) have addressed resistance. Behavior therapy, which was the precursor of CBT, attributed resistance to the therapist's inadequate conceptualization of the conditions that control the behaviors. Cognitive therapists (e.g., Beck, Rush, Shaw, & Emery, 1979) regard resistance as providing information about a client's distorted thinking and beliefs. For example, when a depressed client in cognitive therapy doesn't comply with homework assignments, cognitive therapists search for the beliefs and schemas that may cause such resistance, such as pessimism about change.

In contrast to MI, CBT is a fairly didactic approach that emphasizes teaching clients new behaviors and ways to correct dysfunctional beliefs. The use of the phrase "homework assignments" in CBT highlights the role of therapist as more of a teacher in the change enterprise. The CBT therapist is regarded as an expert who can provide direction for the client in facilitating change. By contrast, MI involves more of an equal partnership than an expert–patient relationship.

MI has the potential for enhancing the effectiveness of CBT and other therapies. For example, Arkowitz (2002), Engle and Arkowitz (2006), and Miller (1988) have discussed how CBT can be conducted in the context of the MI spirit. Strategies of both CBT and psychoanalytic therapies (such as structuring between-session activities in the former and giving interpretations in the latter) can be conducted in the context of a relationship that is more consistent with MI rather than in a manner that is more expert-driven. Potentially, using an MI style can reduce resistance and defensiveness and encourage internal attributions for change. As a result, MI has the potential to enhance the outcomes of other therapies.

HOW EFFECTIVE IS MI?

How well does MI work, for what, and for whom? Across three decades, a large body of research has accumulated to answer these questions. We summarize this literature here in three sections: (1) the efficacy of MI in clinical trials; (2) the relative efficacy of MI when compared with other approaches; and (3) studies of clinical effectiveness—how well the method holds up in community practice, outside the controlled conditions of clinical research. The MI website includes a cumulative bibliography of this literature (see *www.motivationalinterview.org*).

Efficacy Trials

Many consider the randomized clinical trial to be the gold standard in demonstrating treatment efficacy. Participants in such trials agree to be randomly assigned to receive or not receive the treatment being tested. People in the comparison condition may receive no treatment, treatment as usual, or a different type of treatment. As we completed this chapter, more than 100 randomized clinical trials of MI had been published, along with a number of reviews summarizing research findings (Britt, Hudson, & Blampied, 2004; Burke et al., 2003; Dunn, Deroo, & Rivara, 2001; Hettema et al., 2005; Moyer, Finney, Swearingen, & Vergun, 2002; Rubak, Sandbaek, Lauritzen, & Christensen, 2005).

Several general conclusions can be drawn from this literature. There is strong evidence that MI can be effective in triggering change. A large number of studies show significantly greater behavior change by people who received MI, relative to those not receiving MI. At the same time, it is clear that MI does not always work, and its effectiveness has varied across studies, locations, counselors, and clients. In the sections that follow we will consider possible reasons why MI may work in some contexts and not others.

The impact of MI may vary, depending on the type of problem being addressed. Figure 1.1 shows the average effect sizes of MI with different target problems, based on research to date (Hettema et al., 2005), at shorter intervals (up to 3 months) and all follow-ups combined (up to 12 months or longer). In general, MI yields significant effect sizes that by statistical standards would be called small (0.3) to medium (0.5), although there are some large effects (≥ 0.70) as well. Most of the effects are largest within the first few months after MI and tend to decrease over time. Usually this is not due to a decrease in the impact of MI but to the fact that the comparison groups catch up, showing more change over time (consistent with results from other psychotherapy studies). An interesting exception is that MI continues to show a sizable effect (0.6) that holds up over time when MI is added to another treatment (Hettema et al., 2005). MI and other treatment methods seem to

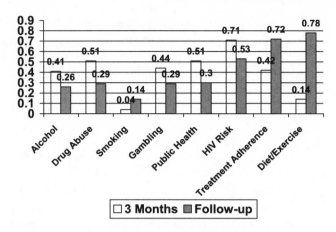

FIGURE 1.1. Average effect size (*d*) of motivational interviewing.

have a synergistic effect, each reinforcing the impact of the other. It appears that MI may increase the efficacy of other methods by enhancing treatment adherence.

Relative Efficacy of MI

What happens when MI is compared directly with other treatment methods? Here, MI is not added to another approach, but instead clients are assigned at random to receive MI or a different treatment. Across studies, people receiving MI tend to show more change relative to those given educational, didactic, or persuasive interventions. When MI is compared with other active treatment approaches (such as CBT), outcomes tend to be similar, with MI achieving its effects in fewer sessions (Hodgins, Currie, & el-Guebaly, 2001; Marijuana Treatment Project Research Group, 2004; Project MATCH Research Group, 1997).

Clinical Effectiveness

Most though not all (Miller, Yahne, & Tonigan, 2003) published studies show significant positive effects of MI on behavior change under the highly controlled conditions of a randomized clinical trial. This does not guarantee effectiveness when MI is applied by frontline clinicians under ordinary conditions of community practice with diverse populations. Nevertheless, several aspects of the clinical trial literature are encouraging in this regard (Hettema et al., 2005). MI has shown efficacy across a wide range of target problems, populations, providers, and nations. U.S. studies of MI with ethnic minority populations have shown, on average, substantially *larger* effects than those with primarily white Anglo-American populations. MI may offer advantages in cross-cultural counseling, particularly because of the therapist's focus on understanding the client's unique context and perspective. Furthermore, studies in which clinicians delivered manual-guided MI showed *smaller* effects than those observed when MI did not follow the constrained guidelines of a manual (Hettema et al., 2005). This is consistent with an emphasis on the overall approach or spirit of MI rather than on specific techniques, and manuals run the risk of decreasing therapist flexibility in a way that disadvantages effective use of the method. In any event, across multiple trials these findings indicate that MI may be used with a variety of groups and problems and does not require the structure of a procedural manual and adherence monitoring.

Several large studies of MI in treating drug abuse are being conducted within the national Clinical Trials Network (CTN) created and coordinated by the National Institute on Drug Abuse. CTN trials are conducted in frontline community programs, with study treatments delivered by the regular clinical staff to ordinary clients of the agency. The first of these to be completed (Carroll et al., 2006) evaluated the impact of a single 20-minute segment of MI delivered within the programs' normal intake interviews. Consistent with prior trials (Hettema et al., 2005), clients given MI attended significantly more subsequent treatment sessions, compared with those receiving normal intake procedures. Other studies have demonstrated significant clinical benefits of MI when delivered by frontline providers for problems including alcohol (Senft, Polen, Freeborn, & Hollis, 1997) and drug abuse (Marijuana Treatment Project Research Group, 2004), hypertension (Woollard et al., 1995), and health promotion (Resnicow et al., 2001; Thevos, Quick, & Yanduli, 2000).

HOW DOES MI WORK?

When the effectiveness of a therapy varies across providers and programs, it suggests the need to understand the critical elements that contribute to its effects. One component of MI regarded by its progenitors (Miller & Rollnick, 2002) as central to its efficacy is the therapist quality of *accurate empathy* (Rogers, 1959; Truax & Carkhuff, 1967). Sometimes misunderstood as having had similar life experience, accurate empathy actually refers to a learnable clinical skill for identifying and reflecting the client's own experiencing. In research preceding the introduction of MI, therapist interpersonal skill in this domain was found to be related to subsequent client change (Miller, Taylor, & West, 1980; Truax & Carkhuff, 1967; Valle, 1981).

As practiced within MI, accurate empathy blends with other interpersonal skill components to comprise an underlying MI spirit, assessed by global ratings of clinician–client interactions (Baer et al., 2004; Miller & Mount, 2001). Observers' ratings of clinicians on this global scale predict more favorable client responses during an MI session (Moyers, Miller, & Hendrickson, 2005) as well as better client outcomes (Miller, Taylor, & West, 1980). Thus there seems to be an interpersonal quality of relationship that contributes to the effectiveness of MI, characterized by collaboration, respect for client autonomy, and evocation of the client's own wisdom and resources (Rollnick & Miller, 1995).

Consistent with this approach, Miller (1983) hypothesized that MI would work by causing clients to verbalize their own arguments for change. Client ambivalence is resolved in the direction of change as clients express aloud the disadvantages of the status quo and the advantages of change and the ability and intention to change (Miller & Rollnick, 1991). Such client statements came to be termed "change talk," and the strategic eliciting of client change talk differentiated MI from more general client-centered counseling (Miller & Rollnick, 2002).

It follows that client change talk during MI sessions should predict the probability of subsequent behavior change. Testing this hypothesis, psycholinguist Paul Amrhein differentiated change talk into statements of desire, ability, reasons, need, and commitment to change. In a study of MI with drug abuse (Miller et al., 2003), he found that only client commitment statements ("I will . . .") predicted abstinence from drugs. Verbalizing the other four types of change talk—desire ("I want to . . ."), ability ("I could . . ."), reasons ("I should because . . ."), and need ("I have to . . .")—led to increasing strength of commitment, which in turn presaged behavior change. These findings parallel the above-mentioned differentiation of MI into two phases (Miller & Rollnick, 1991, 2002). In the first phase the goal is *enhancing motivation for change* by exploring desire, ability, and the reasons and need for change from the client's perspective. Phase 2 follows naturally and focuses on *strengthening commitment to change.*

In contrast, client speech that defends the status quo ("sustain talk") predicts a lack of subsequent change (Amrhein et al., 2003; Miller et al., 1993). The more a client argues against change, the less likely it is to happen. This is not particularly surprising in itself ("Resistant clients don't change"). The implications for practice come from findings that the degree of client resistance is strongly influenced by the clinician's own counseling style (Miller et al., 1993; Patterson & Forgatch, 1985).

Understanding the mechanisms underlying MI still remains a challenge. Our current understanding of how MI works is this: if the clinician counsels in a way that elicits the client's resistance and defense of the status quo, change is unlikely to follow; if, on the other hand, the clinician provides accurate empathy and counsels in a way that elicits the client's own motivations, commitment to change strengthens and behavior change often follows. A more complex question would be "Why or under what conditions does commitment talk lead to change?"

Are there clients for whom MI is particularly indicated or contraindicated? Here the evidence base is thin, but a trend is apparent. The more resistant (oppositional, angry) a client, the greater seems to be the advantage of MI relative to more prescriptive approaches (e.g., Babor & DelBoca, 2003). MI was specifically developed for clients who are ambivalent and less ready to proceed with change. Conversely, MI is unnecessary and may be counterproductive for people who are ready and *eager* for change. If a client is already champing at the bit to take action and finds a recommended approach acceptable, why spend time contemplating the pros and cons of doing so?

HOW DO CLINICIANS LEARN MI?

Understanding how and why a treatment method works is helpful in knowing how to help clinicians learn it. This section focuses on what is known about how counselors learn the method of MI.

Eight Skills in Learning MI

Miller and Moyers (2006) have described eight skills by which clinicians acquire proficiency in MI. The first of these involves at least openness to the underlying assumptions and spirit of the method: a collaborative rather than prescriptive approach, eliciting motivation from the client rather than trying to install it, and honoring client autonomy rather than taking a more prescriptive or confrontational stance. Internalization of this overall spirit increases with practice, but one is un-likely to learn MI (or want to) without first being willing to entertain the feasibility of this approach. Learning MI is, in our experience, par-ticularly difficult for those with a directive-expert perspective on the helping process.

A next task, and a challenging one in itself, is to develop profi-ciency in the interpersonal skills of client-centered counseling, particu-larly accurate empathy. A skillful clinician makes reflective listening look easy, but it is a proficiency that is developed and honed over years of practice. To take the next steps in MI, the clinician needs skill and comfort in forming accurate reflections that move the client forward, encouraging continued exploration.

MI differs from client-centered counseling, particularly in its focus on ambivalence and in particular on change talk. A third skill in learn-ing MI, then, is for the counselor to learn to recognize change talk when hearing it and to distinguish it from other forms of client speech. Amrheim's recent work also suggests the need to differentiate commit-ment language from other forms of change talk, because the former is an especially important predictor of change (Amrhein, Miller, Yahne, Knupsky, & Hochstein, 2004).

Being able to recognize change talk, the clinician next learns how to elicit and reinforce it. In other words, the counselor employs specific strategies to evoke change talk and responds differentially in order to increase and strengthen it. This is linked to a fifth skill, namely, learning how to counsel in a manner that minimizes resistance and how to re-spond to clients' "sustain talk" so as not to increase it.

The exploration of client ambivalence can continue almost indefi-nitely, and there is another skill in knowing when the client is ready to discuss a change plan. Helping clients to formulate change plans repre-sents a sixth skill in learning MI. Prematurely pursuing a change plan, however, can elicit resistance and actually backfire, increasing client commitment to the status quo. In MI, the change-planning process con-tinues to be one of negotiation. With a change plan developed, the counselor must still enlist client commitment to the plan—a seventh task in acquiring MI skillfulness.

Finally, there is the skill of flexibly blending MI with other thera-peutic methods. MI was never intended to be a comprehensive treat-ment, displacing all others. In fact, some of its most consistent beneficial effects are in combination with other forms of treatment. Counselors who develop a high level of skill in MI sometimes have difficulty switching back and forth flexibly with other styles when needed. There is an art to smooth transitioning from MI to a more prescriptive or didactic approach (Rollnick, Miller, & Butler, in press).

Initial Training

From the foregoing set of skills, it is apparent that there is only so much a practitioner could learn from a one-time workshop on MI. Even a 2- to 3-day initial workshop led by a proficient MI trainer is likely to provide only an introduction to the basic style and spirit of MI, first steps toward learning reflective listening, and an ability to recognize change talk. A workshop is not the means but rather only the *beginning* of learning MI. Some ambitious learning goals for a 2-day introductory workshop include:

1. To understand the underlying spirit and approach of MI.
2. To recognize reflective listening responses and differentiate them from other counseling responses.
3. To be able to provide at least 50% reflective listening responses during a conversation.
4. To recognize change talk and be able to differentiate commitment language from other types of change talk.
5. To list and demonstrate several different strategies for eliciting client change talk.

A workshop without follow-up, however, is unlikely to make a significant difference in practice. Although, as indicated above, clinicians may be able to demonstrate some skills on demand after an introductory workshop, the effects on ongoing practice are minimal (Miller & Mount, 2001). More tellingly, there tends to be no change in how clients respond to their therapists (e.g., change talk) after a workshop (Miller, Yahne, Moyers, Martinez, & Pirritano, 2004).

What does seem to help in initially learning MI is a combination of ongoing feedback and coaching. This is sensible in that these two components—personal feedback and performance coaching—are helpful in learning most any new skill. To yield a significant gain in clinical skill in MI, an introductory workshop should be followed by some ongoing individual feedback on actual practice and coaching for performance improvement (Miller et al., 2004). Graduate training affords an opportunity for such ongoing shaping of clinical skillfulness. For example, the University of Arizona clinical psychology graduate program currently offers a year-long practicum on MI that involves lectures and discussion, demonstrations, role-playing exercises, and ongoing supervision of clinical cases referred from the community.

Continuing to Learn

Excellent introductory training in MI, even with a few months of coaching support, still constitutes only an introduction to the clinical method. (Imagine a 2-day workshop to learn psychoanalysis, tennis, piano, or chess!) The real learning is in doing, and that requires ongoing practice with feedback.

As it turns out, the needed feedback is built into the process of MI and depends on knowing what to watch for. In response to a good reflective listening statement, the person keeps talking, reveals a bit more, explores a little further. The very process of reflective listening helps the counselor improve, because clients continually provide corrective feedback. In response to a reflection, a client basically says "Yes" or "No," "Yes, that's right," or "No, that's not quite what I meant," and in either case tends to continue the story and elaborate. This is feedback that is just as reliable as where the golf ball goes after it is hit.

Similarly, once one knows the sequence of client language in successful MI, there is immediate feedback as to how sessions are going. Counselor responses that lead to change talk are the "right stuff." In essence, client change talk becomes a reinforcer for counselor behavior. Counselors also learn what responses evoke sustain talk and resistance. In essence, client sustain talk or resistance serves as an immediate signal not to repeat that response but to try another approach. In this way, clients become teachers, offering ongoing information—much as archers receive immediate feedback after each arrow shot in target practice.

There are other possible aids to continued learning of MI beyond the feedback provided by clients themselves. Videotapes of simulated encounters have been developed to which clinicians can generate responses and receive feedback (e.g., Rosengren, Baer, Hartzler, Dunn, & Wells, 2005). Recording and listening to one's own sessions can be helpful, particularly if using a structured analytic coding system such as the MI Skill Code (MISC; Moyers, Martin, Catley, Harris, & Ahluwalia, 2003) or MI Treatment Integrity code (MITI; Moyers, Martin, Manuel, Hendrickson, & Miller, 2005). Such session tapes can also be reviewed by a supervisor whose task it is to help clinicians develop skill in MI. Some clinicians form peer supervision groups to review session tapes and discuss ongoing challenges in applying MI.

CONCLUSIONS

1. In its relatively brief life to date, MI has made significant impacts on research and practice for helping people change. It has already demonstrated reasonable effectiveness in treating drug and alcohol problems as well as a number of problematic health and lifestyle behaviors.

2. Research is needed to identify those problems and types of people who respond best to MI and those for whom it may be less appropriate.

3. The time is ripe to examine its utility with other clinical problems such as anxiety, depression, eating disorders, and other clinical problems that bring people to seek psychotherapy. In this regard, MI has potential not only as a stand-alone treatment but also as an approach that can be combined (e.g., as prelude) or integrated with other effective therapeutic approaches like CBT. A meta-analysis of treatments (primarily CBT) for depression and some anxiety disorders by Westen and Morrison (2001) has revealed considerable efficacy, with one-half to two-thirds of clients showing significant improvement. However, there is considerable room for improvement when one considers those who drop out, that many of those who are improved still have the problem, and the relatively high relapse rates. Using MI as a prelude, as Westra and Dozois (2006) have done, using MI along with CBT and other treatments, or doing established treatments in the "MI spirit" all have the potential to improve upon these results.

4. Some promising starts have been made in understanding the mechanisms underlying MI, but we still have a long way to go. The more clearly we can identify those factors that most account for the effectiveness of MI, the more we can modify it for greater effectiveness.

5. We also need more research on the most effective methods to teach MI.

REFERENCES

Amrhein, P. C., Miller, W. R., Yahne, C., Knupsky, A., & Hochstein, D. (2004). Strength of client commitment language improves with therapist training in motivational interviewing. *Alcoholism: Clinical and Experimental Research, 28*(5), 74A.

Amrhein, P. C., Miller, W. R., Yahne, C. E., Palmer, M., & Fulcher, L. (2003). Client commitment language during motivational interviewing predicts drug use outcome. *Journal of Consulting and Clinical Psychology, 71*, 862–878.

Anton, R. F., O'Malley, S. S., Ciraulo, D. A., Cisler, R. A., Couper, D., Donovan, D. M., et al. (2006). Combined pharmacotherapies and behavioral interventions for alcohol dependence. The COMBINE study: A randomized controlled trial. *Journal of the American Medical Association, 295,* 2003–2017.

Arkowitz, H. (2002). An integrative approach to psychotherapy based on common processes of change. In J. Lebow (Ed.), *Comprehensive handbook of psychotherapy: Vol. 4, Integrative and eclectic therapies* (pp. 317–337). New York: Wiley.

Arkowitz, H., & Westra, H. (2004). Integrating motivational interviewing and cognitive behavioral therapy in the treatment of depression and anxiety. *Journal of Cognitive Psychotherapy, 18,* 337–350.

Babor, T. F., & DelBoca, F. K. (2003). *Treatment matching in alcoholism.* Cambridge, UK: Cambridge University Press.

Baer, J. S., Rosengren, D. B., Dunn, C. W., Wells, W. A., Ogle, R. L., & Hartzler, B. (2004). An evaluation of workshop training in motivational interviewing for addiction and mental health clinicians. *Drug and Alcohol Dependence, 73*(1), 99–106.

Beck, A. T., Rush, A. J., Shaw, B. E., & Emery, G. (1979). *Cognitive therapy of depression.* New York: Guilford Press.

Bien, T. H., Miller, W. R., & Boroughs, J. M. (1993). Motivational interviewing with alcohol outpatients. *Behavioural and Cognitive Psychotherapy, 21,* 347–356.

Brehm, S. S., & Brehm, J. W. (1981). *Psychological reactance: A theory of freedom and control.* New York: Academic Press.

Britt, E., Hudson, S. M., & Blampied, N. M. (2004). Motivational interviewing in health settings: A review. *Patient Education and Counseling, 53*(2), 147–155.

Brown, J. M., & Miller, W. R. (1993). Impact of motivational interviewing on participation and outcome in residential alcoholism treatment. *Psychology of Addictive Behaviors, 7,* 211–218.

Burke, B., Arkowitz, H., & Menchola, M. (2003). The efficacy of motivational interviewing: A meta-analysis of controlled clinical trials. *Journal of Consulting and Clinical Psychology, 71,* 843–861.

Carroll, K. M., Ball, S. A., Nich, C., Martino, S., Frankforter, T. L., Farentinos, C., et al. (2006). Motivational interviewing to improve treatment engagement and outcome in individuals seeking treatment for substance abuse: A multisite effectiveness study. *Drug and Alcohol Dependence, 81,* 301–312.

Cofer, C. N., & Apley, M. H. (1964). *Motivation.* New York: Wiley.

Connors, G. J., Walitzer, K. S., & Dermen, K. H. (2002). Preparing clients for alcoholism treatment: Effects on treatment participation and outcomes. *Journal of Consulting and Clinical Psychology, 70,* 1161–1169.

Davison, G. C., Tsujimoto, R. N., & Glaros, A. G. (1973) Attribution and the maintenance of behavior change in falling asleep. *Journal of Abnormal Psychology, 82,* 124–133.

Davison, G. C., & Valins, S. (1969). Maintenance of self-attributed and drug-attributed behavior change. *Journal of Personality and Social Psychology, 11,* 25–33.

Dunn, C., Deroo, L., & Rivara, F. P. (2001). The use of brief interventions adapted from motivational interviewing across behavioral domains: A systematic review. *Addiction, 96,* 1725–1742.

Engle, D. E., & Arkowitz, H. (2006). *Ambivalence in psychotherapy: Facilitating readiness to change.* New York: Guilford Press.

Frank, J. (1974). Therapeutic components of psychotherapy: A 25-year progress report of research. *Journal of Nervous and Mental Disease, 159,* 325–342.

Hettema, J., Steele, J., & Miller, W. R. (2005). Motivational interviewing. *Annual Review of Clinical Psychology, 1,* 91–111.

Hodgins, D. C., Currie, S. R., & el-Guebaly, N. (2001). Motivational enhancement and self-help treatments for problem gambling. *Journal of Consulting and Clinical Psychology, 69,* 50–57.

Leahy, R. L. (2002). *Overcoming resistance in cognitive therapy.* New York: Guilford Press.

Lepper, M. R., Greene, D., & Nisbett, R. E. (1973). Undermining children's intrinsic interests with extrinsic reward: A test of the "overjustification" hypothesis. *Journal of Personality and Social Psychology, 28,* 129–137.

Mahoney, M. J. (2001). *Human change processes.* New York: Basic Books.

Marijuana Treatment Project Research Group. (2004). Brief treatments for cannabis dependence: Findings from a randomized multisite trial. *Journal of Consulting and Clinical Psychology, 72,* 455–466.

Miller, W. R. (1983). Motivational interviewing with problem drinkers. *Behavioural Psychotherapy, 11,* 147–172.

Miller, W. R. (1985). Motivation for treatment: A review with special emphasis on alcoholism. *Psychological Bulletin, 98,* 84–107.

Miller, W. R. (1988). Including clients' spiritual perspectives in cognitive behavior therapy. In W. R. Miller & J. E. Martin (Eds.), *Behavior therapy and religion: Integrating spiritual and behavioral approaches to change* (pp. 43–55). Newbury Park, CA: Sage.

Miller, W. R. (Ed.). (2004). *Combined Behavioral Intervention manual: A clinical research guide for therapists treating people with alcohol abuse and dependence* (COMBINE Monograph Series, Vol. 1; DHHS No. 04-5288). Bethesda, MD: National Institute on Alcohol Abuse and Alcoholism.

Miller, W. R., Benefield, R. G., & Tonigan, J. S. (1993). Enhancing motivation for change in problem drinking: A controlled comparison of two therapist styles. *Journal of Consulting and Clinical Psychology, 61,* 455–461.

Miller, W. R., & Mount, K. A. (2001). A small study of training in motivational interviewing: Does one workshop change clinician and client behavior? *Behavioural and Cognitive Psychotherapy, 29,* 457–471.

Miller, W. R., & Moyers, T. B. (2006). Eight stages in learning motivational interviewing. *Journal of Teaching in the Addictions, 5,* 3–17.

Miller, W. R., & Rollnick, S. (1991). *Motivational interviewing: Preparing people to change addictive behavior.* New York: Guilford Press.

Miller, W. R., & Rollnick, S. (2002). *Motivational interviewing: Preparing people for change* (2nd ed.). New York: Guilford Press.

Miller, W. R., Sovereign, R. G., & Krege, B. (1988). Motivational interviewing with problem drinkers: II. The drinker's check-up as a preventive intervention. *Behavioural Psychotherapy, 16,* 251–268.

Miller, W. R., Taylor, C. A., & West, J. C. (1980). Focused versus broad spectrum behavior therapy for problem drinkers. *Journal of Consulting and Clinical Psychology, 48,* 590–601.

Miller, W. R., Yahne, C. E., Moyers, T. B., Martinez, J., & Pirritano, M. (2004). A randomized trial of methods to help clinicians learn motivational interviewing. *Journal of Consulting and Clinical Psychology, 72,* 1050–1062.

Miller, W. R., Yahne, C. E., & Tonigan, J. S. (2003). Motivational interviewing in drug abuse services: A randomized trial. *Journal of Consulting and Clinical Psychology, 71,* 754–763.

Miller, W. R., Zweben, A., DiClemente, C. C., & Rychtarik, R. G. (1992). *Motivational enhancement therapy manual: A clinical research guide for therapists treating individuals with alcohol abuse and dependence* (Project MATCH Monograph Series, Vol. 2). Rockville, MD: National Institute on Alcohol Abuse and Alcoholism.

Moyer, A., Finney, J. W., Swearingen, D. W., & Vergun, P. (2002). Brief interventions for alcohol problems: A meta-analytic review of controlled investigations in treatment-seeking and non-treatment-seeking populations. *Addiction, 97,* 279–292.

Moyers, T. B., Martin, T., Catley, D., Harris, K. J., & Ahluwalia, J. S. (2003). Assessing the integrity of motivational interventions: Reliability of the Motivational Interviewing Skills Code. *Behavioural and Cognitive Psychotherapy, 31,* 177–184.

Moyers, T. B., Martin, T., Manuel, J. K., Hendrickson, S. M. L., & Miller, W. R. (2005). Assessing competence in the use of motivational interviewing. *Journal of Substance Abuse Treatment, 28,* 19–26.

Moyers, T. B., Miller, W. R., & Hendrickson, S. M. L. (2005). How does motivational interviewing work?: Therapist interpersonal skill predicts involvement within motivational interviewing sessions. *Journal of Consulting and Clinical Psychology, 73,* 590–598.

Patterson, G., & Chamberlain, P. (1994). A functional analysis of resistance during parent training. *Clinical Psychology: Research and Practice, 1,* 53–70.

Patterson, G. R., & Forgatch, M. S. (1985). Therapist behavior as a determinant for client noncompliance: A paradox for the behavior modifier. *Journal of Consulting and Clinical Psychology, 53,* 846–851.

Prochaska, J., & Norcross, J. (2004). *Systems of psychotherapy: A transtheoretical analysis* (5th ed.). New York: Wadsworth.

Prochaska, J. O. P., & Prochaska, J. M. (1991). Why don't people change? Why don't continents move? *Journal of Psychotherapy Integration, 9,* 83–102.

Project MATCH Research Group. (1997). Matching alcoholism treatments to client heterogeneity: Project MATCH posttreatment drinking outcomes. *Journal of Studies on Alcohol, 58,* 7–29.

Resnicow, K., Jackson, A., Wang, T., De, A. K., McCarty, F., Dudley, W. N., et al. (2001). A motivational interviewing intervention to increase fruit and vegetable intake through black churches: Results of the Eat for Life trial. *American Journal of Public Health, 91*(10), 1686–1693.

Rogers, C. R. (1951). *Client-centered therapy.* Boston: Houghton Mifflin.

Rogers, C. R. (1959). A theory of therapy, personality, and interpersonal relationships as developed in the client-centered framework. In S. Koch (Ed.), *Psychology: The study of a science: Vol. 3. Formulations of the person and the social contexts* (pp. 184–256). New York: McGraw-Hill.

Rollnick, S., & Miller, W. R. (1995). What is motivational interviewing? *Behavioural and Cognitive Psychotherapy, 23*, 325–334.

Rollnick, S., Miller, W. R., & Butler, C. C. (in press). *Motivational interviewing in health care*. New York: Guilford Press.

Rosengren, D. B., Baer, J. S., Hartzler, B., Dunn, C. W., & Wells, E. A. (2005). The video assessment of simulated encounters (VASE): Development and validation of a group-administered method for evaluating clinician skills in motivational interviewing. *Drug and Alcohol Dependence, 79*, 321–330.

Rubak, S., Sandbaek, A., Lauritzen, T., & Christensen, B. (2005). Motivational interviewing: A systematic review and meta-analysis. *British Journal of General Practice, 55*, 305–312.

Senft, R. A., Polen, M. R., Freeborn, D. K., & Hollis, J. F. (1997). Brief intervention in a primary care setting for hazardous drinkers. *American Journal of Preventive Medicine, 13*, 464–470.

Sorrentino, R. M., & Higgins, E. T. (Eds.). (1996). *Handbook of motivation and cognition: Vol. 3. The interpersonal context*. New York: Guilford Press.

Thevos, A. K., Quick, R. E., & Yanduli, V. (2000). Application of motivational interviewing to the adoption of water disinfection practices in Zambia. *Health Promotion International, 15*, 207–214.

Truax, C. B., & Carkhuff, R. R. (1967). *Toward effective counseling and psychotherapy*. Chicago: Aldine.

Valle, S. K. (1981). Interpersonal functioning of alcoholism counselors and treatment outcome. *Journal of Studies on Alcohol, 42*, 783–787.

Westen, D., & Morrison, K. (2001). A multi-dimensional meta-analysis of treatments for depression, panic, and generalized anxiety disorder: An empirical examination of the status of empirically supported therapies. *Journal of Consulting and Clinical Psychology, 69*, 875–899.

Westra, H. A., & Dozois, D. J. A. (2006). Preparing clients for cognitive behavioral therapy: A randomized pilot study of motivational interviewing for anxiety. *Cognitive Therapy and Research, 30*, 481–498.

Woollard, J., Beilin, L., Lord, T., Puddey, I., MacAdam, D., & Rouse, I. (1995). A controlled trial of nurse counselling on lifestyle change for hypertensives treated in general practice: Preliminary results. *Clinical and Experimental Pharmacology and Physiology, 22*, 466–468.

CHAPTER 2

Integrating Motivational Interviewing into the Treatment of Anxiety

Henny A. Westra
David J. A. Dozois

Motivational interviewing (MI; Miller & Rollnick, 2002) has been widely used and supported in the treatment of substance abuse (see Arkowitz & Miller, Chapter 1, this volume), However, its application to anxiety disorders is a relatively recent development. Existing effective treatments for anxiety (see Barlow, 2002) typically require the individual to take active steps toward enacting change. Yet, many individuals, even those presenting for treatment, are ambivalent about change and implementing change strategies. Given its central focus on the resolution of ambivalence about change, applications of MI for anxiety hold promise for engaging individuals with effective treatments.

In this chapter, we discuss existing treatments for anxiety, outline the rationale for adapting MI for anxiety, present an overview of this approach (with clinical illustrations), outline the clinical challenges in this work, and present the results of a pilot study using this application of MI as a prelude to cognitive-behavioral therapy (CBT) for anxiety disorders. Given that other chapters in this volume deal with specific anxiety disorders (posttraumatic stress disorder, obsessive–compulsive disorder), we focus on other common anxiety disorders including generalized anxiety disorder (GAD), social phobia, panic disorder, and agoraphobia.

ANXIETY AND ITS USUAL TREATMENT

Anxiety disorders are the most common of all mental disorders, with up to 25% lifetime prevalence (Kessler et al., 1994). Without treatment, anxiety disorders tend to be chronic and recurrent, and are associated with significant personal distress and suffering (Dozois & Westra, 2004). The reduced quality of life reported in individuals with anxiety disorders is comparable to and in some instances worse than with other major medical illnesses (Rubin et al., 2000). Anxiety disorders are also costly. In the United States alone, the direct and indirect costs attributable to anxiety disorders are approximately $42 billion a year (Greenberg et al., 1999).

Exposure-based behavioral interventions such as CBT have been the most well-investigated and well-supported treatments for anxiety disorders. In fact, various treatment guidelines now recommend CBT as the first-line approach to treating anxiety disorders (National Institute for Clinical Excellence, 2004). Although CBT typically consists of multiple intervention strategies (breathing retraining, self-monitoring), most researchers agree that exposure to feared situations/stimuli is a critical ingredient in effective psychological intervention for anxiety. Although the specific focus of exposure varies, depending on the type of anxiety being treated, the theoretical principle is the same: by facing anxiety-provoking stimuli, fears become extinguished (through the process of habituation), new coping skills are developed, and significant adaptive cognitive change occurs. Change in threat-related cognitions occurs as new evidence is accumulated that is discrepant from one's catastrophic beliefs, thereby providing an opportunity for new learning to take place.

The efficacy of CBT for anxiety disorders of all types is well established. The highest success rates have been achieved for the treatment of panic disorder. For example, 63% of patients with panic disorder are significantly improved at the end of treatment (Westen & Morrison, 2001), and these gains tend to be maintained at follow-up assessments (Craske & Barlow, 2001). A meta-analysis of 43 controlled studies demonstrated that CBT for panic disorder showed the largest effect sizes and the smallest dropout rates as compared to psychotropic medications or the combination of drug and psychological treatments (Gould, Otto, & Pollack, 1995). In the case of social anxiety, few differences exist between CBT and medication in terms of initial treatment response (Rodebaugh, Holaway, & Heimberg, 2004), but CBT tends to provide a superior prophylaxis against relapse versus pharmacotherapy alone (Hofmann & Barlow, 2002). Although CBT is effective for GAD (Borkovec

& Ruscio, 2001), this population is regarded as the least CBT-responsive anxiety disorder. For example, Fisher and Durham (1999) reanalyzed data from six controlled CBT outcome studies for GAD and reported an overall recovery rate of less than 40%.

RATIONALE FOR USING MI FOR ANXIETY

Enhancing response rates to existing effective treatments is emerging as an important priority for clinical research. It is now clear that when response is defined using stringent recovery criteria, a significant number of individuals fail to respond to CBT. For example, in their meta-analysis of treatments for depression, panic disorder, and GAD, Westen and Morrison (2001) found that 37–48% of completers and 46–56% of the intent-to-treat sample were not improved at follow-up.

Achieving higher recovery rates may, at least in part, be a function of engaging individuals with existing effective treatments (see Collins, Westra, Dozois, & Burns, 2004). Dropout in psychotherapy is common, with 23–49% of clients failing to attend more than one session and two-thirds terminating treatment prematurely (Garfield, 1994). Moreover, homework noncompliance is a commonly acknowledged issue among CBT practitioners (Huppert & Baker-Morissette, 2003), and rates of compliance show much individual variability throughout CBT (e.g., Burns & Spangler, 2000). Given that involvement in treatment is an important predictor of psychotherapy outcome (Henry & Strupp, 1994), enhancing our ability to fully engage individuals in therapy is important to improving and broadening response rates to treatment.

Fluctuating involvement in treatment may be related to high levels of ambivalence about change. In the area of GAD, for example, researchers have identified conflicting beliefs about worry. Borkovec and Roemer (1995) found that, while those with GAD see their worry as a problem, they also hold positive beliefs about their worry (e.g., worry is motivating) and are therefore ambivalent about relinquishing worry. Research with other anxiety populations, such as panic disorder (Dozois, Westra, Collins, Fung, & Garry, 2004) and OCD (Franklin & Foa, 2002), suggest that many individuals enter treatment with significant reservations about engaging with therapy. Finally, motivation for change has also been found to be an important predictor of psychotherapy outcome in anxiety (GAD; Dugas et al., 2003).

Engle and Arkowitz (2006) suggested that much of what is considered resistance or noncompliance in psychotherapy is a reflection of ambivalence about change. In addition, recent research suggests that the way a therapist responds to client ambivalence may be critical to treatment outcomes. For example, Huppert, Barlow, Gorman, Shear, and Woods (2006) reported that high treatment protocol adherence in panic control therapy was associated with poor outcomes in those low in motivation for change. This result concurs with other work and implies that rigid adherence to manualized protocols may interfere with outcome in some contexts (see Castonguay, Goldfried, Wiser, Raue, & Hayes, 1996).

As such, flexibility in treatment, such as recommendations for the judicious use of empathy and a focus on ambivalence in the presence of resistance, emerges as an important therapeutic direction (Burns & Auerbach, 1996). Thus, a combination of MI and CBT may be particularly promising for the treatment of anxiety, with MI directed at increasing motivation and resolving ambivalence about change and CBT directed at helping the client achieve the desired changes (Arkowitz & Westra, 2004).

CLINICAL APPLICATION
OF MI TO ANXIETY DISORDERS

Overview

This application of MI was based on the work of Miller and Rollnick (1991, 2002) and generalized to be applicable specifically to anxiety (see Arkowitz & Miller, Chapter 1, this volume, for a basic description of MI). Our application of this treatment for anxiety embodies all of the core strategies and principles of MI and focuses on ambivalence about changing the overall problem (i.e., anxiety) and applying coping methods for managing anxiety (e.g., avoidance, doing exposure exercises). Following a discussion of ambivalence as encountered in anxiety disorders, which is the cornerstone of work with motivation, we detail each of the core MI principles as applied to anxiety and provide clinical illustrations throughout.

Ambivalence

Ambivalence about change and/or the steps needed to implement change is ubiquitous in clinical practice and indeed in our day-to-day lives. Every clinician has heard clients "talk out of both sides of their mouth" about the issues they are struggling to address. Work with anxiety is no exception. The first author (Westra) can recall reading Miller and Rollnick's (1991) first edition of MI for enhancing motivation in addictions treatment in the late 1990s and inserting "anxiety" for the term "substance abuse," recognizing that ambivalence was no less of an issue for her clients with anxiety disorders.

Clients with anxiety often have strong and mixed reactions to the idea of homework, particularly exposure. In many respects this is not surprising, as exposure in any form is the phenomenological antithesis to nearly every coping effort (typically avoidant) the client has initiated (and may have had some short-term success with) to deal with overwhelming anxiety. Consequently, individuals vary in their receptivity to the treatment rationale, and this receptivity in turn has been demonstrated to predict CBT outcome (Addis & Jacobson, 2000). Clients rarely express change ambivalence openly but nonetheless can communicate this in many ways, such as passivity, lateness or canceling sessions, noncompliance, arguing ("yes-butting"), frustrating the therapist's helping efforts, and so on (Newman, 2001).

The therapist's recognition and integration of change ambivalence (one wants change, yet one resists change simultaneously) as normal can significantly assist the client in working through this dilemma. Creating space to hear, process, validate, integrate, and even honor these different parts of oneself can be crucial to successfully resolving ambivalence. Clients (even those with multiple failed treatment experiences) often enter treatment being zealous about the reasons for change. However, if efforts to change have been repeatedly thwarted or there is a history of struggles engaging with treatment, such articulations may only partially capture the client's more complex views on change.

The decisional balance, done either explicitly or implicitly, is the main framework that guides our work with ambivalence. In our practice, we often do this formally by having clients draw a line down the middle of a sheet of paper to capture both sides of ambivalence (i.e., the pros and cons of change vs. the pros and cons of the status quo), and this is framed as a method of capturing the "tug of war" with respect to change. Consistent with the suggestion of Burns (1989), we propose that clinicians begin with the arguments for "not making a change." In our experience, many clients can beautifully articulate the "good reasons for change" (e.g., "I know this anxiety makes no sense. It's making me depressed and ruining my life to be so avoidant. I'm missing out on so many things I want to have."). We contend that if this type of "change talk" were sufficient in getting clients to move forward, they would have done so already!

Consequently, in our application of MI, we explore change statements only after there has been significant validation and understanding of the side of the ambivalence that is not often articulated or fully appreciated—the part of the person that resists change. To not explore this fully would be to fail to give the person a chance to appreciate that he or she is not acting "irrationally" by resisting change and would miss an opportunity to allow greater self-compassion for the difficulty and often tumultuous nature of the change process. That is, there are important and powerful needs driving the client's resistance that need to be heard and attended to (e.g., the need for control, predictability, safety, freedom from negative consequences such as rejection, etc.). Moreover, when the barriers to change are empathically explored, reasons to change often emerge naturally and spontaneously in the client's verbalizations.

Clients are often far too quick to jump to what seems more acceptable or what they believe others (including therapists) want to hear (i.e., good reasons to change) without fully appreciating the often powerful counterarguments for this position that surface when individuals set out to implement change. In our experience, clients often appreciate this more balanced perspective, since most people already know that they need to change and may even have specific ideas for what is needed to accomplish this. For example, one client with whom we worked and who was struggling in an abusive relationship noted: "I know I need to get out of this relationship. You're the only one who doesn't insult me by telling me what I already know. What I really need to figure out is why I stay."

The basic idea in elaborating the pros of the status quo is to genuinely hear and validate the functional aspects of the "problem." The primary vehicle for exploring these functions is empathy and validation (discussed more fully later). It is important that the therapist cultivate a nonpejorative view of resistance to change. People often fail to appreciate that they are only doing what makes the most sense, given their perspective on their problems. The goal is to help the client hear and "appreciate" the positive motives underlying their seemingly senseless problem. One use of MI, then, can be to validate that the ends are highly desirable and basic to human needs. It is the means by which they have learned to achieve those ends (or when those means no longer work) that are problematic. As Mahoney (2003) notes, every current problem was a solution to a previous problem. Importantly, the goal of exploration is to help the person understand that his or her hesitation about change makes sense when seen from his or her perspective. The goal is also to generate greater self-compassion. When the therapist is open to seeing the value in the client's disavowed aspects of the self, and empathically resonates with these basic needs and desires, he or she models a compassionate approach, one that is allowing and open rather than self-critical and dismissive.

Consider an example of an interaction with a client with social anxiety:

THERAPIST: It's striking that since you've spent so much time attending to what other people think and need, you don't have a strong sense of what it is that you need.

CLIENT: It's dangerous for me to recognize that.

THERAPIST: There's something frightening about going there. If you're willing, can you say more about what is dangerous? What might happen?

CLIENT: Well, others would be hurt. I would end up being mean.

THERAPIST: And that is certainly not a way you like to be. It's important to please other people and look after them. I can understand why you wouldn't want to go there.

CLIENT: But at the same time, I have to. There are so many things I want to do that I've never done, because I give in to others all the time. As I think about it now, I feel like I've been pickpocketed.

THERAPIST: Yeah, like people took things that didn't belong to them. And I didn't even notice. Then you wake up one day and say, "Hey—where's my life?"

CLIENT: Exactly!

THERAPIST: And I'm guessing you might be somewhat angry about that.

CLIENT: Yes. Like the other day my wife told me she wants to do some renovations to our house. There are things that I would like to do with any extra money. I thought, "That's not fair. You never think about what *I* might want."

In terms of content, the person is prompted to consider not only the "value" of staying the same (e.g., familiar, predictable, free from rejection, help in being prepared, etc.) but also freedom from the price of change (e.g. "easier" than doing the hard work of changing, less risk than having to do exposure, don't have to risk failing or hurting others by being assertive, etc.). For example, an individual with GAD may be reluctant to give up reassurance seeking for fear that this will exacerbate worry or lead to other undesirable outcomes such as loss of control or putting loved ones in jeopardy. Or individuals with social phobia may be highly reluctant to do social exposures such as eating in a crowded restaurant or asking a question in class or in a meeting for fear that they may fail, thus leaving them feeling more helpless.

One of the advantages of MI is that it encourages the client—rather than the therapist—to articulate the reasons for change. In exploring the other part of the decisional balance, the therapist helps the client to articulate and elaborate the cons to anxiety or staying the same, and the benefits to change. This is best done when the individual begins to articulate "change talk" (as often happens in the exploration of good reasons to resist change). The therapist facilitates the client's exploration and elaboration of the arguments for change, addressing both the downsides of anxiety/avoidance as well as the possible upsides to change. Increasing change talk (or talk in the direction of change) is the proximal goal of MI here.

In some cases, people may have limited awareness of the costs of not changing. For instance, anxious parents may not wish to be fully cognizant of the impact of their anxiety disorder on their young children. The young man with social anxiety may not fully or frequently consider the limitations this imposes on his career and relationship prospects. Consider the following illustration:

THERAPIST: There are many useful aspects to worrying—yet, you also mentioned some downsides. What are some reasons that you are considering changing it?

CLIENT: Well, it gets in the way and leads to a lot of tension with other people.

THERAPIST: So, worry adds strain to relationships and is an obstacle in other ways as well. How does it get in the way? What specifically are you thinking about?

CLIENT: I feel constantly caught up with worry. I can't concentrate on anything, because I'm worried all the time. And I hate the way it makes me feel—tired, depressed, exhausted.

THERAPIST: So, worry reduces your concentration and takes a lot out of your energy and mood. You're thinking that you would be able to function better if you were less worried.

CLIENT: Yes. I could get more done at work, for example, and I would get along better with other people.

THERAPIST: And both of those things are important to you.

CLIENT: Yes, I feel that I'm only half the person I want to be, and the anxiety has a lot to do with that. It's depressing.

THERAPIST: And if another 6 months or a year went by and your worry was at the same level it is today, what would that be like for you?

CLIENT: Terrible. I would be even more unhappy and feel even more out of control.

It is important to recognize and differentially explore the client's reasons for change. That is, some costs articulated by the client may be more important than others, depending on the person's values and valued life directions. In the example above, the theme of anxiety interfering in relationships might be explored at greater length if it seems more significant for the client (e.g., "Can you give me an example of a time when worry unfavorably impacted your relationships? What hurts the most about that?"). One can also use affect to guide this process—either negative affect at contemplating certain costs or positive affect in contemplating certain aspects of what change would represent. For example, the parent who becomes sad when considering the impact of avoidance on his or her children could be invited to elaborate more on the current and potential future consequences of this. Similarly, the individual who brightens up when discussing how having less social anxiety would make friendships more enjoyable could be invited to differentially elaborate on this possibility (e.g., "What would you like to see in your relationships in the future? What would that give you?").

Core Principles of MI

Express Empathy

Empathy is a complex construct that has vastly differentiated meanings among various theorists (Bohart & Greenberg, 1997). In its most basic form, empathy in psychotherapy refers to the intention to understand the client from the client's frame of reference (Rogers, 1959). Empathy means far more than a friendly, kindly attitude toward the client—it is bringing one's full attention, interest, and intention to understanding the client from the client's own point of view. This is not for the purpose of judging or changing the client, but for fully knowing the client and helping him or her make sense of his or her experience. Empathy involves shared attention (Bohart & Tallman, 1997) on the concerns, hopes, fears, aspirations, expectations, meanings, and beliefs of the client. This means carefully trying to catch the client's meanings, taking the client's responses seriously and nonjudgmentally (i.e., not seeing these from an external frame of reference or regarding them as defensiveness, rationalization, denial, and so forth), continually checking one's understanding and the client's perception of your communications, and getting a feel for what it is like to be the client (Bohart & Tallman, 1997). The therapist also actively puts aside his or her own hopes, biases, theories, preformed categories, values, agendas, and so on in order to experience the client and the uniqueness of the client's reality (Geller & Greenberg, 2002).

Accordingly, what seems important is not so much the correctness of the therapist's understanding but the therapist's curiosity about the client or desire to know the client. When successful, empathic resonance has a quality of "vibrating in harmony with" the client. One element of this resonance, which many definitions of empathy incorporate, is the idea of making the implicit *explicit*, or articulating what was previously left unarticulated. The therapist's responses can build on or carry forward the client's articulations to expand a shared understanding or promote exploration (Greenberg & Elliott, 1997). Consider the following exchange with a client with panic disorder who was ambivalent about marrying her fiancé:

CLIENT: He's great. I don't know what I'm so anxious about. He has so many positive qualities. A gal could do a lot worse.

THERAPIST: On paper, he looks great. It's all really, really good . . . except for your feelings.

CLIENT: (*long pause*) Even though he's a good guy, I don't feel connected to him. I don't feel I know him, and he doesn't know me (*looking very sullen*).

THERAPIST: And that's not OK with you.

CLIENT: No. I don't want to be in a loveless marriage. There has to be more intimacy.

A related concept is Linehan's (1997) concept of validation. Empathy is a prerequisite for validation, and empathic communication is itself validating, but validation also goes beyond empathy. Validation involves explicitly communicating an understanding of the wisdom of a response, belief, feeling, or behavior on either a logical or functional level. It is a process of affirming the inherent validity or worth of the person and his or her responses. Here, the therapist searches for, identifies, communicates, and may even amplify that the responses are understandable, reasonable, functional, logical, or fit with learning history or current circumstances (Linehan, 1997). Statements such as "Naturally," "How could it be otherwise?," or "That makes so much sense" are common when reflecting the validity of the client's experience.

Importantly, empathy is also not synonymous with "technique." Rogers considered empathy to be fundamentally an attitude—of respect, nonjudgment, prizing, and collaboration—that pervades every interaction (Bozarth, 1997). In MI, this attitude is referred to as "spirit." Working with MI techniques in the absence of an empathic attitude or spirit is considered ineffective. Moreover, the therapist believes in the individual—in his or her innate capability. Research in social psychology has supported the existence and influence of such interpersonal expectancy effects. That is, the individual's confidence in the other's ability is associated with actual elicitation of greater ability on the part of the recipient (Rosenthal, 1994). Thus, empathy is a fundamental attitude toward the client that is communicated both verbally and nonverbally.

When successful, empathy fosters safety and open communication. It can create an environment that allows clients to explore dimensions of themselves or their problems that are avoided or that are difficult to tolerate, admit, or explore. Moreover, the therapist's willingness to know the client, ability to embrace difficult feelings, and confidence in the client may promote self-compassion and integration/exploration of disavowed aspects of oneself. This approach may also pave the way toward greater integration of the therapist's ideas and suggestions. Put simply, one is more willing to hear what the other has to say if one is first heard.

Consider the following initial encounter with a client who was not working due to GAD:

CLIENT: I don't know what I'm doing here. My psychiatrist said something about having negative thoughts and I have to think more positively, but I don't agree.

THERAPIST: It's all well and good for your psychiatrist to tell you that you have a problem, but there's no problem here.

CLIENT: Yes and no. I don't think it's that bad really. But I guess there's a reason I've been off work.

THERAPIST: There may be something going on, some trouble, but you're not sure that it's serious enough to seek therapy for. You probably feel "I've managed pretty well so far."

CLIENT: Yes, I'm the kind of person that can simply tell myself "there's no problem here," and that's worked for me, for the most part . . . until recently.

THERAPIST: Sounds like it's been a pretty effective coping strategy, and understandably you're reluctant to give that up. However, now you're wondering whether it might be time to develop some other ways of coping.

CLIENT: Yes. It takes too much energy to keep denying that the way I think is a problem, and it drives other people crazy that I just refuse to hear that there are any problems to deal with.

Developing Discrepancy

Reflecting and even amplifying the discrepancy between what one desires or values more broadly and one's present behavior can enhance motivation for change (Miller & Rollnick, 2002). It does so by revealing a gap between what one strongly desires, or one's preferred direction, and discontent with the present behavior. Having clients identify and articulate what they value in various domains can provide opportunities to help them resolve ambivalence by bringing together what they want and how the problem fits within that vision. The client might be invited to respond to the question "What are the things that are most important to you in your life?" or "What do you dream about? If your future turned out ridiculously well, what would this look like?" Then, the client is asked to reflect on the extent to which his or her current behavior fits or does not fit with this direction.

Similarly, the therapist can also consider building discrepancy between pros and cons identified as the decisional balance unfolds. As with all techniques, inviting the client to consider such discrepancies is offered in a client-centered spirit as food for thought rather than judgmentally or with criticism. Empathic reflection is used to facilitate and help the client process the material that arises.

Consider the examples below of therapist dialogues with various clients, all aimed at developing discrepancies in working with anxiety.

Note that all the material in these vignettes originated in what the client said earlier in the session, not with the therapist.

> [To a client with GAD] "So, on the one hand, worrying provides a sense of protecting other people from harm. And isn't that fantastic to want to do that. Yet, it seems that protecting people by worrying about them is also hurtful to them, because they get the message that you don't trust them. What do you make of that?"

Or

> [To a client, a social worker, who discloses that she feels like she is cheating her clients because her social anxiety prevents her from approaching colleagues for information that would help her clients or from attending workshops] "How does 'cheating' your clients fit with the importance you place on being good at your job? Or to what degree does not going to workshops fit or not fit with your desire to do a good job?"

Or

> [To a client with agoraphobia] "You mentioned that freedom and adventure are very important to you. How does someone who loves freedom feel about staying home all the time?"

Or

> [To a client with GAD] "So, worrying is important in that it keeps you prepared when bad things inevitably happen. Yet you mentioned that worry also paralyzes you too. How does that fit together?"

This style may be familiar to CBT therapists as "examining the evidence." In MI these socratic skills can be integrated within a client-centered spirit. Here, the goal is not to "refute" the ideas or identify them as dysfunctional (they do serve the client) so that they can be replaced with more adaptive ideas, but rather to "observe" them in the service of the client. Importantly, all statements aimed at developing discrepancies are not done with the intent of "changing" the person's thinking but rather in a spirit of curiosity and exploration. That is, consistent with the spirit of MI, the therapist is not allied with an agenda of having the client change or having to see the limits of the problem but rather facilitating the client's own exploration of the problem.

Roll with Resistance

Resistance is one of the most important phenomena in clinical practice, yet one of the least well understood or investigated (Engle & Arkowitz, 2006). Studies of resistance have suggested that it can be toxic to good outcomes (Miller, Benefield, & Tonigan, 1993) and very clinically challenging to navigate for both client and therapist (Burns & Auerbach, 1996). In general, the evidence on resistance suggests that a teach/confront style is associated with greater client noncompliance than a facilitative, supportive style (Miller et al., 1993). Generally, being sensitive to the presence of resistance and adopting a supportive and exploratory style seems critical to effectively navigating resistance.

In MI, resistance is considered relational. Just as empathy can be a shared or co-constructed phenomenon (Bohart & Tallman, 1997), so too is resistance. This can be one of the most challenging ideas to embrace, since it is tempting to attribute resistance solely to such client characteristics as defensiveness, obstructiveness, uncooperativeness, or other personality factors. MI considers that resistance is a product of the degree of client ambivalence, as well as how the therapist responds to this ambivalence (Moyers & Rollnick, 2002). By adopting an empathic stance, the overall presence of resistance can be minimized. In general, the approach in MI is to roll with resistance, or get alongside of it, rather than confronting it directly. Specific strategies are identified that all have the goal of siding with resistance in order to diffuse it (e.g., reframing, amplified and double-sided reflection, emphasizing personal choice and autonomy).

Consider the examples below of responding to resistance. First, we offer illustrations of resistance amplification (therapist error) and then offer an illustration of rolling with resistance.

CLIENT(with social anxiety): It's depressing to be living with your parents and not have a job when you're 30.

THERAPIST: And if you were still living with your parents and without a job a year from now, what do you imagine that would be like? Would your depression ever get any better? [amplifying resistance]

CLIENT: I don't know. (*Shuts down.*)

As this example illustrates, the communication of the therapist's agenda can be quite subtle but nonetheless picked up by the client. Here, the therapist "wants" the client to say, "I will be depressed if I am still in the same situation" (wanting to increase change talk). Now consider the alternative response the therapist made upon recognizing resistance through seeing the client shut down.

CLIENT: I don't know.

THERAPIST: So, if your situation were the same in a year, what would that be like? Good thing, not so good thing? What pros and cons do you see?

CLIENT: I think I'd be quite depressed.

Here the therapist communicates that the client is an autonomous individual who is free to decide how he or she would react to any given circumstance. By using more balanced language the therapist opens up the response options for the client, who then is able to articulate his or her true response free of the therapist's control.

Consider another example of a client with social anxiety, who in this instance is considering being assertive with her husband:

CLIENT: I suppose I could say something, but maybe it's just me. Maybe it's just my problem, and it will just go away.

THERAPIST: That's a nice idea, but what is the evidence that that's true? Has the problem gone away so far by not saying anything? [amplifying resistance]

CLIENT: But if it's my problem, it's not fair to cause more conflict for my husband.

Now consider an alternative response, rolling with resistance.

CLIENT: I suppose I could say something, but maybe it's just me. Maybe it's just my problem, and it will just go away.

THERAPIST: Maybe it will just go away! That would be ideal. Why cause more trouble? Maybe you're just making mountains out of mole hills. [rolling with resistance]

CLIENT: That's exactly what my husband says all the time.

THERAPIST: And what do you think of that? True, not so true?

CLIENT: I think he's wrong. I do have issues that need to be discussed, and he minimizes my concerns all the time.

In each instance, when the therapist gets alongside of the resistance and fosters the client's autonomy in making choices, the client can then move in an unobstructed way to processing the issue. If this correction were not made on the part of the therapist, one can envision how therapeutic communication could easily deteriorate into argument or contribute to the client's shutting down. Interestingly, even when clients agree with us (e.g., this client did agree that something needed to be said to her husband), no one wants to feel coerced. That is, it is not a question of accurate conceptualization but of process. It is also important to observe that this style may seem superficially similar to a strategy employing paradox (see Haley & Richeport-Haley, 2003). The strategic frame of mind of the therapist in using paradox, however, is incompatible with the spirit of MI, as it implies that the therapist is attempting to control the client, to trick him or her into being more motivated or changing. In this example of MI, the therapist is empathically resonating with the client's expressed dilemma (trying to understand her from her perspective).

Explicitly emphasizing choice and autonomy is another method used in MI when resistance is encountered. Consider the following illustration of an adolescent who presents at the first session with health anxiety:

CLIENT: You're the third therapist my parents have taken me to see. I don't want to be in therapy. I can solve this on my own.

THERAPIST: You're almost 16, right?

CLIENT: Yes, 15¾.

THERAPIST: Well, I certainly agree that you are capable of making your own decisions and that your preferences for how to approach this should be respected. After all, you're the one who has to deal with this at the end of the day. We have an hour or so together. We could end here. Or, if you like, we could spend this time talking a bit about the anxiety. And at the end of that time, I could offer an opinion as to whether I might have anything that would help you. Sounds like you're in good hands already, but given that this is my specialty, I might be able to steer you toward something that would be useful to you as well, or at least help you to work through your plan. What would you prefer to do?

CLIENT: I'd like to stay. Where should we start?

Even the best of therapeutic intentions, such as wanting to reinforce a client's progress or wishing to convey optimism, can be met with resistance. Consider the examples below:

CLIENT (with anxiety about speaking in front of others): I don't think I can speak at my friend's AA anniversary, even though I would really like to. That would just be too hard.

THERAPIST: (*drawing on the client's numerous previous successful exposures*) That sounds familiar. You've said "I can't" many times before when doing exposures. Right?

CLIENT: Yes.

THERAPIST: And how many times in the past has that thought "I'll never be able to do this" been correct?

CLIENT: That was then, this is now.

Or

CLIENT: Do you think I'll ever get over this anxiety?

THERAPIST: (*trying to convey hope*) I certainly do! Anxiety is quite treatable.

CLIENT: I doubt it. I've had this problem my whole life.

Or

CLIENT (with agoraphobia, who was chronically unemployed): I got a job.

THERAPIST: That's great! Good for you.

CLIENT: Actually, I don't think it's that great.

In each of these illustrations, the therapist is well intentioned and seems to operating with the principles of good therapy in mind—supporting the client's abilities, expressing confidence in the client or confidence in the possibility of recovery, offering positive reinforcement. As a colleague of ours once observed, "Praise can be coercive." It seems to depend on whose agenda is being served. In each case, the therapist has some well-meaning agenda for the client to view the situation in a certain helpful manner. Yet, on another level, the statements can imply judgment or contingencies for regard based on the therapist's frame of reference—that is, "I will only approve and like you if you do things that move therapy forward," or "It is clearly better to have a job than not have a job," etc. Positive reinforcement or facilitating hope are not wrong in and of themselves and, when well timed, can be very useful in advancing movement toward the client's goals. The key seems to be the ability to read the client's receptivity moment by moment and respond flexibly.

In our experience, these are among the most difficult skills to master. It's easy to be warm and have positive regard for your client when things are going well. The trickier terrain is to continue prizing and seeking to understand the client when we encounter resistance.

Support Self-Efficacy

MI is divided into two main phases: management and resolution of ambivalence and developing confidence in one's ability to initiate and carry out a change plan (Miller & Rollnick, 2002). Phase 2 strategies are only utilized when the client has sufficiently resolved ambivalence about change and begins to articulate preparation-for-change statements. Examples of such statements might include "I've been thinking more about doing things differently," "I just need some advice and suggestions," or "I think it's a good time to make some changes."

As Miller and Rollnick (2002) as well as other theorists (Linehan, 1997; Prochaska, 2000) observe, it is important to switch into an action-based mode of being with the client when the client is ready for change. Not doing so could be experienced as withholding. And continuing to use primarily reflection and validation at this stage will not advance the client's progress. Here one needs to collaborate with the client toward brainstorming change strategies, developing a change plan, and enhancing self-efficacy for change. When the client expresses preparation language, the therapist can use a variety of resources to develop and build self-efficacy and help the client prepare for change. The client remains the expert on what will or won't work and is free to make choices about methods, timing, and preferred strategies for change.

Importantly, Phase 2 work is also done in a client-centered spirit, one that preserves the client's autonomy and construes the therapist as operating as a consultant to the client—volunteering ideas, offering options based on what has worked with other clients in the past, challenging the client, and so forth. If one maintains this spirit of respect and belief in the expertise of the client, then the probability of productive movement forward is enhanced. As well, the therapist must continue to be prepared to roll with resistance. The person may have a fledgling intention to change, and moving too quickly to develop a change plan (falsely assuming that this is a well-consolidated intention to take action) could also retard the client's movement. As such, empathy should not be thought of as stopping here or as being a mere precondition to action. Rather, empathic reflection, in the sense of seeing action and preparation for action through the frame of the other, can be very useful in supporting the client in the effective implementation of change strategies.

Enhancing self-efficacy and developing a change plan could include evocative questions such as "Where would you start if you decided to make a change?," "What previous experiences have you had with changing something that might be relevant in considering this change?," or "What other people or resources might help in making a change, if that's what you decided to do?" (Miller & Rollnick, 2002).

Dabbling with Change

In our experience, a common indication that the client is preparing to change is that he or she begins to "dabble" with change without full immersion in the change process. That is, the client begins to move toward change in a graduated way by implementing some "small" changes. In anxiety, clients typically begin to carve out and initiate exposure tasks (e.g., a client with social phobia reports being assertive in a mildly threatening context, a client with agoraphobia calls a friend who lives out of town to make plans for a visit). The therapist needs to be open to hearing these spontaneous change efforts, to realize that not all change is initiated by the therapist's suggestions, and to have a focus that allows novel fledgling efforts at change to be articulated.

In these situations, the therapist might explore the example as an illustration of the client's potential for change and as an opportunity to enhance self-efficacy and commitment to making change. For instance, if an individual mentions that he or she has done an exposure exercise, the therapist might ask what led up to that attempt, what he or she liked and didn't like about it, what the client learned about him- or herself or about anxiety, and what can be generalized to other instances where this same anxiety theme emerges.

The spirit of curiosity seems critical here. The therapist becomes intensely curious about how and why the client embarked on this deviation from his or her usual style. The therapist might explicitly say (or at least keep in mind) that, as an autonomous individual, the client can choose to continue with the old or avoidant style as a perfectly acceptable option. The emphasis is on the client's own decision making, not forcing particular desirable behavior from the therapist's perspective. Any therapist affirmation or reaction should come after the client has fully explored and evaluated the change from his or her own perspective.

The Elicit–Provide–Elicit Style

Miller and Rollnick (2002) introduce a basic style that is typically thought of in the context of providing feedback (see Zuckoff, Swartz, & Grote, Chapter 5, this volume, for an illustration of this feedback style in the treatment of depression). This style, however, can also be used more broadly in treatment, such as when introducing the therapist's ideas for change strategies. The basic style consists in first asking for permission, offering the information, and then asking for the client's response (Rollnick, Mason, & Butler, 1999).

As just one illustration, a point at which resistance typically occurs in CBT for anxiety is when the therapist introduces highly anxiety-provoking tasks, such as interoceptive exposure, shame attacking, or worry exposure. Here, MI offers an alternative to a more "convincing" style or therapist-driven style. Both may be effective, but the "elicit–provide–elicit" approach may be less likely to be met with resistance. Consider an example in working with a client with panic disorder:

THERAPIST: You've had some nice success with getting better control of the panic, yet your score on the Anxiety Sensitivity Index is still higher than normal. This may mean that, even though you aren't having panic attacks anymore, you are still somewhat afraid of the symptoms of panic.

CLIENT: Yes, that's right. I still get scared when my heart beats fast or I feel dizzy.

THERAPIST: And reducing that fear can often be critical to avoiding relapse. Now, this may or may not be useful to you, but would you care to hear about a technique can be used to put that fear to rest once and for all? [elicit]

CLIENT: Sure.

THERAPIST: Well, it's a bit challenging and will seem kind of strange at first. Sometimes, what other people do who are in similar situations to yours, and what research supports as effective in reducing relapse, is to actually bring on the very symptoms you are afraid of, in order to prove once and for all that heart racing or dizziness won't lead to death or insanity. This is something that may or may not work or fit for you right now, and a lot of people have a really hard time with this idea because it's pretty scary. It's certainly something that we can talk about further if you feel it worth exploring or you would just like to hear more about it. [provide] But it's entirely up to you to decide what might work best. What do you think of that? [elicit]

The therapist strives to preserve the client's freedom of choice. The client is not instructed that he or she must do this (or any technique), but it is merely offered as part of the process of collaboration. The client has a problem, and the therapist draws on his or her resources and "expertise" and offers these to the client, who is free to accept or reject them. Anecdotally, since using this style, we have found that clients' willingness to embrace such suggestions has increased greatly. If the client seems receptive, one can then help the client strengthen commitment or build self-efficacy, using other MI strategies outlined earlier. If he or she is not receptive, the therapist can acknowledge this and shift the focus to exploring other alternatives.

PROBLEMS AND SUGGESTED SOLUTIONS

There are three main difficulties we have encountered in applying motivational interviewing to work with anxiety. These include specification of a problem focus, identifying "good things" about anxiety, and remaining within the client-centered "spirit" of MI. Each of these three will be discussed in turn, together with ways in which we have attempted to address these issues.

Defining a Problem Focus

In anxiety disorders, comorbid problems are the norm, with common comorbidities such as mood disorders, substance abuse, other anxiety disorders, and relationship problems. Each of these may be a focus of concern for the person, and there may be varying levels of motivation to address each. Furthermore, the client-centered nature of MI, with its focus on the client as expert and evoking client agency in treatment, suggests that a rigid predetermined focus on the part of the clinician is not appropriate. Moreover, the client's focus may shift, and frequently does, in clinical practice. It is not uncommon to begin with one focus (e.g., worry) to find that the client may shift his or her interest to a different domain (marital problems) of greater current concern.

There is no easy resolution to these issues, and empirical research is needed. We have found it helpful, and most consistent with the spirit of MI, to consider relevant foci for work with anxiety but also to allow the specific focus to be client-determined and fluid. Consistent with the thinking of Arkowitz and Burke (Chapter 6, this volume) and Burns (personal communication, November 2003), we outline a number of specific foci that could be targets of work on enhancing motivation. With respect to anxiety-specific foci, we consider that an individual could be ambivalent on two levels:

1. Anxiety change itself: What would life look like without panic or worry? Who would I be? Would there be other demands?
2. Use of existing avoidant coping methods and, conversely, implementation of alternative means of managing anxiety—exposure, reducing reassurance seeking, being less overprotective, taking interpersonal risks, etc.

We suggest that early in their relationship the clinician and the client collaboratively seek to understand the major idiographic ways in which the client has attempted to cope with his or her anxiety (e.g., "I procrastinate," "I sleep to avoid thinking," etc.). With this understanding, the decisional balance exercise is then conducted under the broader rubric of pros and cons of "staying the same." This permits some fluidity in the focus but also enables the clinician to bring in specific coping behaviors that the client is ambivalent about relinquishing. For example, the clinician may start with "What are the good things about staying the same?" and then ask related questions more specific in focus, such as "What are the good things about being anxious? . . . about being overprotective? . . . about worrying? . . . about not taking time for yourself? . . . about avoiding people?" Thus, the focus remains on exploring ambivalence and enhancing motivation, but this breadth permits a freedom that seems important in working with multiproblem populations and also helps to avoid a clinician-centered interaction. Additionally, it allows the clinician to avoid the "premature focus trap" (Miller & Rollnick, 2002) by not deciding in advance what is of greatest concern to the client.

Supporting the Client in Identifying "Good Things" about Not Changing

Initially, clients are often taken aback (or sometimes offended) that there may be good things about the problem from which they are seeking relief. In the case of anxiety or worry, this can be challenging for both clients and therapists to conceptualize. It is not uncommon for individuals to insist that there is "nothing good about my anxiety." It is important to retain a client-centered focus here. The clinician should avoid arguing about this point or insisting that there are unrecognized benefits. This tacit point requires considerable clinical skill and a stance that honors both the clients' understandable reluctance that there can be good things about their condition, as well as a nonpejorative view of the dynamics and beliefs about anxiety that may serve clients in important ways.

At this juncture, we offer a number of suggestions to clinicians. These include:

- Offer brief psychoeducation about the process of change.
- Validate the part of the person that wants change while simultaneously gently opening the door to hear the part of the person that thwarts his or her efforts to change.
- Make a suggestion or two about a possible advantage of not changing.
- Frame the issue as "barriers to change" or saboteurs of change (e.g., "What good reasons does your anxiety come up with to talk you out of change?").
- Resonate with and validate, especially early on, the intelligence behind the status quo.

A critical aspect of MI is to make it OK and safe for people to articulate these advantages. Typically, clients consider such information unacceptable (especially to themselves or to therapists). It is not socially acceptable to state "Anxiety is really working well for me" or "I really like the control I feel over people by being anxious." And all too often we as therapists can hold pejorative views of "secondary gain." Consider the following illustration of a client with agoraphobia:

THERAPIST: What are the good things about not leaving your home?

CLIENT: There's nothing good about it. It's a problem.

THERAPIST: Absolutely, I hear loud and clear that this is something you are keen to be without—and good for you. Sometimes—and this may or may not be the case for you—people tell us that staying close to home gives them some sense of safety or control. Would that fit at all for you?

CLIENT: Yes. By not going out, I think I can make sure that nothing bad will happen to me.

THERAPIST: So, staying at home protects you. And we all need a sense of safety in order to function. You probably don't feel all that confident that you could deal with bad things that might happen.

CLIENT: Yes, that's true. I worry that if I go out I might have a panic attack and not be able to control it.

THERAPIST: So, by staying home, you feel better because you don't have to risk inheriting more difficult problems than you already have. Sounds pretty smart. What else motivates you to stay home?

Staying in the "Spirit" of MI

The seamless movement between promoting acceptance and facilitating action may be among the most formidable challenges to using MI effectively, and to the wider adoption of MI. Working with this dialectic is particularly challenging if one (such as the authors) is more experienced with action-oriented, or more structured, methods for facilitating anxiety management. In these cases, one has the dual task of making the MI-consistent response but also of inhibiting the MI-inconsistent response (Miller & Mount, 2001). If this is not effectively accomplished, therapists can find themselves saying the right words (e.g., "you get to decide") while communicating the very opposite. Miller and colleagues' work on training others in MI (Miller, Yahne, Moyers, Martinez, & Pirritano, 2004) also suggests that training emphasizing the spirit of MI, rather than a focus on technique, is more effective. MI, and indeed empathy, seems deceptively simple but can be enormously challenging in practice.

Empathy and related concepts such as alliance, have garnered much empirical support in contributing to positive psychotherapy outcomes (see Bohart & Greenberg, 1997). As such, they hold great promise as points of fuller integration, through methods such as MI, with action or change-based models. Yet, greater integration of these ideas is not always smooth or easy. That is, stronger integration of MI spirit, for example, can be a source of challenge to foundational assumptions about how change emerges, the source of change, the processes and mechanisms of change, the role of the therapist, and so on. The essence of human encounter is not an easy concept to integrate in this age of relative emphasis on technologies of change. Being truly empathic requires a fundamental shift in frame that is not always easily accomplished. Put differently, using MI as a clever technology to facilitate change is antithetical to the very foundations of the model. In a reciprocal manner, it is often difficult for therapists from empathy-based models to seamlessly integrate action-based methods (Bohart, 2001). This dialectic of acceptance and change, way of being and technique, directive and nondirective, may be worthwhile to wrestle with but is also precarious.

In our experience, fear often arises in therapists when trying to shift from a change agenda to an acceptance frame. Therapists may fear (and perhaps clients as well) that validating the part of the person that resists change will be "giving permission to not change" and may make change less likely. Or, if we view our role primarily as change agents, then coming alongside of resistance may feel as though we are "giving up" on the client (and of course we resist that!). One can realize the limits of exhortation for change but still struggle to let go of these methods in the moment. In short, accommodating alternative and divergent ways of being can be unfamiliar and uncomfortable for us as well as our clients.

RESEARCH: RANDOMIZED PILOT STUDY

Although applications of MI are being increasingly applied to various mental health problems, to date no controlled studies of MI have been conducted with anxiety populations. This is certainly an area worthy of greater empirical attention. In adapting MI for work with anxiety, we conducted a series of controlled case studies with CBT nonresponders, some of which have been published elsewhere (e.g., Arkowitz & Westra, 2004; Westra, 2004; Westra & Phoenix, 2003).

Westra and Dozois (2006) have conducted a randomized pilot study of MI adapted for anxiety (Westra & Dozois, 2003) and offered as a prelude to CBT. Prior to group CBT (GCBT), 55 individuals with a principal anxiety diagnosis (45% panic disorder, 31% social phobia, and 24% generalized anxiety disorder) were randomly assigned to receive either three sessions of MI adapted for anxiety or no pretreatment (NPT). Results demonstrated that the MI pretreatment group showed significant increases in positive expectancy for anxiety change from pre- to post-MI, compared with the NPT (i.e., the passage of time; effect size

= 0.60). This result is interesting in view of theoretical speculation that resolution of change ambivalence should be associated with increased optimism about change (Miller & Rollnick, 2002). Moreover, early positive expectancy has received considerable empirical support as an important variable associated with positive outcomes in CBT (Arnkoff, Glass, & Shapiro, 2002).

Throughout group CBT, the MI pretreatment group, compared to NPT, reported significantly greater homework compliance (effect size = 0.96). Some 84% of the MI pretreatment group completed group CBT, compared with 63% of the NPT group. Although this trend was in favor of greater retention in the MI group, this difference was not statistically significant but, if replicated, may be clinically noteworthy. Both groups demonstrated significant anxiety symptom improvements from pre- to post-CBT. However, using criteria to assess clinical significance, the MI pretreatment group had a significantly higher number of CBT responders (75%) as compared to NPT (50%). At 6-month follow-up, both groups evidenced maintenance of gains.

In summary, these results provide preliminary evidence that MI may enhance engagement with and outcome from subsequent treatment. The strongest effects were observed for self-reported homework compliance in CBT, suggesting that one possible advantage of the MI may be as a catalyst, promoting enhanced involvement in subsequent action-based treatment procedures. The promising results also justify the future investigation of these effects using more powerful designs that may discern whether the effects are specific to MI (or resolution of change ambivalence) or to some type of pretreatment. Moreover, these results are consistent with MI research in other domains supporting the use of MI as a prelude to other interventions. Other types of treatment will form important comparison groups in subsequent clinical trials. Conceivably, other types of treatment preludes merit investigation as treatment catalysts such as expectancy enhancement (Constantino, Greenberg, & Aptekar, 2005) or engagement therapy (Zuckoff et al., Chapter 5, this volume). Investigating the means of identifying ambivalence about change, and thus matching the use of MI to those higher on ambivalence about change, may also be a worthwhile pursuit.

CONCLUSIONS

Given the prevalence of ambivalence about change in individuals with anxiety, MI may hold promise as an adjunct to, or context for, existing

Treatment outcome and long-term follow-up. *Journal of Consulting and Clinical Psychology, 71*, 821–825.

Engle, D. E., & Arkowitz, H. (2006). *Ambivalence in psychotherapy: Facilitating readiness to change.* New York: Guilford Press.

Fisher, P. L., & Durham, R. C. (1999). Recovery rates in generalized anxiety disorder following psychological therapy: An analysis of clinically significant change in the STAI-T across outcome studies since 1990. *Psychological Medicine, 29*, 1425–1434.

Franklin, M. E., & Foa, E. B. (2002). Cognitive behavioral treatments for obsessive–compulsive disorder. In P. E. Nathan & J. M. Gorman (Eds.), *A guide to treatments that work* (2nd ed., pp. 367–386). London: Oxford University Press.

Garfield, S. L. (1994). Handbook of psychotherapy and behavior change. In A. E. Bergin & S. L. Garfield (Eds.), *Research on client variables in psychotherapy* (pp. 190–228). New York: Wiley.

Geller, S., & Greenberg, L. (2002). Therapeutic presence: Therapists' experience of presence in the psychotherapy encounter in psychotherapy. *Person-Centered and Experiential Psychotherapies, 1*, 71–86.

Gould, R. A., Otto, M. W., & Pollack, M. H. (1995). A meta-analysis of treatment outcome for panic disorder. *Clinical Psychology Review, 15*(8), 819–844.

Greenberg, L. S., & Elliott, R. (1997). Varieties of empathic responding. In L. S. Greenberg & A. C. Bohart (Eds.), *Empathy reconsidered: New directions in psychotherapy* (pp. 167–186). Washington, DC: American Psychological Association.

Greenberg, P. E., Sisitsky, T., Kessler, R. C., Finkelstein, S. N., Berndt, E. R., Davidson, J. R., et al. (1999). The economic burden of anxiety disorders in the 1990s. *Journal of Clinical Psychiatry, 60*, 427–435.

Haley, J., & Richeport-Haley, M. (2003). *The art of strategic therapy.* London: Taylor & Francis.

Henry, W. P., & Strupp, H. H. (1994). The therapeutic alliance as interpersonal process. In A. O. Horvath & L. S. Greenberg (Eds.), *The working alliance: Theory, research and practice* (pp. 51–84). New York: Wiley.

Hofmann, S. G., & Barlow, D. H. (2002). Social phobia (social anxiety disorder). In D. H. Barlow, *Anxiety and its disorders* (2nd ed., pp. 454–476). New York: Guilford Press.

Huppert, J. D., & Baker-Morissette, S. L. (2003). Beyond the manual: The insider's guide to panic control treatment. *Cognitive and Behavioral Practice, 10*, 2–13.

Huppert, J. D., Barlow, D. H., Gorman, J. M., Shear, M. K., & Woods, S. W. (2006). The interaction of motivation and therapist adherence predicts outcome in cognitive behavioral therapy for panic disorder: Preliminary findings. *Cognitive and Behavioural Practice, 13*, 198–204.

Kessler, R. C., McGonagle, K. A., Zhao, S., Nelson, C. B., Hughes, M., Eshleman, S., et al. (1994). Lifetime and 12-month prevalence of DSM-III-R psychiatric disorders in the United States: Results from the National Comorbidity Survey. *Archival of General Psychiatry, 51*, 8–19.

Linehan, M. M. (1997). Validation and psychotherapy. In L. S. Greenberg & A. C. Bohart (Eds.), *Empathy reconsidered: New directions in psychotherapy* (pp. 353–392). Washington, DC: American Psychological Association.

Mahoney, M. J. (2003). *Constructive psychotherapy: Theory and practice.* New York: Guilford Press.

Miller, W. R., Benefield, R. G., & Tonigan, J. S. (1993). Enhancing motivation for change in problem drinking: A controlled comparison of two therapist styles. *Journal of Consulting and Clinical Psychology, 61,* 455–461.

Miller, W. R., & Mount, K. A. (2001). A small study of training in motivational interviewing: Does one workshop change clinician and client behavior? *Behavioral and Cognitive Psychotherapy, 29,* 457–471.

Miller, W. R., & Rollnick, S. (1991). *Motivational interviewing: Preparing people to change addictive behavior.* New York: Guilford Press.

Miller, W. R., & Rollnick, S. (2002). *Motivational interviewing: Preparing people for change* (2nd ed.). New York: Guilford Press.

Miller, W. R., Yahne, C. E., Moyers, T. B., Martinez, J., & Pirritano, M. (2004). A randomized trial of methods to help clinicians learn motivational interviewing. *Journal of Consulting and Clinical Psychology, 72,* 1050–1062.

Moyers, T. B., & Rollnick, S. (2002). A motivational interviewing perspective on resistance in psychotherapy. *Journal of Clinical Psychology, 58,* 185–194.

National Institute for Health and Clinical Excellence. (2004). *Anxiety: Management of anxiety (panic disorder, with or without agoraphobia, and generalized anxiety disorder) in adults in primary, secondary and community care.* London: Author. Retrieved July 13, 2005, from *www.nice.org.uk/CG022quickrefguide*

Newman, C. F. (2001). A cognitive perspective on resistance in psychotherapy. *Journal of Clinical Psychology, 58,* 165–174.

Prochaska, J. O. (2000). Change at differing stages. In R. E. Ingram & C. R. Snyder (Eds.) *Handbook of psychological change: Psychotherapy processes and practices for the 21st century* (pp. 109–127). New York: Wiley.

Rodebaugh, T. L., Holaway, R. M., & Heimberg, R. G. (2004). The treatment of social anxiety disorder. *Clinical Psychology Review, 24*(7), 883–908.

Rogers, C. R. (1959). A theory of therapy, personality, and interpersonal relationships as developed in the client-centered framework. In S. Koch (Ed.), *Psychology: The study of a science.* New York: McGraw-Hill.

Rollnick, S., Mason, P., & Butler, C. (1999). *Health behaviour change: A guide for practitioners.* Edinburgh, UK: Churchill Livingstone.

Rosenthal, R. (1994). Interpersonal expectancy effects: A 30-year perspective. *Current Directions in Psychological Science. 3,* 176–179.

Rubin, H. C., Rapaport, M. H., Levine, B., Gladsjo, J. K., Rabin, A., Auerbach, M., et al. (2000). Quality of well-being in panic disorder: The assessment of psychiatric and general disability. *Journal of Affective Disorders, 57,* 217–221.

Westen, D., & Morrison, K. (2001). A multidimensional meta-analysis of treatments for depression, panic, and generalized anxiety disorder: An empirical examination of the status of empirically supported therapies. *Journal of Consulting and Clinical Psychology, 69,* 875–899.

Westra, H. A. (2004). Applications of motivational interviewing to mixed anxiety and depression. *Cognitive Behavior Therapy, 33,* 161–175.

Westra, H. A., & Dozois, D. J. A. (2003). *Motivational interviewing adapted for anxiety/depression*. Unpublished treatment manual. Available at *hwestra@ yorku.ca*

Westra, H. A., & Dozois, D. J. A. (2006). Preparing clients for cognitive behavioural therapy: A randomized pilot study of motivational interviewing for anxiety. *Cognitive Therapy and Research, 30*, 481–498.

Westra, H. A., & Phoenix, E. (2003). Motivational enhancement therapy in two cases of anxiety disorder: New responses to treatment refractoriness. *Clinical Case Studies, 2*, 306–322.

CHAPTER 3

Enhancing Combat Veterans' Motivation to Change Posttraumatic Stress Disorder Symptoms and Other Problem Behaviors

Ronald T. Murphy

THE CLINICAL POPULATION AND USUAL TREATMENTS

Soldiers have exhibited emotional and behavioral problems related to their wartime experiences throughout the history of warfare. The problems that Vietnam veterans experienced upon their return home helped precipitate the inclusion of posttraumatic stress disorder (PTSD) as an Axis I diagnosis in the third, fourth, and current versions of the *Diagnostic and Statistical Manual of Mental Disorders* (American Psychiatric Association, 2000). PTSD includes three main categories: Reexperiencing, Persistent Avoidance, and Persistent Arousal. Reexperiencing symptoms typically include recurrent images, flashbacks, and nightmares, while Persistent Avoidance refers to efforts to avoid exposure to aversive cues related to traumatic experiences. Persistent Arousal includes hypervigilance, irritability, and startle reactions, all signs of a general hyperalertness to danger. In daily life, these symptom labels more commonly are associated with anger problems, social isolation, mistrust, and emotional numbness. Common comorbidities include substance abuse and depression.

Health professionals, especially in the Veterans Administration (VA) hospital system, have long dealt with Vietnam veterans whose long-standing PTSD symptoms are labeled "chronic," with many Vietnam veterans still seeking treatment for combat-related PTSD symptoms caused by traumatic events that occurred almost 40 years ago. Treatment of chronic PTSD among war veterans typically includes cognitive-behavioral approaches and psychiatric medication, particularly in VA treatment programs. These programs often provide a broad range of interventions, including exposure/extinction approaches designed to reduce anxiety and training in coping and social skills to reduce anger, depression, and social isolation. For example, in the New Orleans VA PTSD Clinic, patients participate in month-long groups that differ in focus (e.g., anger management, relationship skills, and stress management). There is also a group module that reviews lifespan events, including combat experiences.

Clinicians and researchers labor to develop more effective treatments, and professional conferences are replete with presentations about new cognitive-behavioral, drug, and alternative interventions. Yet, treatment effectiveness of combat-related PTSD remains in doubt due to findings of poor treatment outcome in two major studies (Fontana & Rosenheck, 1997; Schnurr et al., 2003). Related to this issue, but often not seen as connected to it, is the reputation of veteran patients with PTSD as being reluctant and difficult participants in therapy. This chapter addresses an important aspect of the treatment of long-standing combat-related PTSD that treatment providers have neglected or used confrontational methods to address but that any clinician working with this population can recognize: the reluctance of patients with PTSD to acknowledge the need to change PTSD symptoms and related maladaptive coping styles.

RATIONALE FOR USING MOTIVATIONAL INTERVIEWING FOR COMBAT-RELATED PTSD

Seeking and accepting help is problematic for veterans with PTSD. One report indicates that 38% of these veterans are not receiving Veterans Affairs services (Rosenheck & DiLella, 1998). In a study of recent Operation Iraqi Freedom and Operation Enduring Freedom (Afghanistan) returnees, Hoge and colleagues (2004) found that only 38–45% of those soldiers who met screening criteria for a mental disorder indicated an interest in receiving help. In addition, returnees meeting the screening criteria for a mental disorder were twice as likely as those not meeting criteria to report concern about being stigmatized and about other barriers to services. Finally, a sample of veterans with PTSD who had not received services in the prior year reported experiencing barriers to treatment seeking, including unfavorable views of mental health care (McFall, Malte, Fontana, & Rosenheck, 2000).

Even when they seek treatment, these veterans frequently do not fully engage in treatment and question the need to change their defensive approach to life, including hyperalertness to danger, social isolation, frequent anger, and mistrust of others. Unfortunately, the author has witnessed therapists (including himself!) arguing with patients about the best way to handle situations involving social interactions with family, friends, and strangers (e.g., "road rage"). In fact, many PTSD treatment programs included confrontational components derived directly from Synanon-style approaches to denial of alcohol problems. Argumentation and other confrontational approaches lead to increased resistance and are less effective than more supportive approaches like motivational interviewing (MI; Miller, Benefield, & Tonigan, 1993). The ineffectiveness of such approaches provided some of the impetus for applying MI (Miller & Rollnick, 2002) to PTSD treatment.

Recently studies have provided some support for the notion that veterans in PTSD programs are ambivalent about the need to change important symptoms and related problem behaviors. Murphy, Cameron, and colleagues (2004) asked veterans with combat-related PTSD in an inpatient program to report any problems that they "Might Have." These were defined as problems either that they wondered if they had or that other people told them that they had but they disagreed. These "Might Haves" were listed separately from any problems that patients were sure that they had ("Definitely Have") or sure that they did not have ("Don't Have"). Results indicated that the patients reported a wide range of categories of PTSD symptoms and related behaviors as "Might Have" problems, with the highest percentage of patients (48%) classifying anger-related behaviors as "Might Have." Approximately one-third of the patients labeled isolation, depressive symptoms, trust, and health as a "Might Have," and about one-fourth reported conflict resolution, alcohol, communication, relationship/intimacy, restricted range of affect, and drugs as "Might Haves." Other types of PTSD-related problems (e.g., hypervigilance) were reported as "Might Haves" by 15–21% of the patients.

to be consistent with the MI approach of evoking statements conducive to change, and patients are never told that they should adopt this way of thinking. This component seemed critical to add, since the patients treated in typical VA programs frequently have a general externalizing coping style that inhibits their ability to problem-solve and examine their role in the difficulties they experience in daily life.

In another departure from standard MI applications, homework is assigned at the end of each group session, including reading sections from the patient workbook and completing decision-making tasks (see below). Patients are encouraged to complete these assignments as a way to get maximum benefit out of the group. It is hoped that the disadvantages of being fairly directive in this component of the PME Group may be outweighed by the value of extra preparation time, rehearsal, and active information processing in increasing the comprehensibility and effectiveness of the cognitive-oriented tasks presented.

Finally, the PME Group also includes a session addressing the identification of cognitive and emotional "roadblocks" to change. Often people do not acknowledge a problem because they are avoiding some type of fear (Newman, 1994). DiClemente and Vasquez (2002) discuss reluctance, rebelliousness, resignation, and rationalization as reasons why precontemplators do not change, in addition to the factors characterizing individuals in each of the stages of change (e.g., lack of information for precontemplators, negative consequences of change outweighing positive consequences for contemplators). In their explanatory framework for addressing treatment adherence with MI, Zweben and Zuckoff (2002) note that lack of problem acceptance may be due to misunderstandings or uncertainties about the significance of a problem, fears about the unintended consequences of change, and doubts about whether or not change is possible or within reach. Other obstacles to acknowledging the need to change are discussed below. This is an area of MI that would benefit from more discussion and research, with the goal of developing methods for assessing obstacles to change and devising specific techniques for addressing them more directly within the MI model or outside the model (e.g., cognitive therapy).

INTEGRATION OF THE PME GROUP WITH OTHER TREATMENTS

The goal of the PME Group is to enhance the effectiveness of whatever PTSD treatment program the patient is involved in, by increasing awareness of problems that need to be addressed. The desired outcome of participation in the PME Group is increased patient engagement in therapeutic tasks and skills rehearsal, which in turn promotes symptom reduction and adaptive functioning. Therefore, it may best be implemented at the beginning of a treatment program so that patients are clear about what problems they need to focus on in subsequent skills-oriented groups. The PME Group has usually been utilized in this fashion.

Another way the PME Group might be used is to help combat veterans decide whether they need to enroll in a PTSD program. The PME Group might be offered to veterans who are experiencing difficulties coping with daily life but are unsure about the need for treatment, the source of their difficulties, or possible negative aspects of treatment participation. In this context, the PME Group might be offered in a briefer workshop format or as the regular four-session group without asking veterans to commit to further treatment.

OVERVIEW OF THE PME GROUP: RATIONALE, STRUCTURE, AND TECHNIQUES

The PME Group protocol currently consists of four 90-minute modules (with each module conducted in one session) that focus on the use of decision-making skills to help patients recognize the need to change any unacknowledged PTSD-related problems. The PME Group is best implemented with eight patients and one or two group leaders. The group leaders work from a manual with a detailed script, and patients use a workbook that contains an explanatory introduction, the format for each group module/session (matching the leaders' manual), and therapeutic activity blank forms and example forms.

The first session and the initial part of subsequent sessions consist of a review of the purpose, rationale, and specific goals of the group (described in the Module 1 section below), presented in a question-and-answer format in which the group leader asks a question and invites participants to respond. This format is used as a cognitive rehearsal technique in which the patients should be able to give the appropriate response more quickly by the end of the four sessions, and thereby recall and understand the point of participation in the group more easily. Repetition was necessary due to the frequency and extent of cognitive and memory deficits among the patients. There are a number of causes for these deficits, including long histories of substance abuse, sleep problems, brain injury, depression, and concentration and attention problems that are themselves hyperarousal symptoms of PTSD.

The rationale for the PME Group is that increased recognition of the need to change specific PTSD symptoms and other problems will lead to better treatment adherence and outcome, because patients will perceive coping skills learned in treatment as more personally relevant to them. In one sense, the goal is to prevent relapse to PTSD symptoms and related problems. As explained to the patients, the purpose of the group is to help them avoid being "blindsided" by unrecognized problems after treatment. In the jargon of the group, unidentified problems are called "blindsiders."

In addition, a key part of the intervention, assessment of possible unrecognized problems, occurs in this first session. Patients generate a list of behaviors or beliefs that might be a problem for them, called "Might Have" problems, using an open-ended worksheet called Form #1 (see Appendix 3.1). Participants then use decision-making tools taught in subsequent sessions of the PME Group to help them decide if these "Might Have" problems are actually problems they definitely have.

Modules 2, 3, and 4 provide specific tools and activities for deciding if a possible unrecognized problem ("Might Have") is definitely a problem or definitely not a problem. Module 2 employs a basic decisional-balance technique, and Module 3 consists of a norm-comparison exercise. Module 4 is aimed at identifying cognitive and emotional roadblocks to acknowledging unrecognized problems. Homework is also given after each of the first three sessions, including reading in preparation for the next session and completion of additional session-specific decision-making activities.·

Module 1: Group Review and Possible Problem Identification

In the first module, the purpose and potential value of the group are reviewed in detail, and target problems are identified. The rationale presented is that posttreatment relapse may not be due to inadequate treatment or "unfixable" patients but rather to unacknowledged problems that lead to the gradual or sudden return to old coping styles. Topics include what the group is about, the purposes of the group, and how it might be useful to the client (e.g., preventing relapse due to the posttreatment emergence of unidentified problems).

As presented to group participants, the purpose of the group is to help patients make decisions about problems that they *might* have that are either definitely or definitely not a problem requiring change. A clear distinction is drawn between problems listed as "Might Have" and behaviors and cognitions that they definitely are convinced they need to change. The reasons why it might be useful to make decisions about problems they might or might not have are elicited from the group and expanded upon by the group leaders. At the end of the rationale review, the therapist points out that the ultimate goal of the group is to help patients to avoid getting "blindsided" by unacknowledged problems following discharge.

As mentioned earlier, a recent modification to the PME Group addresses the general externalizing cognitive style frequently encountered among veterans in treatment for chronic PTSD. This style often takes the form of blaming other people or the state of society for provoking strong reactions like anger or necessitating isolation, hypervigilance, and mistrust. Frequently the government is blamed for symptoms and difficulties. In all these cases, there is a general relinquishing of responsibility for coping with difficult situations or controlling their symptoms and reactions. The section of the PME Group addressing this issue attempts to walk a fine line between being overly directive and yet providing encouragement for taking responsibility for controlling symptoms (often not viewed as symptoms, e.g., mistrust, isolation, being "controlling" or perfectionistic). Specifically, one goal of the PME group is to help participants consider that unacknowledged problems may contribute to their difficulties, that their past traumatic experiences may be influencing their reactions to situations that trigger or exacerbate symptoms or cause difficulties for them, and that they may need to take more responsibility for handling difficult situations. Patients are given a list of self-statements that would be consistent with this new attitude. Reproduced below is a sample self-statement excerpted from the manual covering this point. As in all parts of the review of group rationale and purpose, group leaders ask patients for responses and feedback to the question prompts and also read aloud the desired response.

The new general attitude is that whenever you experience problems, you are self-reflective about the possibility that how you are reacting or thinking is contributing to some degree (a little or a lot) to your problems, even if you have not caused the problem. Part of this attitude is believing that you are not responsible for the fact that you were put in combat situations that changed you, but you are responsible now for handling situations and your PTSD symptoms in a way that is based on the reality of situations and not on your past experiences.

We want you to be open to saying "There's something about the way I'm looking at, reacting to, or handling the situation rather than the situation itself that is causing me to have difficulties." In other words, you always look for "blindsiders" when you are having difficulties. This is a hard attitude to accept, and may not seem fair because of what you went through. But it may save your life, improve your health and relationships, reduce stress, and give you the opportunity to have more satisfaction in different areas of your life.

Each group participant also reads one of the statements aloud from the "Self-Talk Checklist for Continued Progress after Treatment." This checklist is presented in Appendix 3.2.

Identification of Target "Might Have" Problems

The remainder of this first session is spent having patients generate a list of behaviors or beliefs that might be a problem for them, that is, that they may be unaware of or ambivalent about changing. Patients fill out the Form #1 worksheet (see Appendix 3.1), which is divided into three columns: "Definitely Have," "Might Have," or "Definitely Don't Have." The "Might Have" column is further divided into two categories: "Problems you have wondered if you have" and "Problems other people say you have but you disagree." "Might Have" problems are defined in these two ways to elicit not only problem areas that they have considered as possibly needing change (contemplation stage) but also problems that they might be unaware of or unwilling to change (precontemplation stage). Patients are asked to consult a prompt list of PTSD symptoms and other problems and examples of completed worksheets that are contained in the patient workbook. The goal is for patients to eventually sort items listed under "Might Have" into the "Definitely Have" or "Definitely Don't Have" categories.

The advantages of using an open-ended format where patients use their own language to describe possible problems quickly became apparent. Our target population is prone to check off many problems when they are presented on a checklist, partly because they are often receiving or applying for service-related compensation and feel the need to document their difficulties as thoroughly as possible. Also, patients often do not equate certain behaviors or attitudes with categories as presented in assessment checklists. Another manifestation of this is that patients can consider certain trauma-based behaviors or attitudes as adaptive when they are not labeled as symptoms. For example, the author has seen patients endorse anger as a problem on a questionnaire and yet later report that they disagree with others' complaints that they are short-tempered or irritable, rationalizing the behavior with statements like "You've got to be hard on people, because they just won't do things right."

After being given some time to complete the worksheet, the participants are asked to read aloud what they have listed in each of the four columns. This allows group members to hear possible problems that they may not have considered and makes them feel more at ease about raising issues that they may feel embarrassed or anxious about revealing as possible problems. As always with these patients, they feel less alone or "crazy" when they hear other patients discuss issues that they may have never spoken about with anyone, or at least never admitted might be problematic for them.

Finally, some general points about successful participation in the group are made. Below are some examples from the workbook:

What Is the Goal of the Group?
  —Move Might Have Problems to either Definitely Have or Definitely Don't Have
  —DECIDE if Might Have Problems really are problems that I need to change

What Do You Learn in the Next 3 Weeks (PME Group Sessions 2, 3, & 4)?
  —Decision-Making Tools to help decide if Might Have problems are Definitely Have or Don't Have

Who Decides If a Might Have Problem Is Really a Definitely Have or Don't Have?
  —It's completely up to the patient, program staff doesn't decide, it's the patient's responsibility

What Is Needed to Make This Group a Success?
  —Honesty, Participation, and . . . an Open Mind about possible problems

Does Success in This Group Mean You Have to Move All the Might Haves out of the Middle Columns?
  —Success doesn't equal the number of items moved. As long as you are considering that you may have some problems you haven't recognized before, the group is a success. Deciding if you have unrecognized problems might be a long and continuing process

What Do You Do with Problems You Have Identified as Definitely Haves?
With Definitely Don't Haves?
—I bring the Problems I Definitely Have to the other groups in the Trauma Recovery Program and PTSD treatment, where I can work on them. Problems I Definitely Don't Have—I don't have to worry about them or do anything about them

Homework is assigned before the group ends; specifically, it is suggested that patients read sections in the patient workbook reviewing this first session and also the upcoming session on decisional balance.

Module 2: "Pros and Cons"

In this second PME Group session, decisional balance methods are reviewed and practiced to help patients decide about the need to change "Might Have" behaviors that they agree they do but are not sure are actually problematic. In this technique, patients weigh the advantages and disadvantages of various PTSD symptoms and other behaviors listed as "Might Have" problems, such as gun ownership, continued alcohol use, and hypervigilance. For example, a patient may list isolation as a "Problem others say I have, but I disagree." "Pros" might include "Feel safer," "When I want to do something, I can just do it," "Don't have to deal with other people's problems," and "Don't get into hassles with other people." The "cons" listed could be "Distant from children," "I get depressed," "I think more about bad things that happened in the war," and "Think more about using drugs." After a general example is reviewed, using input from the entire group, patients are asked to list the pros and cons to one of their own "might have" problems, using a decisional balance worksheet. Patients are also instructed to give a value weight to each pro and con, using a scale of 1–10 in terms of personal importance. Individual patient examples are then reviewed with the whole group, with all participants asked to offer any suggestions for additional pros and cons that may apply to each individual analysis. After each individual pros and cons analysis is reviewed, patients are asked if they had come to a conclusion about the need to change the "might have" problem.

For homework, patients are encouraged to finish any pros and cons analysis they worked on in the group session and also to complete a new pros and cons analysis as applied to another "might have" problem. This homework, as with the next week's assignment, is reviewed at the beginning of the following session.

Module 3: Comparison to the Average Guy

The third module, "Comparison to the Average Guy," is aimed at helping patients compare their behavior to estimated age-appropriate but non-PTSD "norms" in order to help them judge how problematic their behavior might be. A thorough review of this rationale is presented to the patients. The specific decision-making tool involves categorizing a possible problem behavior along a range of problem severity categories including "Average," "Moderate Problem," and "Extreme Problem." At each of these levels, three dimensions of behavior are examined: frequency, severity of consequences, and purpose. Group leaders guide members in analyzing what a particular behavior would look like at each of the three levels on each of the three dimensions. For example, if hypervigilance were the behavior selected (see Appendix 3.3), group leaders would elicit a description of normative levels of safety awareness, which might include checking to make sure doors are locked at night and installing motion-sensitive lights outside the house. At this level consequences are mild, such as the additional cost of the lights. The purpose of the average level of safety awareness may be to feel reasonably safe. At the moderate problem level, behaviors might include the frequent checking of doors and windows at night and installing more elaborate alarm systems, with the consequences including more time expended and money invested. Here, the purpose begins to take on more of an anxiety-reduction role. At extreme levels of hypervigilance, behaviors may include checking the perimeter of the house all night, keeping a gun under the bed, and setting booby traps. Consequences are a great deal of time and energy spent and risk to children and others from the gun, with the purpose of the behavior more about survival and a feeling of "life or death." The key point is determining where one's own behavior fits in this range of problems in order to help patients consider that they might have a problem they had not previously recognized. After an example is reviewed, using input from the entire group (usually the hypervigilance example described above), patients are asked to apply a "Comparison to the Average Guy" analysis to a behavior from their own list of "Might Have" problems. Common examples given by patients during this activity include isolation, trust, lack of emotional expressiveness, and alcohol use. Individual patient examples are then reviewed with input from the whole group, with patients asked to consider where their own behavior fits in the range of problem severity for the particular "Might Have" problem they examined.

The assigned homework is completion of the "Comparison to the

Average Guy" analysis worked on in the group session and preparing another comparable form applied to another "Might Have" problem.

Module 4: Roadblocks

In the final module, leaders discuss the concept of "roadblocks" as beliefs, fears, or situations that make it difficult to even consider whether a behavior is problematic and in need of change. Often people do not acknowledge a problem because they are avoiding some type of fear (Newman, 1994). Common roadblocks include guilt, shame, fears, cognitive distortions, and inaccurate stereotypes about what it means to have a problem. In this context, veterans have often reported fears of being perceived as weak, or shame about the distress they have brought to loved ones. Some of the roadblocks reviewed include fears of being overwhelmed by problems or being rejected if problems are acknowledged. Cognitive distortions include "all-or-nothing thinking," such as "If I admit to having one more problem, I will have to acknowledge being a complete failure." Consideration of the presence of a problem can elicit "internal stereotypes," or incorrect perceptions of what it means to have a particular disorder. An alcoholic may not want to admit to a drinking problem or seek treatment because his or her stereotypes of people so labeled involve images of the town drunk, a homeless person, or some other extreme or inaccurate depiction (Cunningham, Sobell, & Chow, 1993; Cunningham, Sobell, Sobell, & Gaskin, 1994). A veteran may want to avoid being perceived as a "crazy Vietnam veteran." Patients often report that they want to avoid thinking that they have the same problems as a specific person in their past, such as a father with an alcohol problem or violent temper or a family member who had been put into a mental hospital because of a "nervous breakdown." After the group generates a variety of possible roadblocks, participants are instructed to list on a worksheet only those that they feel apply to them. In addition, for each problem they have identified as a "Might Have," they are instructed to list any roadblocks that could prevent them from acknowledging it as a problem needing change. Patients are prompted to use a list of possible roadblocks (see Appendix 3.4).

CLINICAL ILLUSTRATIONS

Patients respond very positively to the PME Group in terms of its value and helpfulness (Franklin et al., 1999). During the group, individual patient responses to the goals and methods vary. It would be ideal to report that recognition of the need to change a specific problem is always clearly and immediately evident after patients engage in the use of the decision-making tools (Pros and Cons, Comparison to the Average Guy, and Roadblocks analysis). Although this often does occur, some patients tend not to make decisions about the need to change specific problems until near the end of the group, almost as if they are "softening" in their attitudes about examining the need to change. Two case examples might be useful in illustrating the various ways that patients respond to the group and take advantage of the specific techniques for decreasing ambivalence.

Albert was a 52-year-old Marine veteran in a VA outpatient PTSD treatment program who saw heavy combat during a 1-year tour of duty in Vietnam. He initially presented as quiet and stern-looking, and was irritable and defensive when attempts were made to engage him in group discussion and activities. On his Form #1 worksheet, he had listed many "Definitely Have" problems, among them anger, depression, isolation, trust, and sleep problems. For "Might Haves: Problems you have wondered if you have," he listed socializing, loneliness, and impatience. For "Might Haves: Problems other people say you have," he listed relationship problems, control, hypervigilance, and asking for help. He listed drinking and drug use as problems he didn't have.

Albert participated in the group activities, initially somewhat grudgingly. He was easily angered by any perceived lack of clarity on the group leaders' part regarding scheduling of questionnaire completion, group rules, and assignments. He did not report any particular dramatic recognition of the need to change any of his "Might Haves" immediately after using the specific decision-making tools in each group session.

As the group progressed, he appeared to respond well to a reflective listening approach when he expressed frustration, concerns, or confusion about the group or, as is very common with these patients, anger about how he had been treated by the military, the government, and the VA. It takes a delicate balance of empathy and limit setting when this issue arises, as the patients tend to get very upset quickly and as a group want to talk at length about their bitterness and resentment, to the exclusion of group activities. When handled appropriately, as in Albert's group, patients feel that the group leaders are understanding and willing to listen, and at the same time important group activities can still be accomplished. Over time, Albert became slightly friendlier in his manner toward the group leaders. In the review of roadblocks to acknowledging the need to change, Albert seemed to be struck by group discussion of how military training and social expectations for males make it shameful to admit the need for help or that someone can't handle his own problems. This is particularly true for Marines, who see participation in any activity related to help seeking, including problem acknowledgment, as a sign of weakness, since self-reliance was so heavily emphasized as a Marine virtue. Group process—specifically, seeing peers engage in the self-examination activities of the group—also seemed to encourage Albert to consider the need to change. By the end of the group, Albert had changed the "Might Have" problems on his Form #1 to "Definitely Have" problems. Albert went on to complete the entire 1-year treatment program.

Other patients have more of an "aha" experience in problem recognition during the group sessions, as the next case illustrates. Jack was an Army veteran in his early 50s who had been a helicopter doorgunner in Vietnam. He was new to PTSD treatment, having been referred from a drug treatment program where he had sought help for addiction to painkillers and alcohol. His main problems centered around avoiding people and difficulties in relationships, as he was very mistrustful of others and had remained isolated for many years. He initially identified "hard to get along with" as a "Might Have: A problem other people say you have but you disagree." During Session 2, he said that he would like to address "not trusting others" in a pros and cons analysis even though he had not initially listed it anywhere on his Form #1. He used the pros and cons decisional-balance form in Module 2 to address the possible need to change this approach to people. For pros, he listed feeling safe, don't get hurt, and don't get used. For cons, his list included not easy to let people in my life, isolation, makes other people angry, makes day-to-day living difficult, and becoming paranoid from being alone. His list of pros and cons was put up on a whiteboard as part of the group format, which also includes getting feedback from other group members about additional items for a patient to consider. As with a number of PME Group participants seeing their decisional-balance form displayed, Jack became quiet and appeared thoughtful. He then said that seeing the cons of being mistrustful so clearly delineated and outnumbering the pros made him consider for the first time that he had to change this way of approaching relationships with people. During Session 4, he talked about one of his roadblocks to being honest with himself as being "fear of facing the truth." At the end of the group, he had changed "hard to get along with" from "A problem other people say you have but you disagree" to a "Definitely Have" problem.

PROBLEMS AND SUGGESTED SOLUTIONS

There are some problems that have arisen in the application of MI principles in the PME Group with veterans. One somewhat surprising issue was that treatment providers in some VA programs have been hesitant to use an MI-based approach because of their concerns about giving patients an opportunity to express their true feelings about the value or credibility of the treatment program. Therapists also may not want to allow patients to raise doubts about the behaviors and beliefs identified by therapists as treatment targets. Generally, veterans are often uncomfortable with the level of control and directiveness of typically highly structured VA programs. Also, as described above, PTSD patients are frequently defensive about their mistrustful, isolative, hyperalert, and anger-prone styles of dealing with daily life. Some treatment providers feel that there is little clinical benefit to allowing patients to vent their feelings about these matters and that treatment time would be better spent on educating patients about the nature of their problems and teaching them new coping styles. This suggests that dissemination efforts must pay special attention to providing data to clinicians on the benefits of an MI approach and, using the MI approach in dissemination itself, giving plenty of opportunity for treatment providers to express and process their doubts and concerns about adopting this new approach.

Similarly, many patients are reluctant to engage in the PME Group because they do not see the value of "trying to find more problems," as some PTSD patients have put it. They often feel overwhelmed by the problems they already have, and coming up with more problems appears to be too much to face. Related to this, various patient characteristics make participation in the PME Group difficult, particularly patients with all-or-nothing thinking styles, so that dealing with ambiguity about the presence of a problem is anxiety-provoking. Also, many patients who are very narcissistic, proud, or highly self-reliant often feel that it would be a sign of weakness or stupidity to admit that they may have missed identifying a problem. In these cases, the patient will not list any possible "blindsiders" in the two "Might Have" columns. In addition to reflective listening to patients' thoughts about their inability to identify "Might Haves," further discussion of the rationale for the group, particularly avoiding future difficulties after treatment by identifying "blindsiders," usually has some impact on patients' willingness to consider possible problems. Also, it is hard for most patients to avoid finding at least one "Might Have" problem that other people have told them they have but with which they disagree.

Therapists, too, have their blind spots when implementing the PME Group, sometimes falling into the "expert trap" (Miller & Rollnick, 2002) by giving in to old conceptions of the "helper" (or worse, as the "expert") as someone who gives advice in response to patient questions or complaints. The supervision and training of group leaders must include emphasis on the importance of building therapeutic trust through reflective statements or by asking other group members to respond to concerns raised by patients, and how this frequently outweighs the benefits of a more directive information-giving approach, no matter how tempting it might be. In the author's experience in training clinicians, cognitive-behavioral therapists, even (and often particularly) skilled and experienced ones, frequently have difficulty in "rolling with resistance," or letting go of technique or goal-oriented approaches in the face of patient dissatisfaction or overtly oppositional or uncooperative behavior. They still tend to see these patient reactions to therapy as obstacles—as opposed to opportunities to address important patient concerns, fears, expectations, doubts, and misunderstandings. It may be that the critical nature of the therapeutic relationship and a patient-centered viewpoint in maximizing treatment outcome has still not been comfortably integrated into cognitive-behavioral theory and practice (see Newman, 1994, for an excellent guide to MI-consistent approaches to resistance in the context of cognitive-behavioral therapy).

Also, patients sometimes have a difficult time understanding the concepts and therapy tasks of the PME Group. The author and other colleagues using the PME Group have often been surprised by patients who appear to understand a basic decisional balance task when first introduced but eventually show their lack of understanding of what they are being asked to do. The group format often aids in patient comprehension of this and the other tasks by allowing patients to witness others' process in completing the task and the more assertive patients to model asking questions. Also, in the PME Group, half of each session is devoted to review of the purpose and methods of the group, but therapists must still be vigilant that patients may not necessarily demonstrate their lack of comprehension of group activities.

RESEARCH

The first outcome study of the PME Group involved a single group who received the procedure (Murphy, Cameron, et al., 2004). Subjects were

243 veterans who were also participating in inpatient PTSD treatment. By the end of the group, significantly more veterans reclassified the following "Might Have" problems to "Definitely Have" than to "Don't Have" problems: Anger, Isolation, Anxiety, Authority, Guilt, Emotional Masking, Relationship/Intimacy, Smoking, and Trust. The lack of a control group in this feasibility study prevents attributing these outcomes specifically to the PME procedure.

Early unpublished results are also available from an ongoing randomized trial of the PME Group. The goal of this study is to determine whether the PME Group will improve combat veterans' treatment adherence (higher rates of attendance at all treatment-related groups and lower dropout rate) in a year-long outpatient PTSD program. The rationale is that increased problem recognition will lead to better PTSD program treatment adherence because patients will perceive treatment as more relevant to them. Furthermore, increased perception of treatment relevance should lead to better skills learning, thereby resulting in better PTSD treatment outcomes.

Participants are veterans with combat-related PTSD, mainly male Vietnam veterans, admitted to the New Orleans VA PTSD Clinic's Trauma Recovery Program (TRP). The year-long TRP consists of a sequence of 12 separate month-long (four-session) group interventions that vary in focus (e.g., PTSD education, anger management, lifespan review). Study participants are randomly assigned to receive four sessions of the PME Group or the usual PTSD Psychoeducation Group in the second month of their participation in the TRP. Measures of readiness to change PTSD problems, perceived treatment relevance and satisfaction, and PTSD-related functioning are assessed before and after the intervention phase (PME or Psychoeducation Group) and then monthly for the duration of patient's year-long PTSD program participation. At this time, attendance data for the full 10-month follow-up period are available on 71 subjects, which is about half the number needed for adequate power to detect group differences in this study. PME Group participants and controls were compared on the percentage of scheduled PTSD program sessions attended for each of the 10 months of their PTSD program participation after the intervention phase of the study (PME Group or PTSD Psychoeducation Group). The analysis reported here includes only patients who had attended 75% or more of the PME Group (n = 32) or control intervention (n = 28). This was deemed necessary because of variations in attendance at the study interventions and to examine the effectiveness of the PME Group at "full dose." A 2 (treatment condition: PME Group vs. control) × 10 (time: 10 follow-up months) analysis of variance with repeated measures yielded a significant treatment condition × time interaction ($p < .01$), with the results suggesting higher treatment attendance for PME Group participants in the middle of their PTSD program participation, although not near the beginning or end (see Figure 3.1).

In terms of process, there are also data available for analysis for 54 study participants on questionnaire items developed for this study assessing attitudes toward the need to change and treatment satisfaction and relevance (Murphy, Thompson, Rainey, & Murray, 2004). The measures available for analysis at this time were those obtained before and immediately after the intervention phase. Briefly, analyses indicated that, in contrast to controls, the PME group participants showed significantly increased agreement with items concerning the need to consider others' feedback, importance of considering behavior pros and cons, helpfulness of comparing behavior to norms, and taking responsibility for handling difficult or anger-provoking situations. There were no differences on treatment satisfaction and relevance after the intervention phase due to a ceiling effect, as patients generally report being very satisfied in the well-run TRP program.

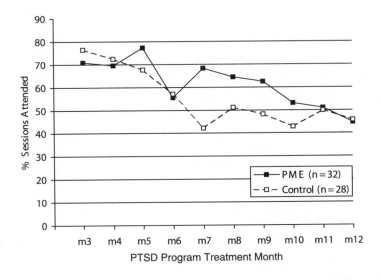

FIGURE 3.1. PTSD program attendance for PME Group participants and controls.

These preliminary results are only suggestive that the PME Group is having intended effects on readiness to change and treatment adherence, but they are encouraging. More definitive conclusions about the PME Group's effectiveness await the forthcoming results of analyses with adequate power that examine all measures of treatment adherence, readiness to change, and PTSD-related functioning.

CONCLUSIONS

Application of the MI approach to PTSD is still a developing area, requiring more research to support the rationale and clinical techniques described in this chapter. At this time, there appears to be support for continuing this work. As described above, a case can be made for the applicability of MI principles to the treatment of chronic combat-related PTSD. One indirect indicator of this is the response of clinicians to the PME Group. The author has been cautious about promoting the use of this intervention because of the lack of clear evidence for its effectiveness. Yet, providers of treatment for PTSD who attend conference presentations or read articles about the ongoing work on the PME Group are highly enthusiastic about it and have employed it in their clinical work. This enthusiasm for the intervention is due solely to clinicians' familiarity with the common but rarely documented (or addressed by clinical researchers in the trauma field) ambivalence of veteran patients with PTSD about the need to change important PTSD symptoms and related problems. The patients' responses also have been positive, and they often report that it was of great help to them to take a closer look at what might be contributing to their difficulties. It may be too, that the supportive, empathic stance employed in MI allows them to take an honest look at themselves in a way that is much less painful and anxiety-provoking than they had imagined.

Despite patients' and clinicians' enthusiasm for introducing MI-based techniques to PTSD treatment, results from an ongoing randomized trial of the PME group will be critical for making decisions about the value of incorporating a motivation enhancement approach into PTSD treatment. If empirical validation of this method occurs, further studies will be needed as well. These include exploring the value of targeting general externalizing patient cognitive styles; obtaining more data supporting the conceptualization of the need to change PTSD-related problems within the stages-of-change model; and developing more sophisticated cognitive-behavioral models for specifying and understanding obstacles to problem recognition.

Furthermore, it is unknown how the MI approach may benefit soldiers now returning from deployment in Iraq and Afghanistan who are experiencing stress symptoms and adjustment problems following their war-zone experiences. In contrast to Vietnam veterans seeking treatment for stress disorder, these veterans have had difficulties related to their military duty for only a short time. In the author's experience, there are both similarities and differences in readiness to change between these new combat veterans and Vietnam veterans. One difference is that the relatively short duration of their symptoms can contribute to increased ambivalence about the need to change, because fewer negative consequences resulting from their symptoms or trauma-based coping styles have occurred. However, one difference that promotes acknowledgment about the need to change is that soldiers' stress reactions to combat and difficulties in adjusting upon their return home are now frequently depicted in the news media. One striking similarity is that both Vietnam vets and those of Iraq and Afghanistan can still view important PTSD symptoms such as anger, mistrust, and isolation as adaptive coping strategies. Also, both groups of vets can be unaware of the link between their behavior and their traumatic experiences, enhanced by externalizing the cause of their problems to provocative or difficult situations or people. They also have at least some of the same cognitive and emotional obstacles to acknowledging the need to change, with not wanting to appear "weak" by needing help or admitting that one can't handle problems on one's own as a example that has been particularly striking to the author. As a final note, the Iraq and Afghanistan veteran participants in the PME Group also reported that the intervention was very useful to them, and in the group sessions demonstrated increased problem recognition (e.g., one Iraq vet was finally able to admit that anger was a problem in his life that needed change). So, it appears that MI may be of value in helping newly returned veterans to identify and acknowledge unrecognized problems, with the hoped-for but yet unseen result that the effectiveness of their PTSD treatment is improved.

The potential value of this endeavor for improving PTSD treatment outcome among combat veterans with chronic PTSD is enormous but unproven. Certainly, efforts in this direction could not even be attempted without the creativity and volume of the theoretical, clinical, and research work supporting MI. The incorporation of MI principles and methods into PTSD treatment may be one additional item on the list of valuable extensions of this approach.

REFERENCES

American Psychiatric Association. (2000). *Diagnostic and statistical manual of mental disorders* (4th ed., text rev.). Washington, DC: Author.

Cunningham, J. A., Sobell, L. C., & Chow, V. M. (1993). What's in a label?: The effects of substance types and labels on treatment considerations and stigma. *Journal of Studies on Alcohol, 54*, 693–699.

Cunningham, J. A., Sobell, L. C., Sobell, M. B., & Gaskin, J. (1994). Alcohol and drug abusers' reasons for seeking treatment. *Addictive Behavior, 19*, 691–696.

DiClemente, C. C., & Vasquez, M. M. (2002). Motivational interviewing and the Stages of Change. In W. R. Miller & S. Rollnick, *Motivational interviewing: Preparing people for change* (2nd ed., pp. 201–216). New York: Guilford Press.

Fontana, A., & Rosenheck, R. (1997). Effectiveness and cost of the inpatient treatment of posttraumatic stress disorder: Comparison of three models of treatment. *American Journal of Psychiatry, 154*, 758–765.

Franklin, C. L., Murphy, R. T., Cameron, R. P., Ramirez, G., Sharp, L. D., & Drescher, K. D. (1999, November). *Perceived helpfulness of a group targeting motivation to change PTSD symptoms.* Poster presented at the annual meeting of the International Society for Traumatic Stress Studies, Miami, FL.

Hoge, C. W., Castro, C. A., Messner, S. C., McGurk, D., Cotting, D. I., & Koffman, R. L. (2004). Combat duty in Iraq and Afghanistan, mental health problems, and barriers to care. *The New England Journal of Medicine, 351*(1), 13–22.

McFall, M., Malte, C., Fontana, A., & Rosenheck, R. A. (2000). Effects of an outreach intervention on use of mental health services by veterans with posttraumatic stress disorder. *Psychiatric Services, 51*, 369–374.

Miller, W. R., Benefield, R. G., & Tonigan, J. S. (1993). Enhancing motivation for change in problem drinking: A controlled comparison of two therapist styles. *Journal of Consulting and Clinical Psychology, 61*, 455–461.

Miller, W. R., & Rollnick, S. (2002). *Motivational interviewing: Preparing people for change* (2nd ed.). New York: Guilford Press.

Miller, W. R., Sovereign, R. G., & Krege, B. (1988). Motivational interviewing with problem drinkers: II. The Drinker's Check-Up as a preventive intervention. *Behavioural Psychotherapy, 16*, 251–268.

Murphy, R. T., Cameron, R. P., Sharp, L., Ramirez, G., Rosen, C., Drescher, K., et al. (2004). Readiness to change PTSD symptoms and related behaviors among veterans participating in a Motivation Enhancement Group. *The Behavior Therapist, 27*(4), 33–36.

Murphy, R. T., Thompson, K. E., Rainey, Q., & Murray, M. (2004). *Early results from an ongoing randomized trial of the PTSD ME Group.* Poster presented at the annual meeting of the International Society for Traumatic Stress Studies, New Orleans, LA.

Newman, C. F. (1994). Understanding client resistance: Methods for enhancing motivation to change. *Cognitive and Behavioral Practice, 1*, 47–69.

Prochaska, J. O., & DiClemente, C. C. (1983). Stages and processes of self-change in smoking: Toward an integrative model of change. *Journal of Consulting and Clinical Psychology, 40*, 432–440.

Prochaska, J. O., DiClemente, C. C., & Norcross, J. C. (1992). In search of how people change: Applications to addictive behaviors. *American Psychologist, 47,* 1102–1114.

Rosen, C. S., Murphy, R. T., Chow, H. C., Drescher, K. D., Ramirez, G., Ruddy, R., et al. (2001). Posttraumatic stress disorder patients' readiness to change alcohol and anger problems. *Psychotherapy, 38,* 233–244.

Rosenheck, R. A., & DiLella, D. (1998). *Department of Veterans Affairs National Mental Health Program Performance Monitoring System: Fiscal year 1997 report.* Veterans Affairs Connecticut Healthcare System, Northeast Program Evaluation Center.

Schnurr, P. P., Friedman, M. J., Foy, D. W., Shea, M. T., Hsieh, F. Y., Lavori, P. W., et al. (2003). Randomized trial of trauma-focused group therapy for posttraumatic stress disorder. *Archives of General Psychiatry, 60,* 481–489.

Zweben, A., & Zuckoff, A. (2002). Motivational interviewing and treatment adherence. In W. R. Miller & S. Rollnick, *Motivational interviewing: Preparing people for change* (2nd ed., pp. 299–319). New York: Guilford Press.

APPENDIX 3.1. Sample Problem Identification Worksheet (Form #1)

	MIGHT HAVES		
Problems You DEFINITELY *HAVE*	Problems you *might* have: You have wondered if you have	Problems you *might* have: Problems other people say you have but you disagree	Problems You DEFINITELY *DON'T* HAVE
PTSD	Judgmental	Workaholic	Crazy
Anger	Patience	Smoking	Drugs
Depression	Authority	Emotionally numb	Cancer
Alcohol	Weapons	Perfectionistic	Legal
Intimacy	Hypervigilance	Trust	
Isolation	Self-Esteem		

APPENDIX 3.2. Self-Talk Checklist
for Continued Progress after Treatment

If I'm having difficulties after treatment, I will consider or do the following:

____ There might be something about the way I'm looking at the situation (because of my past experiences) rather than the situation itself that is causing difficulties.

____ I need to think if my difficulties might be at least partly due to problems I'm not aware of.

____ Look for "blindsiders": ways I act or think that I don't think are a problem, but really are.

____ Threats to my progress after/during treatment are not just problems I already know I have.

____ I have to consider what other people say when they give me feedback about my behavior or my way of thinking.

____ It is important to consider both the positives and negatives about my behavior or my way of thinking.

____ Comparing myself to guys my age who don't have PTSD will help me decide if I need to change my behavior or way of thinking.

____ I plan on getting more help for my problems.

____ I may not understand myself and my problems as well as I think.

____ I am responsible for handling situations that are difficult, upsetting, or get me angry, even when other people, traumatic situations in my past, or bad luck are part of the problem.

APPENDIX 3.3. "Comparison to the Average Guy"

Sample Behavior: Hypervigilance

	Average	Moderate Problem	Extreme Problem
Frequency	Makes sure the door is locked before going to bed	Checks the locks at least twice a night	Checks the perimeter of the house several times a night
	Installing motion detector lights outside the house	Likely to install motion detector lights and a burglar alarm system	Multiple locks on doors that are checked often
	May own a dog	May own at least one gun	Owns a pit bull
	May think about buying a gun but decides it is too risky		Gun under pillow
			May own high-caliber weapons
Severity of Consequences	If he owns a gun, it makes his family nervous	Limits his relationships with neighbors and others	Has poor relationships with neighbors—sees threats everywhere
	He's out the cost of the lights	Intimidates others with dog	Keeps spending money
		May interfere with sleep and work	Health problems
		More time and money spent on security	Cannot sleep
Purpose	Allows him to feel secure	Tells himself it's better to be safe than sorry	Survival
		Trying to feel safe	Feels "life or death"

APPENDIX 3.4. Roadblocks

This is a list of thoughts, feelings, and beliefs that might prevent someone from taking an honest look at himself or herself. Some may apply to you, and some may not.

Fears

Fear of rejection

Fear of change

Fear of embarrassment

Fear of feeling "weak"

Fear of being seen as weak

Fear of feeling overwhelmed

Fear of emotions coming up

Fear of facing the truth

Fear of crying

Fear of not being able to stop crying

Fear of "I told you so"

Fear of finding out I'm "crazy"

Fear that others will think I'm crazy

Fear of being "locked up"

Fear of being judged

Fear of being seen as "damaged"

Fear of feeling "stupid"

Fear that others will see me as "stupid"

Fear of losing control

Feelings

Guilt

Shame

Beliefs

Admitting problem equals weakness

Shameful to tell other people your problems

Don't deserve help

Shame about past events

Don't want to think about past events

Don't want to have feelings of failure

Don't want to fail

Have to take care of problems yourself

Internal Stereotypes

Belief that alcohol problem = "skid row" type of alcoholic, homeless person

Belief that drug problem = dirty "addict"

Belief that needing help for psychological problems = "crazy mental patient"

CHAPTER 4

Motivating Treatment-Refusing Patients with Obsessive–Compulsive Disorder

David F. Tolin
Nicholas Maltby

THE CLINICAL POPULATION AND USUAL TREATMENTS

Obsessive–compulsive disorder (OCD) is a chronic anxiety disorder marked by recurrent, intrusive, and distressing thoughts (obsessions) and/or repetitive behaviors (compulsions) (American Psychiatric Association, 2000). Factor- and cluster-analytic studies have repeatedly identified dimensions or subtypes of OCD. These include contamination fears and washing compulsions, harm-related thoughts and checking compulsions, compulsive hoarding, and symmetry obsessions and ordering/arranging compulsions (for reviews, see Mataix-Cols, Rosario-Campos, & Leckman, 2005; McKay et al., 2004).

Recent epidemiological data suggest a 12-month prevalence of 1% (Kessler, Chiu, Demler, & Walters, 2005) and a lifetime prevalence of 2% (Kessler, Berglund, Demler, Jin, & Walters, 2005). A survey of individuals with OCD indicated that 20% spent 5–8 hours per day engaged in rituals, with 13% spending over 17 hours per day during the most severe period of the disorder (Gallup Organization Inc., 1990). Not surprisingly, OCD symptoms often severely disrupt social and vocational functioning (Leon, Portera, & Weissman, 1995), and OCD is associated with a 40% unemployment rate (Steketee, Grayson, & Foa, 1987). Self-reported quality of life among patients with OCD has been reported to be comparable to or poorer than that of patients with schizophrenia, depression, and substance dependence (Bobes et al., 2001; Bystritsky et al., 2001; Koran, Thienemann, & Davenport, 1996).

The psychosocial treatment of choice for OCD is cognitive-behavioral therapy (CBT) incorporating exposure and response prevention (ERP). Numerous controlled trials attest to the efficacy of ERP (e.g., Cottraux, Mollard, Bouvard, & Marks, 1993; Fals-Stewart, Marks, & Schafer, 1993; Foa et al., 2005; Lindsay, Crino, & Andrews, 1997; van Balkom et al., 1998). In addition, ERP has also proven effective in clinical settings (Franklin, Abramowitz, Kozak, Levitt, & Foa, 2000; Warren & Thomas, 2001) and with medication-resistant patients (Kampman, Keijsers, Hoogduin, & Verbraak, 2002; Simpson, Gorfinkle, & Liebowitz, 1999; Tolin, Maltby, Diefenbach, Hannan, & Worhunsky, 2004). A recent large-scale controlled trial (Foa et al., 2005) indicated that patients completing ERP alone showed a greater reduction in OCD severity than did patients receiving the tricyclic antidepressant clomipramine. Furthermore, the addition of clomipramine to ERP did not appear to yield treatment effects that were greater than those of patients receiving ERP alone. After treatment discontinuation, treatment responders were followed for an additional 12 weeks (Simpson et al., 2004). Patients receiving ERP with or without clomipramine were less likely to relapse after treatment discontinuation than were patients receiving clomipramine alone; again, there was no apparent benefit of adding clomipramine to ERP. Thus, an expert consensus panel (March, Frances, Carpenter, & Kahn, 1997) wrote, "When available, CBT is recommended for every patient with OCD *except those who are unwilling to participate*" (p. 12; emphasis added).

RATIONALE FOR USING MOTIVATIONAL INTERVIEWING FOR THIS DISORDER/PROBLEM

Despite the clear evidence of the efficacy of ERP, a substantial number of patients refuse this treatment (Franklin & Foa, 1998). In the Foa and colleagues (2005) study, of 521 eligible participants who were screened by telephone, 10% refused to schedule an initial appointment due to an unwillingness to receive ERP (although it is also noted that 11% refused to schedule the appointment due to an unwillingness to receive clomipramine). Upon learning of their treatment condition, 22% of patients withdrew from the ERP condition, and 22% from the combined medication-only conditions (clomipramine or placebo), compared to 6% from the ERP + clomipramine condition. Thus, these proportions hint at a higher acceptability of combined treatment over either medication or ERP alone, although they do not indicate a higher refusal rate for ERP as compared to medication. Among patients who began treatment, 28% dropped out of ERP, 25% from clomipramine, 23% from placebo, and 39% from the combined ERP + clomipramine condition. Thus, although ERP does not appear to be associated with a higher refusal or dropout rate than are medications, a clinically unacceptable 43% of patients assigned to ERP monotherapy either refused or dropped out of this treatment.

The reasons why some OCD patients refuse ERP have not been well documented. However, several potential reasons have been examined for OCD and other anxiety disorders. In their survey of treatment utilization in Australia for anxiety disorders, Issakidis and Andrews (2002) indicated that most treatment-refusing patients cited a preference to manage the disorder without help (58%). In some cases, self-directed treatment has been shown to be helpful for OCD, although the available evidence suggests that it is significantly less effective than is treatment administered by a trained therapist (see Tolin & Hannan, 2005, for a review).

Our clinical experience has been that many OCD patients appear to refuse ERP due to fear or apprehension about the difficulty and intensity of ERP (Maltby & Tolin, 2005). ERP requires considerable effort by OCD patients. They are required to attend lengthy and frequent treatment sessions and are asked to confront anxiety-provoking situations while resisting rituals. Increased fear during exposure sessions is not only an inevitable part of the process; many researchers consider it a necessary element for successful fear reduction (Foa & Kozak, 1986). Some patients have difficulty with this aspect of treatment and prefer to seek out treatments that are less threatening.

Another factor that may influence rates of treatment refusal is patient readiness for change. Transtheoretical models (Prochaska, DiClemente, & Norcross, 1992), initially developed to increase readiness for change in addictive disorders, have recently been applied to the treatment of anxiety disorders (Westra, 2003, 2004; Westra & Phoenix, 2003). Transtheoretical models posit that clinical change involves progression through five different stages of change (SOC): precontemplation, contemplation, preparation, action, and maintenance. Patients in the precontemplation, contemplation, and preparation stages are not yet ready to begin active attempts to change. Thus, it may be that OCD patients in these three SOC are more likely to refuse ERP than are patients in the action or maintenance stages.

Some OCD patients are classified as having poor insight, which may also impact rates of treatment refusal. Indeed, in the DSM-IV field trial (Foa et al., 1995), only a minority of OCD patients were described as having excellent insight (i.e., a firm conviction that feared consequences would not occur if they did not perform their compulsive behaviors); poor insight appeared particularly common among patients with religious or harm-related obsessions (Tolin, Abramowitz, Kozak, & Foa, 2001). Lack of insight into the irrationality of obsessive fears has been associated with poorer outcome in some studies of pharmacotherapy and CBT (Catapano, Sperandeo, Perris, Lanzaro, & Maj, 2001; Erzegovesi et al., 2001; Foa, 1979; Neziroglu, Stevens, & Yaryura-Tobias, 1999), although not in others (Eisen et al., 2001; Foa et al., 1983; Hoogduin & Duivenvoorden, 1988).

Finally, some patients may refuse ERP due to low expectancies for improvement or that ERP will be helpful. Expectancy effects are a strong predictor of treatment outcome (Kirsch, 1990; Lambert, 1992), as well as acceptance of specific interventions (Elkin et al., 1999). In their service utilization study for all anxiety disorders, Issakidis and Andrews (2002) reported that low expectancy was endorsed by 14% of treatment refusers. We have found expectancies for improvement to be fairly high in our OCD clinic samples (Tolin, Diefenbach, Maltby, & Hannan, 2005; Tolin et al., 2004), although it remains possible that some patients who refuse treatment do so because of low expectations for change.

Thus, although ERP does not appear to be associated with higher refusal or dropout rates than are some other treatments, these rates remain high, and many patients who might benefit from ERP ultimately do not complete this treatment due to personal choice factors. Factors that may influence refusal and dropout rates include a belief that professional treatment is not necessary, fear of the ERP procedures, early SOC, poor insight, or low expectancies for improvement with treatment. Motivational interviewing (MI) principles (Miller & Rollnick, 2002) appear promising to address these potential obstacles to OCD treatment. MI was initially developed to enhance motivation for change and resolve treatment ambivalence for the addictive disorders, but it has been recently applied to anxiety disorders that are similarly characterized by ambivalence about change. MI involves the use of a cluster of principles to increase intrinsic motivation, including being nonjudgmental, expressing empathy, avoiding argumentation, using reflective listening, exploring ambivalence, developing discrepancy, avoiding confrontation, and supporting self-efficacy. Among military veterans with PTSD, interventions incorporating MI principles have led to increased action on problems that had previously gone unaddressed (Murphy, Chapter 3, this volume). MI also appears to be helpful as an adjunctive treatment for anxiety disorders, leading to improved outcomes for some patients who were initially nonresponders to CBT (Westra & Dozois, Chapter 2, this volume). In a recent study of a mixed sample of non-OCD anxiety patients who were not treatment refusers, brief pretreatment with MI as a prelude to CBT appeared to increase expectancies for change and increased CBT efficacy; there was also a nonsignificant trend toward reduced dropout rates (Westra & Dozois, Chapter 2, this volume). In this chapter, we describe a brief readiness program developed for treatment-refusing OCD patients that incorporates elements of MI in hopes of resolving ambivalence and preparing patients to enter ERP treatment.

CLINICAL APPLICATION OF MI TO THIS DISORDER/PROBLEM

We (Maltby & Tolin, 2005) developed a brief (four-session) readiness intervention (RI) for patients with OCD who, after an initial assessment, declined to enter ERP for reasons other than practical obstacles to care (e.g., lack of transportation, living too far away from the clinic, etc.). As described above, we speculated that there might be several reasons why patients refuse treatment, of which early SOC, low expectancies, and fear of ERP seemed most likely, given our informal discussions with these patients. Thus, we included in these four sessions specific interventions to address these issues. These interventions included the following.

Psychoeducation

This component included a brief discussion of OCD, encompassing its epidemiology, symptoms, and biological and behavioral models of the disorder. OCD was presented as both a neurobiological and behavioral condition that could be treated with medications or with ERP. One aim of this component was to provide corrective information for low expectations of change. Thus, we reviewed empirical data demonstrating the positive effects of ERP. In the spirit of MI, we also discussed the potential limitations of this knowledge as well as the potential "downsides" of ERP (e.g., time commitment, anxiety elicited by exposures). Psychoeducation was also hoped to begin the process of reducing fear by educating participants about the components of ERP and the rationale for their use.

Motivational Interviewing

MI targets patients' ambivalence about change that could influence fear of treatment and beliefs that ERP is too much work. MI might also influence insight, as it emphasizes a nonjudgmental examination of the positive and negative impacts of the disorder on functioning. While MI was explicitly used in two of these four sessions, MI principles guided therapist–patient interactions throughout the RI condition. Thus, therapists were nonjudgmental, empathic, developed discrepancy, and encouraged self-efficacy throughout the RI program. For example, while psychoeducation was intended to counter fears of ERP, low expectations of improvement, and lack of information about available treatment options, it was not presented in the same way as with an OCD patient who had initially accepted ERP. This discussion was deliberately as neutral-to-change as possible, with efforts to minimize external pressures to change. Examining the pros and cons of all options, including doing nothing, was encouraged. Throughout the process, patients were encouraged to consider the decisional balance of changing in general as well as enrolling in ERP specifically. When participants raised concerns or expressed ambivalence, therapists were instructed to use empathic listening skills (e.g., reflection) rather than provide counterarguments.

Viewing a Videotape of ERP

The videotape of a simulated ERP session (with an actor playing the role of the patient, a fact of which participants were made aware) was hoped to reduce fears and modify expectancies by providing a concrete example of ERP, within- and between-session habituation to fear cues, and patient–therapist interactions. Our experience has been that, before beginning ERP, OCD patients often have misconceptions as to how exposures are conducted, frequently believing that they will be forced to engage in very difficult exposures. The video provided an example of the cooperative nature of exposures in ERP. Again, MI principles were utilized during this task. Thus, critical thinking and examination of the pros and cons of elements of ERP were encouraged as patients were asked to discuss their cognitive and emotional responses to the video-tape.

Constructing a Sample Exposure Hierarchy

With assistance from the therapist, participants constructed an exposure hierarchy that would be used if the participant were to enter ERP. Consistent with the spirit of MI, participants were told that they would not be pressured to actually do any of these exposure exercises and that the hierarchy was being constructed for educational purposes only. This step was included for two reasons. First, it was hoped to enhance fear reduction by providing concrete examples of what ERP would entail, and demonstrate the graded nature of exposures. Second, constructing an exposure hierarchy was a means to shape successive approximations toward ERP as patients began to engage in steps associated with treatment.

A Telephone Conversation with a Patient Who Had Completed ERP

Participants spoke anonymously by telephone with a former patient from our clinic who had received ERP. Efforts were made to match patients according to OCD symptom presentation (e.g., we would try to have a patient with washing compulsions speak with a prior patient with washing compulsions). The phone conversation with a successful ERP patient was complementary to the video but added several specific elements. It was confidential. The therapist was not in the room and was not informed of what occurred during the conversation. Thus, the participant was free to ask any questions and to be critical of ERP (or the therapist) without concern about affecting his or her relationship with the therapist. The two could talk for any length of time and on any topic. The aim of this activity was to provide a real-life example of the effects of ERP. It also encouraged active steps to understand OCD treatment and engage in early change processes, as it was unscripted and required the patient to take an active role. This encouraged a highly personalized dialogue about fears of treatment and expectations about change. Thus, the belief that ERP involves personal control of treatment decisions was enhanced, as was the implicit process of shaping successive approximations to engage in treatment.

As should be evident from the foregoing description, our use of MI differed from that of Miller and Rollnick (2002) in several ways. Though efforts were made to minimize therapist expectations of entry into ERP, patients were aware that the purpose was ultimately to increase acceptance of ERP. The RI program was more action-oriented than is traditional MI, with the therapist setting a specific agenda for each session. Greater emphasis was placed on treatment-targeting beliefs about ERP than on beliefs about change in general. Homework assignments, which are not a traditional element of MI, were used. Lastly, the four-session readiness intervention was more constrained than standard MI. Patients engaged in specific treatment elements at each session, as opposed to utilizing specific MI principles as appropriate to the context of the therapy session.[1]

CLINICAL ILLUSTRATION

Linda is a 35-year-old Caucasian woman with a history of OCD since late adolescence. She presented at the Anxiety Disorders Center with the rather unusual fear that she would be contaminated by objects or people that were from, or had been to, Japan. If she accidentally became "contaminated" (e.g., an object she touched was later found to be from Japan), Linda went through a lengthy cleaning ritual in which the item was discarded and items that came into contact or could possibly have come into contact with it were repeatedly washed. She checked new items extensively for information about their country of origin. At the time of intake, her fear of objects from Japan had caused her to be highly avoidant to the point where she limited her time spent outside of her home. She also reported some concerns with general contamination and ordering/arranging, but these were clearly secondary to her primary obsessions about Japan. On the Yale–Brown Obsessive–Compulsive Scale (Y-BOCS; Goodman et al., 1989), she received a total score of 27, hich placed her in the severe OCD category. On the Clinician's Global Impression scale (CGI; Guy, 1976) she was rated as being "markedly ill." Using the Structured Clinical Interview for DSM-IV (SCID; First, Spitzer, Gibbon, & Williams, 1995), she was diagnosed with OCD and major depressive disorder.

After reviewing the cognitive-behavioral model of OCD and the rationale behind ERP, Linda was offered a program of ERP to treat her OCD. Linda refused this treatment and stated that her reasons for refusing ERP were that

1. ERP was too difficult, and she wanted an easier treatment.
2. She didn't believe that any treatment could help her.
3. She believed that going to therapy was embarrassing.
4. She had other things in her life she wanted to focus her energies on.

When asked how scared she was to start treatment, she indicated that her fear of ERP was a 95 on a 100-point scale, where 100 = "I am so afraid to start therapy that I could not stand it" and 0 = "I am not at all afraid to start therapy." On the University of Rhode Island Change Assessment Questionnaire (URICA; Greenstein, Franklin, & McGuffin, 1999), her scores were consistent with being in the contemplation stage of change.

Linda was then offered our four-session readiness program designed to promote patients' readiness to enter into ERP. This was described to her as having five components:

1. Education about OCD and its treatment.
2. Building a model exposure hierarchy.
3. Viewing a videotaped example of ERP.
4. Having a phone conversation with a former OCD patient who had completed ERP.
5. Procedures derived from MI, including encouraging her to discuss her ambivalence, and a review of the costs and benefits of entering treatment.

She was assured that the readiness intervention was free of pressures to enter into treatment and would not involve engaging in actual exposure activities. Linda then agreed to participate in the readiness intervention.

All of the RI strategies were delivered in the spirit of MI. During the first session, it was stressed that the readiness intervention was collaborative, and Linda was encouraged to ask questions and to follow up with areas of uncertainty. With her therapist she discussed the cognitive-behavioral model of OCD, with particular emphasis on the role of avoidance in maintaining the disorder. She also discussed the etiology of OCD and the different treatment options available for OCD as well as with expected treatment outcomes. Linda was an active participant in this process and asked follow-up questions. At the end of this session, her fear of beginning ERP was slightly decreased from intake and was an 85 on a 0–100 scale. Her score on the Expectancies Rating Form (ERF; Borkovec & Nau, 1972) indicated that she expected ERP to be moderately efficacious. For homework she was asked to read several handouts about OCD and CBT.

During the second session, Linda and the therapist reviewed any questions she had from the reading assignments. In order to gauge her understanding of the cognitive-behavioral model of OCD and to encourage elaborative processing, the therapist encouraged Linda to verbalize her understanding of how OCD is maintained and treated. Linda had read both handouts and demonstrated that she had a working knowledge of these factors. With the therapist's help, she constructed a sample exposure hierarchy in order to learn what ERP would entail for her, to encourage fear reduction, and to shape successive approximations toward ERP. Her hierarchy (see Figure 4.1) included a number of items that were associated, directly or indirectly, with her fear of contamination from Japanese objects. For instance, until her husband showered, she feared that he had had incidental or direct contact with items from Japan and was therefore contaminated. Similarly, she avoided public tables, chairs, and so on, because she could not confirm that they were free of "contamination" from Japan.

Linda and her therapist then discussed how she might approach exposures. This discussion was introduced by the therapist as being hy-

Anxiety Rating	Exposure
100	Touch items from Japan
90	Hugging husband when he comes home from work
85	Have someone else sit on her bed
75	Touching chairs in public areas
70	Put dirty clothes on bed
65	Place her combs in the dirty sink and then put them away
55	Touching door handle to bedroom
40	Touching husband when he comes home from work

FIGURE 4.1. Linda's exposure hierarchy.

pothetical, and that Linda would not actually be required to do the exposures they discussed. In this way, Linda was able to imagine exposing herself to feared stimuli and to engage in an open discussion about exposure therapy without feeling pressured to do exposures. Linda stated that she felt she could not touch an object from Japan, but could start with lower-level items such as touching her husband when he came home from work. She suggested that she might touch him lightly on the shoulder when he got home, since she thought his shoulder would be the least likely area to be contaminated. This led to a discussion of how fear reduction is achieved, using examples from simple phobias such as fear of dogs, with which she did not have a problem. Linda was able to recognize that fear reduction would require multiple repetitions and that, although she could begin with lower level items, she would need to confront the highest items in order to have significant symptom reduction. For instance, drawing on the dog phobia analogy, the therapist asked how she might get over being scared of German shepherd dogs. Linda thought that she could do so by having increasing contact with smaller, quieter dogs but acknowledged that she did not think she would get over being scared of large dogs like German shepherds unless she actually had contact with them. She was able to relate this process to her primary fear of Japan but did not think it would be possible to actually handle items from Japan. At the end of this session, her fear of beginning ERP, at 85 on a 0–100 scale, was unchanged from her previous session. Her ERF score was also unchanged and indicated that she expected ERP to be moderately efficacious.

During the third session, Linda watched a videotape of an ERP session. The therapist remained in the room to answer any questions and encouraged Linda to view the videotape critically and to discuss any issues that arose from viewing it. The videotape, focusing on contamination concerns, was well matched to her main symptoms of OCD. However, Linda wondered if it would be as easy for her as for the patient in the videotape. For instance, in the video the patient habituated to touching a doorknob relatively rapidly (up to four repetitions). Linda thought this would be unrealistic for her, leading to a discussion of individual differences in changing OCD fears. She wondered if it was possible to fail to habituate. This also led to a conversation of the elements that can block habituation (avoidance, safety cues, failure to repeat, not remaining in the situation until anxiety levels are reduced). During this session, Linda appeared to take more control, and her questions, such as the ones above, implied an increased curiosity about, and perhaps willingness to engage in, exposure exercises.

During this session, the therapist began using MI to explore Linda's ambivalence about beginning treatment, starting with an analysis of the pros and cons of her current behaviors. The therapist started with the benefits of engaging in OCD behaviors so as to avoid beginning with a potentially confrontational subject. Under pros, Linda listed the fact that avoidance reduced her anxiety and made her fear of Japan more tolerable. Staying home and limiting contact with others significantly reduced her anxiety. However, consistent with the MI principle of developing discrepancy, this discussion led Linda to spontaneously list the costs of OCD. For instance, she felt that she was rarely anxiety-free, since she was regularly concerned about her husband being contaminated when he was outside the home. Additionally, the mail terrified her, because she worried that her mail or packages had come into contact with items from Japan. As a result, she avoided dealing with the mail and had gotten into financial trouble in the past when she had not paid bills. Although her husband now had the responsibility of paying the bills, this was often made more difficult by her insistence that he not bring the mail into the house. She also recognized that she was socially isolated, since she did not want other people to visit her house and was uncomfortable visiting others due to contamination fears. This was particularly bothersome to her, because she typically viewed herself as an outgoing person. During this conversation the therapist elicited and supported spontaneous change statements while avoiding an argumentative or didactic style. At the end of this session, Linda's fear of beginning ERP, 70 on a 0–100 scale, was reduced from her previous session; her ERF was unchanged and continued to suggest that she expected ERP to be moderately efficacious.

During the fourth session, Linda had a phone conversation with a former OCD patient from our clinic who had completed ERP. Efforts were made to match OCD symptoms; however, fear of contamination by a country or place is relatively rare, so the ex-patient was selected for having more typical contamination fears. During this phone conversation the therapist was not present, so as to encourage an open interchange of ideas and to allow a critical examination of ERP. While the therapist does not typically ask questions about the phone conversation, Linda spontaneously reported that the phone conversation was extremely valuable to her. She was able to talk to someone who had similar concerns and was as scared of exposures as she was. She stated that the ex-patient helped her see the benefit of efforts to overcome her OCD and helped her believe that she could change.

After the phone conversation, the therapist continued the use of motivational interviewing principles. At this point, Linda was more willing to consider beginning exposures and was able to develop discrepancy on her own between her fears of treatment and her wishes to have her OCD symptoms improve. She appeared to be leaning toward more active efforts to change OCD, as evidenced by her increased verbalization of change statements, such as "You know, it's really silly of me to avoid working on this; I mean, if not now, when?" At the end of this session, the therapist asked Linda if she wanted to begin ERP. Linda stated that she now felt that she wanted to, though she was still quite scared to try it. Figure 4.2 presents Linda's changes in fear of ERP and expectancy ratings during the readiness intervention. At the end of the readiness intervention, her fear of beginning ERP, now at 50 on the 100-

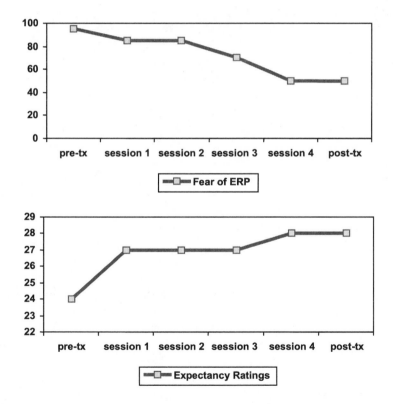

FIGURE 4.2. Linda's changes in fear of ERP and expectancy ratings during the readiness intervention.

point scale (indicating moderate fear of starting ERP), was significantly reduced from her pretreatment score of 95, and her ERF score was slightly improved from her pretreatment score. In addition, on the URICA, her scores were still consistent with being in the contemplation stage of change. Thus, while Linda was now willing to begin ERP, this decision was associated with a moderate but incomplete reduction in fear of ERP and with a minimal improvement in her expectancy ratings of ERP. However, she did not advance to a more action-oriented stage of change.

When Linda began ERP, she had difficulty progressing due an initial reluctance to engage in exposures fully, thus reducing habituation and her sense that ERP could be effective for her. However, during the fifth session, the therapist had her skip ahead to one of the top items on her hierarchy, handling an item from Japan. She was able to habituate to this item and became confident that she could do so with her other feared items. She began actively engaging in exposures, bringing items from Japan into her home and contaminating otherwise "clean" possessions. At the end of 15 sessions, she was rated as "borderline ill" and "very much improved" on the CGI severity and improvement scales. In addition, her Y-BOCS score of 3 was consistent with subclinical OCD. Thus, in her case, there is evidence that an initial reluctance to begin ERP does not have to negatively impact outcomes during later treatment.

RESEARCH

We conducted a small pilot study of the RI with 12 treatment-refusing OCD patients (see Maltby & Tolin, 2005, for a complete description of the study). All patients, after an initial diagnostic assessment, had refused to enter ERP for other than logistical reasons. Seven of these patients were assigned at random to receive the RI (four sessions over 4 weeks); five were assigned to a 4-week wait-list (WL) condition.

Participants randomized to RI completed a 4-session intervention consisting of individual visits with a therapist. As described in the case example above, the sessions included psychoeducation, motivational interviewing, viewing a videotape of ERP, constructing a sample exposure hierarchy, and a telephone conversation with a patient who had completed ERP. Participants assigned to the WL condition did not receive any intervention but returned to the clinic for assessment 1 month later. At the completion of the RI/WL period, patients were reassessed by an examiner blind to treatment condition and offered the chance to enter into ERP. Those accepting ERP underwent 15 sessions of intensive ERP. At the completion of ERP, patients were assessed again to examine the efficacy of ERP on patients who initially refused treatment.

Participants' reasons for refusing ERP can be inferred from the pretreatment assessment data. Unexpectedly, participants' highest scores on the URICA were in the contemplation or action stages of change. Similarly, participants rated themselves on the ERF as moderately confident that ERP would successfully reduce their OCD symptoms, suggesting that treatment refusal was not a function of lack of credibility of the treatment. However, fear of beginning ERP was high, as measured by the numeric scale added to the ERF, with the average patient rating his or her fear as a 75 on a 0–100 scale. Thus, to the extent that the URICA and ERF accurately capture the constructs of ambivalence about changing and expectancy of positive treatment outcome, the pretreatment data suggest that the primary reason for treatment refusal was fear of the treatment procedures rather than other such factors as lack of awareness of the problem or low expectancies of treatment efficacy.

Using the Y-BOCS, we determined that OCD symptom severity was unchanged for participants completing the RI and WL conditions, suggesting that the interventions did not influence OCD symptoms directly. However, The RI condition led to a significantly greater proportion of participants agreeing to begin ERP than did the WL condition. Figure 4.3 presents rates of accepting, entering, and completing ERP for both groups. Six of the seven (86%) RI participants and one of the five (20%) WL participants chose to begin ERP after the 4-week intervention period, a significant difference. Thus, the RI appeared to lead to a significantly higher rate of treatment acceptance among patients who had previously refused treatment.

In order to determine factors associated with the decision to enter into treatment, we analyzed change scores (pre-RI/WL vs. post-RI/WL) on the URICA, ERF, and the fear of ERP item on the ERF. Only one significant difference was found: the RI condition led to significantly greater decreases in fear of ERP than did the WL condition. Thus, the primary mechanism of the RI appeared to be one of fear reduction, although the precise mechanisms behind the fear reduction (e.g., habituation, modeling, self-efficacy, information, etc.) are not clear.

The secondary research question was whether, once they decided to enter ERP, patients who had previously refused treatment would fare as well as do patients who accept treatment immediately. Three of the

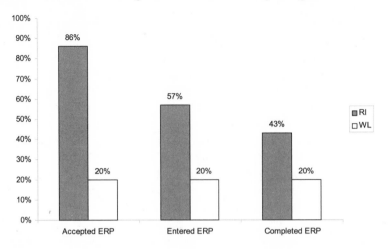

FIGURE 4.3. Rates of accepting, entering, and completing exposure and response prevention following a readiness intervention (RI) or wait list (WL). From Maltby and Tolin (2005). Copyright 2005 by Taylor & Francis. Reprinted by permission.

six (50%) RI participants who initially accepted ERP dropped out of treatment prematurely. Two of these dropped out before attending any treatment sessions, citing scheduling delays, an issue that we will discuss in depth later. The third discontinued after completing 6 of 15 ERP sessions. The sole WL participant accepting ERP completed ERP. All three RI participants who completed ERP exhibited substantial improvements in OCD symptoms. The small sample size of ERP completers precluded statistical analysis; however, average Y-BOCS scores dropped from the severe range at baseline to the mild range at post-RI. The average participant in the RI condition exhibited a 59% decrease in their Y-BOCS total score, a rate of improvement consistent with OCD patients who did not initially refuse ERP (Foa et al., 2005; Franklin et al., 2000). Y-BOCS improvement was mirrored in CGI severity and improvement scores. On average, independent evaluators rated these participants as being "markedly ill" at baseline and "mildly ill" and "much improved" at post-RI. The sole WL participant who completed ERP was not a responder to treatment even when using a very liberal criterion of 25% improvement on the Y-BOCS. At post-WL, this participant received CGI severity and improvement ratings indicating that he was extremely ill and unchanged from baseline, respectively. Thus, initial treatment refusal is not associated with a poorer outcome in subsequent ERP trials. This stands in contrast to some cohorts of OCD patients, such as nonresponders to multiple medication trials, who might not do as well in ERP as do medication-naive patients (Tolin et al., 2004).

PROBLEMS AND SUGGESTED SOLUTIONS

Our intervention consisted of a variety of procedures aimed at reducing ambivalence about starting ERP. Although the preliminary data are encouraging, it is not clear which treatment components were responsible for patients' decisions to start treatment. Pretreatment with MI has been demonstrated to enhance the outcomes of subsequent interventions, including treatments such as 12-step programs that, although different from ERP, are nevertheless difficult, directive, and associated with risk of refusal and dropout (Burke, Arkowitz, & Menchola, 2003). Furthermore, the RI program bears some similarity to a "role-induction" strategy that was less effective than was MI for substance use disorders (Connors, Walitzer, & Dermen, 2002). From the data, it appears that the decision to enter ERP treatment was most strongly associated with reduced fear of the treatment. We did not find evidence that the decision to enter ERP was associated with movement from one SOC to another, nor was it associated with increased expectancies for change. A session-by-session evaluation of the key outcome variables would have been beneficial in resolving this issue, as would a comparison between the RI program and a more "pure" MI procedure.

A clear understanding of the impact of MI, however, is impeded by sample characteristics. Of particular note, participants in the present study were characterized by contemplation or action stages of change and moderately confident that ERP would successfully reduce their OCD symptoms. These data suggest that, for these patients at least, treatment refusal was not a function of unwillingness to change or lack of credibility of the treatment. Thus, we would have little reason to expect that the RI would lead to substantial improvements in these variables. This sample might be representative of the broader population of OCD patients who attend an initial evaluation and then refuse treatment. In such a setting, treatment refusal necessarily implies some treatment-seeking behavior (i.e., scheduling and attending an assessment) in the first place. Would the RI also work for patients in the precontemplation or contemplation SOCs or those who had low expectancies for improvement at baseline? Although such patients might be less likely to present to a specialty clinic for assessment, it seems likely that many such individuals exist in nontreatment settings, particularly given the rather low frequency of treatment seeking among individuals with anxiety disorders (Collins, Westra, Dozois, & Burns, 2004). It remains to be seen whether the RI as a whole would be effective for this population and, if so, whether the mechanisms of action would be the same as those seen in the present sample.

We were disappointed to see that 33% of treatment-refusing OCD patients who, after completing the RI, decided to enter ERP did not actually attend any ERP sessions. In both cases, this seemed to be associated with a substantial scheduling delay between agreeing to start ERP and the initial ERP session. We are cautious not to infer a hypothetical counterfactual: we do not know how well these patients would have done in ERP or whether they would have dropped out prematurely, had their treatment started immediately. Nevertheless, these patients appeared to us to be ready to begin ERP immediately after completing RI. Thus, initial decisions to accept ERP after completing the RI appear to be tenuous. Like MI, the RI may present a window of opportunity that must be taken advantage of quickly (Miller & Rollnick, 2002). Overall, without increased efforts to retain treatment accepters, ERP following RI was associated with a higher refusal/dropout rate (50%) than the 20–30% typically observed in ERP studies (Foa et al., 2005; Franklin et al., 2000; Tolin et al., 2004). Miller and Rollnick (2002) suggest that MI is never "over"—rather, once a patient has decided to change, MI principles should be maintained throughout the treatment. This seems to be the case with our OCD patients as well.

CONCLUSIONS

ERP is the first-line psychosocial treatment of choice for OCD; however, it is also time-consuming, difficult, and even frightening to some. Thus, some patients who might otherwise be appropriate for ERP, and for whom ERP is readily available, refuse this treatment. In this chapter, we have described the development of a four-session program (the RI) designed to address the potential concerns of OCD patients who initially refused ERP treatment. Borrowing heavily from MI principles (Miller & Rollnick, 2002), we designed the RI to be nonconfrontational and empathic, presenting information relevant to treatment decision making in a manner that emphasized patients' freedom of choice. Although the program was largely MI-based, it also contained several additional elements known to be instrumental in fear reduction.

Overall, the RI appeared to be useful in terms of increasing patients' likelihood of entering ERP after their initial refusal. It appears from our pilot work that the RI may have affected fear of treatment to a greater extent than it did patients' SOC or expectancies for improvement; however, this may have had more to do with the nature of the sample than with the program itself. Results following the RI suggest that previous treatment-refusing patients can benefit from ERP in the same manner as do patients who did not initially refuse. However, they also underscore Miller and Rollnick's (2002) admonishment to strike while the iron is hot: acceptance of ERP following initial refusal appears to be quite tenuous, and it appears important that the therapist be able to provide treatment immediately once the patient has agreed. In our ongoing work, we are focusing on the use of MI/RI principles not only as a pretreatment augmentation but also as an integral part of the treatment itself. Given the fact that motivation is likely to fluctuate over the course of treatment, employing MI principles in an ongoing manner is likely to be more effective than using the principles solely during pretreatment. Furthermore, although this study specifically targeted patients who had flatly refused ERP, additional consideration might be given to the use of the RI for patients who are uncertain about the treatment or even those who are generally "on board" but remain somewhat fearful.

On a slightly different note, as we were preparing this chapter, we were discussing the process of the research itself. Early in the process, we worried about generating a large enough sample for the study. Frankly, we were having difficulty finding patients who refused ERP. This may have been due in part to the fact that, unlike the participants in most controlled research trials (e.g., Foa et al., 2005), the majority of patients seen in our clinic have tried at least one psychiatric medication, and many have received some form of counseling in the past. Thus, patients may come to our clinic (and perhaps others as well) "premotivated" by the knowledge that they have few remaining viable treatment options. As one patient told us, "I've tried just about everything else, so I guess I don't have much choice but to try this exposure thing." This left us in a bit of a quandary. As we discussed our methods during the intake process, we both noticed that, although perhaps not deliberately, the way we described ERP to prospective patients changed over time. Initially, we had emphasized the gradual nature of exposures, how most patients find it's not that bad, etc. Although we retained this information, we also found ourselves emphasizing the more difficult or aversive aspects of ERP. A typical "challenging" introduction, after reviewing the basics of pharmacotherapy and ERP, might be:

"Compared to medications, ERP is a challenging treatment. In this treatment, you will gradually come into contact with things that are progressively more frightening to you. So, in your case, we might start with doing activities like having you touch a doorknob in this building, and then rub your hands over your clothing, hair, and face so that you feel contaminated. These exposures would get more difficult as you go, and after about six sessions you would progress to touching the toilet seat in a public bathroom, and then rubbing your hands over your clothing, hair, and face. During this time, we would instruct you to refrain from washing your hands or your body for a 3-day period between showers so that you can really give the contamination a chance to 'sink in.' In addition to doing these exercises here with us, you would continue these exposures for at least an hour a day, every day, on your own between sessions. So, as you can see, this treatment isn't for everyone. Lots of people decide that it's easier to just take medications than to do this kind of program. This program is for people who are really fed up with their OCD, are ready to invest some time and energy into the process, and are willing to feel anxious along the way in order to get better. Does this sound like the kind of program you'd like to do?"

As is evident from the above, we unintentionally began describing ERP as if we wanted people to refuse the treatment! Much to our surprise, however, this change did not have the "desired" effect of eliciting more treatment refusals (and thus increasing enrollment in the RI study). In fact, if anything, the change seemed to have the *opposite* effect. Patient after patient, after hearing this description of ERP, would think for a moment and respond, "It sounds really tough, but I think that's exactly what I need. Sign me up." Why would increasing the threat value of the treatment description not only fail to elicit treatment refusals but perhaps even decrease them? Had we "thrown down the gauntlet" in some way to which patients felt compelled to respond? Had our implication that this treatment is only for people who really want to get rid of OCD somehow led patients to rise to the occasion? Had we elicited a cognitive dissonance, resulting in increased subjective sense of motivation (see Draycott & Dabbs, 1998, for a discussion)? Had our "it's not for everyone" rationale emphasized patients' sense of autonomy and choice? We do not know the answers, but our informal observations suggest that there may be multiple ways to reduce treatment refusal among OCD patients and that different patients may well respond to different strategies.

ACKNOWLEDGMENTS

We thank Gretchen Diefenbach and Patrick Worhunsky for their assistance.

NOTE

1. A treatment manual used for this study is available from David F. Tolin.

REFERENCES

American Psychiatric Association. (2000). *Diagnostic and statistical manual of mental disorders* (4th ed., text rev.). Washington, DC: Author.

Bobes, J., Gonzalez, M. P., Bascaran, M. T., Arango, C., Saiz, P. A., & Bousono, M. (2001). Quality of life and disability in patients with obsessive–compulsive disorder. *European Psychiatry, 16*, 239–245.

Borkovec, T. D., & Nau, S. D. (1972). Credibility of analogue therapy rationales. *Journal of Behavior Therapy and Experimental Psychiatry, 3*, 257–260.

Burke, B. L., Arkowitz, H., & Menchola, M. (2003). The efficacy of motivational interviewing: A meta-analysis of controlled clinical trials. *Journal of Consulting and Clinical Psychology, 71*, 843–861.

Bystritsky, A., Liberman, R. P., Hwang, S., Wallace, C. J., Vapnik, T., Maindment, K., et al. (2001). Social functioning and quality of life comparisons between obsessive–compulsive and schizophrenic disorders. *Depression and Anxiety, 14*, 214–218.

Catapano, F., Sperandeo, R., Perris, F., Lanzaro, M., & Maj, M. (2001). Insight and resistance in patients with obsessive–compulsive disorder. *Psychopathology, 34*, 62–68.

Collins, K. A., Westra, H. A., Dozois, D. J., & Burns, D. D. (2004). Gaps in accessing treatment for anxiety and depression: Challenges for the delivery of care. *Clinical Psychology Review, 24*, 583–616.

Connors, G. J., Walitzer, K. S., & Dermen, K. H. (2002). Preparing clients for alcoholism treatment: Effects on treatment participation and outcomes. *Journal of Consulting and Clinical Psychology, 70*, 1161–1169.

Cottraux, J., Mollard, E., Bouvard, M., & Marks, I. (1993). Exposure therapy, fluvoxamine, or combination treatment in obsessive–compulsive disorder: One-year followup. *Psychiatry Research, 49*, 63–75.

Draycott, S., & Dabbs, A. (1998). Cognitive dissonance. 2: A theoretical grounding of motivational interviewing. *British Journal of Clinical Psychology, 37*(Pt. 3), 355–364.

Eisen, J. L., Rasmussen, S. A., Phillips, K. A., Price, L. H., Davidson, J., Lydiard, R. B., et al. (2001). Insight and treatment outcome in obsessive–compulsive disorder. *Comprehensive Psychiatry, 42*, 494–497.

Elkin, I., Yamaguchi, J. I., Arnkoff, D. B., Glass, C. R., Sotsky, S. M., & Krupnick, J. L.

(1999). "Patient–treatment fit" and early engagement in therapy. *Psychotherapy Research, 9*, 437–451.

Erzegovesi, S., Cavallini, M. C., Cavedini, P., Diaferia, G., Locatelli, M., & Bellodi, L. (2001). Clinical predictors of drug response in obsessive–compulsive disorder. *Journal of Clinical Psychopharmacology, 21*, 488–492.

Fals-Stewart, W., Marks, A. P., & Schafer, J. (1993). A comparison of behavioral group therapy and individual behavior therapy in treating obsessive–compulsive disorder. *Journal of Nervous and Mental Disease, 181*, 189–193.

First, M. B., Spitzer, R. L., Gibbon, M., & Williams, J. B. W. (1995). *Structured Clinical Interview for DSM-IV Axis I Disorders—Patient Edition* (SCID I/P, version 2.0). New York: Biometrics Research Department.

Foa, E. B. (1979). Failure in treating obsessive–compulsives. *Behaviour Research and Therapy, 17*, 169–176.

Foa, E. B., Grayson, J. B., Steketee, G. S., Doppelt, H. G., Turner, R. M., & Latimer, P. R. (1983). Success and failure in the behavioral treatment of obsessive–compulsives. *Journal of Consulting and Clinical Psychology, 51*, 287–297.

Foa, E. B., & Kozak, M. J. (1986). Emotional processing of fear: Exposure to corrective information. *Psychological Bulletin, 99*, 20–35.

Foa, E. B., Kozak, M. J., Goodman, W. K., Hollander, E., Jenike, M. A., & Rasmussen, S. A. (1995). DSM-IV field trial: obsessive–compulsive disorder. *American Journal of Psychiatry, 152*, 90–96.

Foa, E. B., Liebowitz, M. R., Kozak, M. J., Davies, S., Campeas, R., Franklin, M. E., et al. (2005). Randomized, placebo-controlled trial of exposure and ritual prevention, clomipramine, and their combination in the treatment of obsessive–compulsive disorder. *American Journal of Psychiatry, 162*, 151–161.

Franklin, M. E., Abramowitz, J. S., Kozak, M. J., Levitt, J. T., & Foa, E. B. (2000). Effectiveness of exposure and ritual prevention for obsessive–compulsive disorder: Randomized compared with nonrandomized samples. *Journal of Consulting and Clinical Psychology, 68*, 594–602.

Franklin, M. E., & Foa, E. B. (1998). Cognitive-behavioral treatments for obsessive–compulsive disorder. In P. E. Nathan & J. M. Gorman (Eds.), *A guide to treatments that work*. New York: Oxford University Press.

Gallup Organization Inc. (1990). *A Gallup study of obsessive–compulsive sufferers*. Princeton, NJ: Author.

Goodman, W. K., Price, L. H., Rasmussen, S. A., Mazure, C., Fleischmann, R. L., Hill, C. L., et al. (1989). The Yale–Brown Obsessive Compulsive Scale: I. Development, use, and reliability. *Archives of General Psychiatry, 46*, 1006–1011.

Greenstein, D. K., Franklin, M. E., & McGuffin, P. (1999). Measuring motivation to change: An examination of the University of Rhode Island Change Assessment Questionnaire (URICA) in an adolescent sample. *Psychotherapy and Psychosomatics, 36*, 47–55.

Guy, W. (1976). *Assessment manual for psychopharmacology*. Washington, DC: U.S. Government Printing Office.

Hoogduin, C. A., & Duivenvoorden, H. J. (1988). A decision model in the treatment of obsessive–compulsive neuroses. *British Journal of Psychiatry, 152*, 516–521.

Issakidis, C., & Andrews, G. (2002). Service utilisation for anxiety in an Australian community sample. *Social Psychiatry and Psychiatric Epidemiology, 37*, 153–163.

Kampman, M., Keijsers, G. P., Hoogduin, C. A., & Verbraak, M. J. (2002). Addition of cognitive-behaviour therapy for obsessive–compulsive disorder patients non-responding to fluoxetine. *Acta Psychiatrica Scandinavica, 106*, 314–319.

Kessler, R. C., Berglund, P., Demler, O., Jin, R., & Walters, E. E. (2005). Lifetime prevalence and age-of-onset distributions of DSM-IV disorders in the National Comorbidity Survey Replication. *Archives of General Psychiatry, 62*, 593–602.

Kessler, R. C., Chiu, W. T., Demler, O., & Walters, E. E. (2005). Prevalence, severity, and comorbidity of 12-month DSM-IV disorders in the National Comorbidity Survey Replication. *Archives of General Psychiatry, 62*, 617–627.

Kirsch, I. (1990). *Changing expectations: A key to effective psychotherapy.* Pacific Grove, CA: Brooks/Cole.

Koran, L. M., Thienemann, M. L., & Davenport, R. (1996). Quality of life for patients with obsessive–compulsive disorder. *American Journal of Psychiatry, 153*, 783–788.

Lambert, M. J. (1992). Psychotherapy outcome research: Implications for integrative and eclectic therapists. In J. C. Norcross & M. R. Goldfried (Eds.), *Handbook of psychotherapy integration* (pp. 94–129). New York: Basic Books.

Leon, A. C., Portera, L., & Weissman, M. M. (1995). The social costs of anxiety disorders. *British Journal of Psychiatry, 166*(Suppl. 27), 19–22.

Lindsay, M., Crino, R., & Andrews, G. (1997). Controlled trial of exposure and response prevention in obsessive–compulsive disorder. *British Journal of Psychiatry, 171*, 135–139.

Maltby, N., & Tolin, D. F. (2005). A brief motivational intervention for treatment-refusing OCD patients. *Cognitive Behaviour Therapy, 34*, 176–184.

March, J. S., Frances, A., Carpenter, D., & Kahn, D. A. (1997). The expert consensus guideline series: Treatment of obsessive–compulsive disorder. *Journal of Clinical Psychiatry, 58*(Suppl. 4).

Mataix-Cols, D., Rosario-Campos, M. C., & Leckman, J. F. (2005). A multidimensional model of obsessive–compulsive disorder. *American Journal of Psychiatry, 162*, 228–238.

McKay, D., Abramowitz, J. S., Calamari, J. E., Kyrios, M., Radomsky, A., Sookman, D., et al. (2004). A critical evaluation of obsessive–compulsive disorder subtypes: symptoms versus mechanisms. *Clinical Psychology Review, 24*, 283–313.

Miller, W. B., & Rollnick, S. (2002). *Motivational interviewing: Preparing people for change* (2nd ed.). New York: Guilford Press.

Neziroglu, F., Stevens, K., & Yaryura-Tobias, J. A. (1999). Overvalued ideas and their impact on treatment outcome. *Revista Brasileira de Psiquiatria, 21*, 209–214.

Prochaska, J. O., DiClemente, C. C., & Norcross, J. C. (1992). In search of how people change. Applications to addictive behaviors. *American Psychologist, 47*, 1102–1114.

Simpson, H. B., Gorfinkle, K. S., & Liebowitz, M. R. (1999). Cognitive-behavioral therapy as an adjunct to serotonin reuptake inhibitors in obsessive–compulsive disorder: An open trial. *Journal of Clinical Psychiatry, 60*, 584–590.

Simpson, H. B., Liebowitz, M. R., Foa, E. B., Kozak, M. J., Schmidt, A. B., Rowan, V., et al. (2004). Post-treatment effects of exposure therapy and clomipramine in obsessive–compulsive disorder. *Depression and Anxiety, 19*, 225–233.

Steketee, G., Grayson, J. B., & Foa, E. B. (1987). A comparison of characteristics of obsessive–compulsive disorder and other anxiety disorders. *Journal of Anxiety Disorders, 1*, 325–335.

Tolin, D. F., Abramowitz, J. S., Kozak, M. J., & Foa, E. B. (2001). Fixity of belief, perceptual aberration, and magical ideation in obsessive–compulsive disorder patients. *Journal of Anxiety Disorders, 15*, 501–510.

Tolin, D. F., Diefenbach, G. J., Maltby, N., & Hannan, S. E. (2005). Stepped care for obsessive–compulsive disorder: A pilot study. *Cognitive and Behavioral Practice, 12*, 403–414.

Tolin, D. F., & Hannan, S. E. (2005). The role of the therapist in behavior therapy. In J. S. Abramowitz & A. C. Houts (Eds.), *Handbook of obsessive–compulsive spectrum disorders* (pp. 317–332). New York: Springer.

Tolin, D. F., Maltby, N., Diefenbach, G. J., Hannan, S. E., & Worhunsky, P. (2004). Cognitive-behavioral therapy for medication nonresponders with obsessive–compulsive disorder: A wait-list-controlled open trial. *Journal of Clinical Psychiatry, 65*, 922–931.

van Balkom, A. J., de Haan, E., van Oppen, P., Spinhoven, P., Hoogduin, K. A., & van Dyck, R. (1998). Cognitive and behavioral therapies alone versus in combination with fluvoxamine in the treatment of obsessive compulsive disorder. *Journal of Nervous and Mental Disease, 186*, 492–499.

Warren, R., & Thomas, J. C. (2001). Cognitive-behavior therapy of obsessive–compulsive disorder in private practice: An effectiveness study. *Journal of Anxiety Disorders, 15*, 277–285.

Westra, H. A. (2003). Motivational enhancement therapy in two cases of anxiety disorder: New responses to treatment refractoriness. *Clinical Case Studies, 2*, 306–322.

Westra, H. A. (2004). Managing resistance in cognitive behavioural therapy: The application of motivational interviewing in mixed anxiety and depression. *Cognitive Behaviour Therapy, 33*, 161–175.

Westra, H. A., & Phoenix, E. (2003). Motivational enhancement therapy in two cases of anxiety disorder. *Clinical Case Studies, 2*, 306–322.

CHAPTER 5

Motivational Interviewing as a Prelude to Psychotherapy of Depression

Allan Zuckoff
Holly A. Swartz
Nancy K. Grote

THE CLINICAL POPULATION AND USUAL INTERVENTIONS

Despite the availability of efficacious therapies, the majority of those who suffer from depression never receive adequate care. Young, Klap, Sherbourne, and Wells (2001), for example, found that only 25% of patients with depressive disorders received either pharmacotherapy or psychotherapy over a 1-year period; among those entering psychotherapy, only half attended at least four sessions.

We have been working with two groups of adults with notably high rates of depression and low rates of treatment: mothers of psychiatrically ill children and economically disadvantaged pregnant women. Swartz and colleagues (2005) found that 61% of mothers bringing their children to a pediatric mental health clinic met DSM-IV (American Psychiatric Association, 1994) criteria for a current Axis I disorder, most commonly depression (35%); two-thirds of those with a psychiatric diagnosis were not receiving psychiatric treatment. Poor women face twice the risk of mood and anxiety disorders as do men, but they rarely receive treatment in mental health settings (Miranda, Azocar, Komaromy, & Golding, 1998).

A variety of interventions to improve engagement in mental health treatment have been described. Psychotherapy preparation strategies have included role induction, vicarious therapy pretraining, and experiential pretraining (see Walitzer, Dermen, & Connors, 1999, for a review). A pretherapy telephone interview and combined telephone-plus-first-session intervention addressing barriers to care increased attendance of inner-city youth at a mental health intake (McKay, McCadam, & Gonzales, 1996), and case management has been employed to engage depressed women in primary care into depression treatment (Miranda, Azocar, Organista, Dwyer, & Areane, 2003). Despite their promise, none of these approaches has been widely used.

RATIONALE FOR ADAPTING MOTIVATIONAL INTERVIEWING TO ENHANCE ENGAGEMENT IN DEPRESSION TREATMENT

There are many possible contributors to limited treatment participation by depressed and vulnerable women. Practical barriers include cost, clinic inaccessibility, and problems with child care. Depressed people suffer, by definition, from low energy, hopelessness, and cognitive slowing, symptoms that may make them more vulnerable to the "time and hassle" factors associated with treatment seeking.

However, psychological and cultural factors also play an important role. Worry or embarrassment about acknowledging their depression and doubts that treatment could be helpful (Scholle, Hasket, Hanusa, Pincus, & Kupfer, 2003) as well as previous negative experiences of mental health services (McKay & Bannon, 2004) inhibit engagement, and feeling misunderstood or unhelped predicts premature discontinuation (Garcia & Weisz, 2002). Mismatches between the type of treatment offered and that desired (McCarthy et al., 2005), incompatible views of the nature of the problem, negative attitudes about the legitimacy of accepting help, disclosing private experiences, or taking care of oneself (e.g., Mackenzie, Knox, Gekoski, & Macaulay, 2004), and negative relationship expectancies are also inhibitory. Cultural insensitivity or ignorance on the part of therapists may also present a significant barrier (Miranda, Azocar, Organista, Munoz, & Lieberman, 1996).

While treatment preparation interventions have educated patients about treatment and/or problem-solved pragmatic barriers, they have rarely attended to patients' agendas—including a wish to tell their story, understand the nature of their problems, and specify the kind of help they wish to receive—or to the psychological and cultural barriers they might face. Motivational interviewing (MI; Miller & Rollnick, 2002) emphasizes the meeting of the treatment aspirations of patient and therapist within a client-centered relationship. Furthermore, many barriers to treatment can be understood in terms of *ambivalence* about accepting and changing the problem to be addressed, participating in treatment, or both. As a method for resolving ambivalence in the context of an empathic understanding of individuals' perspectives, hopes, and concerns, MI provides a promising framework for adherence intervention.

Research in the areas of substance abuse and health behavior change supports this view. Zweben and Zuckoff (2002) reviewed studies reporting positive effects of MI on treatment entry, attendance, and retention, adherence to treatment procedures, and medication compliance. Meta-analyses have found medium-sized effects of MI pretreatments on patient outcomes (Burke, Arkowitz, & Menchola, 2003) and lasting medium-to-large effects on treatment adherence as well as outcomes (Hettema, Steele, & Miller, 2005).

Applications of MI to enhancing engagement in mental health treatment have emerged more recently. Arkowitz and Westra (2004) described the integration of MI into cognitive-behavioral therapy (CBT) of depression and anxiety, and Westra and Dozois (2006) reported that three MI sessions prior to group CBT for patients with panic disorder, generalized anxiety disorder, or social phobia resulted in significantly higher expectancy of anxiety change, homework compliance, and rate of treatment response, compared with group CBT alone. Simon, Ludman, Tutty, Operskalski, and Von Korff (2004) used structured MI exercises to enhance engagement of depressed primary care patients in telephone CBT, and Nock and Kazdin (2005) reported significant effects of three within-session 5- to 15-minute MI-and-overcoming-barriers discussions on the treatment motivation, session attendance, and adherence to treatment procedures of parents participating in treatment for child behavior problems.

CLINICAL APPLICATION OF MI TO ENGAGEMENT OF DEPRESSED WOMEN INTO PSYCHOTHERAPY

Seeking effective yet feasible ways to reach out to difficult-to-engage populations, Swartz, who had developed a brief form of interpersonal psychotherapy for depressed mothers of psychiatrically ill children (IPT-B; Swartz et al., 2004), and Grote, who adapted IPT-B for depressed pregnant women (Grote, Bledsoe, Swartz, & Frank, 2004), initiated a collaboration with Zuckoff, who with colleagues had described (Daley & Zuckoff, 1999; Zuckoff & Daley, 2001; Zweben & Zuckoff, 2002) and pilot-tested (Daley, Salloum, Zuckoff, Kirisci, & Thase, 1998; Daley & Zuckoff, 1998) an MI-based approach to adherence intervention targeting motivation for treatment as well as motivation for change. From ethnographic interviewing (Schensul, Schensul, & LeCompte, 1999), in complement to MI's client-centeredness, we incorporated heightened awareness of the potential for interviewers' culturally specific values, ways of understanding others, and judgments about what constitutes "rational" behavior to interfere with their ability to grasp and support those of the interviewee. From IPT we incorporated psychoeducation about depression, provided in an MI-consistent style: remaining sensitive to the potential for the "labeling trap" but recognizing that the diagnostic language of "major depression" can provide relief through the message that changes in behavior are attributable not to personal weakness or moral failings but to an illness for which patients are not to blame and which can be effectively treated.

The "engagement session" is a single-session pretherapy intervention focused on communicating the therapist's understanding of patients' individual and culturally embedded perspectives, helping patients see how the potential benefits of treatment align with their own priorities and concerns, facilitating identification and resolution of ambivalence, and problem-solving barriers to engagement. The session is semistructured, with five phases: *Eliciting the Story*; *Providing Feedback and Psychoeducation*; *Exploring the History of Distress, Coping, and Treatment, and Hopes for Treatment*; *Problem Solving Practical, Psychological, and Cultural Treatment Barriers*; and *Eliciting Commitment or Leaving the Door Open*. We describe each phase and provide an annotated transcript with a prototypical patient.

Eliciting the Story

The goals of the initial phase are to ensure that the patient feels understood and to elicit talk about the *importance* of change in her state and situation. The therapist begins by inquiring how the patient has been feeling and what things have been like for her lately. If she responds by talking solely about how she feels, the therapist also asks about her situation: "You've been feeling so hopeless lately. . . . What has been going on in your life that might be affecting you?" Similarly, if she responds by talking solely about the circumstances of her life, the therapist also asks about how she has been feeling: "You're stuck with all these bills and busy all the time. . . . Tell me about how you're being affected by the lousy situation you're in." The therapist listens for the patient's perspective on how she is suffering, what she believes is contributing to her suffering, and how it interferes with her daily life, attending specifically to the social and interpersonal context.

In almost all cases, the patient's "story" can be framed as a *dilemma*: a problem that is unsolvable in principle, because each potential solution would exact intolerable costs. This both reflects, and is a source of, feelings of hopelessness inherent to depression. A successful conclusion to this phase comprises a summary that both *crystallizes* the patient's dilemma and highlights her wishes for help in escaping from it.

THERAPIST: Thank you for filling out the questionnaires. We will put them to good use together in the next 45 minutes or so. Before we do that, I wonder if you could tell me how things have been going for you and how you have been feeling lately.

Beginning with an affirmation, then an open-ended question to draw out the story.

PATIENT: My son Johnny is just a terror. He is getting on my nerves so bad. I don't know what I am going to do. I feel like I'm really going to hurt him. He's been getting into trouble at school. He won't let me alone at home. I just don't know what to do.

The patient focuses on how her troubled child is affecting her and conveys her sense of helplessness.

THERAPIST: Johnny's on top of you constantly and creating problems for you. You're starting to worry about the way you feel around him—you might lash out and do something that you would really regret.

The therapist reflects meanings and feelings.

PATIENT: Yeah, it's really affected my whole life. I've been irritable at work and snapping at my coworkers.

THERAPIST: It affects you when you're not with him, too. What else have you noticed about how you've been feeling and acting that are different from the way you usually feel or act?

Reflection, then asking for elaboration to elicit problem recognition.

PATIENT: I'm not enjoying my free time. I'm just angry all the time, and I try to get away from Johnny. I lock myself in my room. I don't want to talk to anyone, and, I'm just . . . I'm never happy anymore.

The patient describes symptoms of depression.

THERAPIST: It doesn't matter where you are or who you're with or what you're doing, you feel the same way . . . this angry, unhappy feeling, and it's really hard because you are trying to deal with Johnny, and no matter what you do it doesn't seem to get any better.

Reflective summary of the patient's complaints.

PATIENT: Yeah, that's about it. I can't, anything I try just doesn't work with him. It's getting worse and worse.

The patient confirms that she feels understood.

THERAPIST: It's been incredibly frustrating for you.

Reflection of feeling.

PATIENT: Yeah, I'm very frustrated with everything.

THERAPIST: And this is a big change from the way things were before.

Looking back.

PATIENT: Yeah, it's just over the past year that he's gotten worse. His father left, and now he's living across the street from me with his girlfriend.

Focusing on the context of her child's problems, she describes sources of current distress.

THERAPIST: That sounds like a very difficult situation.

PATIENT: And before that things weren't too good between his father and me, and he saw a lot of that, but it's been worse since his father left. It seems like he is escalating and it's out of control. He's on the verge of being expelled from school, and I've had conferences with his teachers and his guidance counselor, and they make it seem like it's all my fault.

Is she afraid the therapist will blame her as well?

THERAPIST: You're doing everything you can think of to get Johnny to come around, and not only is it not working, not only is that really hard for you, but you're also feeling blamed by other people who you're looking to for help. (*Patient nods.*) And you're really angry about this.

Affirmation and complex reflections (and identification of possible engagement barrier).

PATIENT: I am. Nobody seems to understand what is going on.

She feels understood.

THERAPIST: You feel pretty much alone in all of this? (*Patient nods.*) No one seems to be able to help, no one seems to really get it.

Reflections of feeling and meaning.

PATIENT: No. Even my mother blames me for the break up. She thinks I should have just stuck it out.

THERAPIST: How did you make that decision? What happened between you?

Eliciting her dilemma . . .

PATIENT: Well, he was being abusive, and I just couldn't take it anymore. He was going to kill me. I felt really bad because Johnny saw all of this. I would try to have him go upstairs so that he wouldn't see it, but he would sneak down and sometimes he would see his father beating on me.

. . . which she describes in terms of her situation and reasons for her actions.

THERAPIST: You came to the point where you felt like you really had no choice. You had to leave or you could be killed. (*Patient nods vigorously.*) Let me see if I'm understanding the situation.

Empathizing with her choice in the face of her dilemma.

You've been dealing with these problems for a while now, even before this past year, but things were getting worse and worse. So you made the decision that you had to get away from this man or else something horrible was going to happen, and you made that decision for yourself but also for Johnny because you were worried about what he was seeing and how that was affecting him. You're trying to do the best thing you know how to do, make the best decision you can, and the result has been that things have seemed to get worse.

Transitional summary, including her view of how she came to be in her current problematic situation, affirmation of her good intentions and efforts . . .

PATIENT: That's right!

THERAPIST: Instead of feeling or acting better, Johnny seems to be acting worse and worse, and you don't know how to get through to him or how to help him or what to do for him. It's like you took this incredibly difficult step, and things have just gone downhill instead of uphill.

. . . acknowledgment of her feelings and her sense of being stuck in a dilemma that has seemed unsolvable . . .

PATIENT: Yeah. I feel like, no matter what I do, I just can't win.

THERAPIST: And you are at the point that you don't know where to turn, you don't know what to do, and you are really worried about what you might be capable of if things don't get better.

. . . and her fears about what will happen if she doesn't get help.

PATIENT: Yeah, I'm afraid I'm just going to lose it. I'm afraid I'm going to lose control, or at work I'm going to lose my job.

Implicit recognition of the need for change.

THERAPIST: And that's really scary, and the bottom could really drop out.

PATIENT: Yeah. And I don't know how to get out of this by myself.

Toward adherence talk.

Providing Feedback and Psychoeducation

The goal of this phase is to offer the patient a different perspective on her current difficulties. The therapist reframes the problems as comprising a recognizable medical condition for which effective treatment is available rather than a hopeless situation or a failure of will or ability. This is not intended to minimize the importance of the contextual factors but rather to suggest that alleviating the mood disorder will allow the patient to cope with these factors more effectively.

The patient is first given individualized feedback on her current condition, using whatever assessment tools the therapist has available. The therapist then offers basic psychoeducation on depression, including the ideas that depression is a "no-fault" illness and thus that the depressed person is not to blame for the troubles she is having; that depression negatively affects people's ability to solve interpersonal problems or manage difficult situations; that depression can be effectively treated; and that when depression is treated successfully, people often begin to see alternative solutions to what had seemed like unsolvable life problems.

The therapist asks the patient's permission before offering information, helping to ensure that she is open to what the therapist has to say and to reduce the likelihood of a resistant response. By eliciting what the patient already knows about depression, providing information objectively, and then eliciting her reaction, the therapist communicates respect for her views and acknowledges that it will be her interpretation of this information that will ultimately determine what she does with it.

Thus, the therapist tailors feedback and psychoeducation to the patient's individual concerns and current knowledge. Should the patient nonetheless object to diagnostic language, express uncertainty as to whether she is really "depressed" (rather than, for example, "stressed out" or "overwhelmed"), or feel reluctant to acknowledge that she needs "treatment," the therapist recognizes the status quo side of the patient's ambivalence and responds empathically and nondefensively. Inquiring about the patient's perspective and emphasizing its legitimacy, the therapist at the same time looks for opportunities to connect troubles the patient describes—painful feelings, problematic thinking patterns, difficulty functioning—to the therapist's ability to help:

> "As you see it, stress is very different from depression, and you're sure that you're stressed rather than depressed. You've also told me that your new situation has been a big source of stress. Would a therapy that could help you find and use some better ways of managing the situation be something you'd find worthwhile?"

THERAPIST: We gave you a questionnaire to give us a first impression of whether or not you seem to be depressed. I'd like to review the questionnaire to let you know what we make of your responses and see what your thoughts are. Is that OK?

Brief structuring statement, introduction of feedback.

Asking permission.

PATIENT: Yes, it sounds good.

THERAPIST: Great. Let me know if there is anything I say that doesn't sound right to you because I really want to know that, as well as anything that does make sense to you. This is the Patient Health Questionnaire. It asks about markers that we use to tell us if somebody is depressed or not, and of the seven markers you agreed with five. For example, you said you had noticed some changes in your sleep. Tell me what you've noticed about how your sleep has changed.

Inviting her to be active in the discussion.

Characterizing the source of feedback, explaining how we arrive at an assessment, providing feedback, and asking for elaboration.

PATIENT: I'm waking up a lot in the middle of the night. I'll have a nightmare about something that I'm worried about, and when it wakes me up, I stay awake.

THERAPIST: So, it's harder to stay asleep, and it's harder to get back to sleep. You also said your appetite is not as good.

Clarifying symptoms.

PATIENT: I've basically been living on junk food. I eat, but not regular meals like I usually do. I don't know why.

THERAPIST: Changes in sleep and appetite are two physical changes we often see when people are depressed. Depression affects people's bodies as well as their thoughts and feelings. You've also been feeling much less interested in things, you don't have the energy you usually

Offering information, in terms of the model of depression, in response to an implicit question.

have, and you've had some thoughts of wanting to die. Can you tell me about that?

PATIENT: Well, Johnny really acts out, and I don't have anybody to talk to. I feel like the reason I am living now is to take care of him, and then when he acts out it makes me feel like there is nothing really worth living for.

THERAPIST: You're exhausted all the time trying to deal with this, and you can't sleep well or eat right and that's taking a toll also. So, you just sometimes reach this point where you just want to give up. You just feel like there is no point in going on.

Collecting summary.

PATIENT: Yeah, why should I do it for him if he's going to treat me like that?

THERAPIST: So, there is an angry part, too. Like, "The hell with you . . . if you're going to act this way, I don't even want to be here."

Reflection of feeling.

PATIENT: Exactly. Isn't that terrible to feel that way toward your son?

THERAPIST: When people have these kinds of problems with sleeping, appetite, energy, interest, and feeling like giving up, we say they have depression. So, from our perspective it looks like you are experiencing depression right now, and that's why you're feeling and acting in ways that aren't normal for you. What are your thoughts about that?

Reframing her mood and behavioral changes, and her self-blame, in terms of the medical model of depression, then eliciting her reaction.

PATIENT: Well, I don't think that I would be depressed if it wasn't for everything going on in my life right now.

A little resistance (defensiveness) emerges.

THERAPIST: Everything that's happening is having a big impact on how you feel and how you're doing.

Rolling with resistance via reflection.

PATIENT: Yeah, if Johnny wasn't acting out, if his father wasn't living across the street with his girlfriend, if I wasn't trying to scrape to get by, I don't think I would feel this way.

THERAPIST: That makes sense. People who are undergoing really stressful situations are more vulnerable to becoming depressed and feeling the way you've been feeling. I think that is very consistent with the way we see things. Do you have any other thoughts about that? (*Patient shakes her head, looking uncertain.*) You're sure?

Reframing her resistance in line with the model of depression, then eliciting her reaction.

Drawing out unspoken resistance.

PATIENT: So, is depression something inside me? Is it like a disease?

THERAPIST: You're wondering what I mean when I use the word "depression." When you hear the word "depression," what is your understanding?

Eliciting the patient's understanding, and the concern she's hinting at.

PATIENT: Well, just feeling sad. Like when my friend broke up with her boyfriend, she was down in the dumps and she said she was feeling depressed.

THERAPIST: People can use the word "depression" to talk about times when they just feel kind of down or sad, something that will probably pass on its own. It sounds like that's how you're thinking about it. Our understanding of depression is that it is a medical illness that people can suffer from but, fortunately, also something that is very treatable and something that we know how to help people with. (*Patient looks thoughtful.*) We

Providing psychoeducation (and hope).

also think that once someone is depressed, stressful situations are more
difficult to deal with. So, each one affects the other—all the stress and difficulties can trigger a depression. Then,
once you're depressed, the difficulties
are harder to deal with. You don't have
the same energy and focus to handle
the stressful situations in your life.   *Eliciting her reaction to*
Does that sound like what has been   *the psychoeducation.*
happening?

PATIENT: So, what you're saying is that the   *More resistance?*
way I'm feeling is because of every-
thing going on, and once I feel this
way it is going to make everything
seem like it is worse than it really is?

THERAPIST: Not that it seems worse than   *Being careful not to*
it really is, but probably more *hopeless*   *minimize the difficulty of*
than it really is. I believe your situa-   *her situation . . .*
tion is very difficult and that it feels
really bad to you. What we find is that
when someone is depressed it becomes   *. . . and reframing in*
very hard to see any kind of solution   *terms of the model of*
to difficult situations. Everything looks   *depression, which offers*
sort of bleak. As people become less   *hope.*
depressed, it doesn't make the situation
get better right away, but they're more
able to see ways to improve the situation and to use the things that they
know how to do to deal with difficult
situations. You're nodding—that makes
sense?

PATIENT: Yes. I could definitely use some   *Adherence talk—the*
help dealing with some of the things   *resistance seems defused.*
that are going on. Because I can't fix
them myself.

THERAPIST: The good news is that if we   *Offering hope.*
can provide that help for you, you will
probably start to feel a little more like

you can deal with the situation, and
that's actually going to help the
depression as well. How does
that sound?

PATIENT: It sounds good. That would be
good.

This phase, in which the therapist shifts focus from the patient's perspective to a professional one, is one place where racial, cultural, or gender-related barriers may arise. Understanding the patient's cultural context and allowing the patient to educate the therapist about unique elements of her background and identity are crucial. However, it is often very difficult for individuals of different backgrounds—most especially, whites and people of color—to frankly discuss issues of mistrust and misunderstanding. Therefore, the therapist should invite and even encourage patients to voice concerns related to aspects of the psychiatric view of depression and its treatment that may be considered culturally unacceptable. These concerns may include reluctance to confide in a therapist of a different race or gender or to reveal sensitive information in a professional treatment context. For example, talking with an African American patient:

THERAPIST: I noticed that you got quiet when I said that this questionnaire shows that you're depressed. Could I ask what you were thinking just then?	*Drawing out unspoken resistance.*
PATIENT: Nothing important (*looking away*).	
THERAPIST: I don't want to put any pressure on you to tell me anything you'd rather keep to yourself. Would it be all right if I asked you one more question? (*Patient nods.*) Sometimes when I've talked with African American patients, they've told me they had some doubts about these kinds of questionnaires. I was wondering if you might feel that way, too.	*Emphasizing personal choice and control, and asking permission.* *Pulling for the negatives.*

PATIENT: I think they made those questionnaires by asking white folks a bunch of questions, and that doesn't necessarily mean it's the same for us.

Cultural resistance.

THERAPIST: The questions we asked might not really apply to you.

Amplified reflection.

PATIENT: Well, some of those are true for me, but that doesn't necessarily mean I have some illness. No offense, but that's what white people have always done to black people—called them sick just because their lives are hard.

Articulation of the patient's concern.

THERAPIST: I really appreciate your being so honest with me. And the last thing I'd want would be for you to feel like I'm putting some label on you that doesn't fit. Putting aside the questionnaire, how would you describe the way you've been feeling lately?

Affirmation, rolling with resistance, and eliciting the patient's perspective.

PATIENT: I don't mind the word "depressed." I just don't think those questionnaires are the last word on how I feel.

The resistance is diminishing.

THERAPIST: I couldn't agree more. Your perspective on what you're going through is definitely what matters the most.

Joining with the patient.

EXPLORING THE HISTORY OF DISTRESS, COPING, AND TREATMENT, AND HOPES FOR TREATMENT

The therapist's goals in this phase include understanding the patient's current difficulties in the context of her relevant history; uncovering potential barriers to engagement related to negative experiences with or beliefs about treatment; understanding her past and present coping efforts and affirming the strengths she has called on in doing so; and eliciting talk about the possibility of positive change (i.e., hope).

The therapist begins by asking whether the patient has previously felt the way she feels now. Discussion of the patient's experience with depression is followed by questions about how she coped with these feelings (if she has been depressed previously) as well as about what she has tried recently to help herself feel better and manage her situation. The therapist looks for opportunities to affirm the patient for her efforts and to support self-efficacy as well as to understand the kinds of interventions she is likely to find plausible or desirable.

If the topic has not come up already, the therapist then shifts explicitly to asking about the patient's perceptions of treatment. These may derive from personal or vicarious (e.g., children's or other family members') experience, or from media portrayals. It is crucial to elicit discussion of both positives and negatives—the former, because they constitute "adherence talk," and the latter, because they potentially constitute the most potent sources of ambivalence or barriers to treatment engagement. The therapist employs empathic reflection to communicate nonjudgmental understanding of negative feelings and/or beliefs about treatment, strategies such as shifting focus and emphasizing personal choice and control if such negativity generalizes to the current therapist or treatment, and reframing to emphasize the potential for the proposed treatment to be more helpful.

Finally, the therapist asks about the patient's hopes and fears for treatment now. Encouraging the patient to describe what she does and does not want from the treatment and from the therapist is both an unusual thing to do and, we believe, among the elements of the session that have the most powerful engagement effect. "Looking forward"— "What would you like to be different at the end of this treatment?" or "If this treatment were to work exactly the way you hope, what would your life be like 2 months from now?"—can further evoke hope that things can be better and that treatment could play an important role in the improvement.

During this discussion, the therapist looks for opportunities to help the patient see how the treatment being offered can provide what she is hoping for. This typically involves briefly characterizing the treatment's basic outlook and principles and noting consistencies between the treatment approach and the patient's wishes. We have found IPT to be a good match for the women with whom we work; the idea that depression is linked to transitions, disputes, or losses in our interpersonal world seems to make intuitive sense to them and almost always fits with the focus of the discussion. Similarly, the stance of the IPT therapist—

warm, active, encouraging, moving flexibly between more and less directive interventions—has great appeal. The effectiveness of the engagement session is tied in part to the acceptability of the treatment in which patients are being asked to engage.

THERAPIST: So, this has been an awful way to feel, so angry and hopeless and just stuck in this situation with Johnny. Have there been times in the past when you have felt like you're feeling now?

Asking for the depression history.

PATIENT: When my dad passed about 2 years ago. It only lasted about a month. Things were bad for a while, and then they gradually got better. This time they seem to be getting worse, and I just don't see an end in sight.

Change talk: recognition that the current problem is different.

THERAPIST: You expect to have difficult periods in your life and then for things to get back to normal. But this time it's not getting back to normal.

Highlighting change talk through reflection.

PATIENT: Yeah, usually I am able to kind of get myself back up.

THERAPIST: How have you done that?

Asking about past coping.

PATIENT: Well, Johnny's father was there for me. Johnny wasn't as bad when he was around. And when my dad was around, if I felt this way I could talk to him. Then after my dad passed I could talk to my mom some and Johnny's father. Now it just seems like I'm taking care of Johnny all by myself, and no one really cares or understands. They can't understand what's going on.

Identifying interpersonal contributors to current depressive episode.

THERAPIST: You really feel like you no longer have anyone to turn to when you are feeling down and when you need someone to understand you or just offer a little support to you. That's the big difference between now and before—you don't have anyone to turn to who could help.

Reflection of meaning . . .

. . . and a subtle reframe.

PATIENT: I hadn't really thought about it that way. Yeah, I don't have anyone now who I can really talk to.

THERAPIST: And you miss that, and you're really feeling the need for it now.

OK—but better to elicit this from the patient.

PATIENT: I've got to do something. I just can't go on feeling like this anymore.

Change talk; not yet adherence talk.

THERAPIST: Have you ever been able to talk to someone outside the family or friends?

Asking about previous treatment experience.

PATIENT: My son used to have a pediatrician that I talked to. She understood the kinds of problems Johnny was having. But she seemed to understand me, too. We talked about how hard it was for me to deal with him. I always felt better after that.

Describing what she wants from a "helper"— beginning adherence talk.

THERAPIST: You said she seemed to understand you. What was it about her that made you feel understood?

Reflection, asking for elaboration.

PATIENT: Well, even though most of the focus was on Johnny, she would take time to ask how I was dealing with things and just listen to me. I feel like I'm taking care of everyone else all the time, and she was just interested in how I was feeling.

More adherence talk.

THERAPIST: You didn't have to worry about taking care of her for once. You could just let her take care of you a little bit, be concerned about you.

Reflection of meaning.

PATIENT: Yeah, I guess so. I mean, she wasn't family, so . . . she never really talked about her problems.

THERAPIST: She listened, she seemed to understand, and she wanted to help. She seemed to care about you and wanted to help you feel better and deal with Johnny better.

Interim (collecting) summary.

PATIENT: She would help me deal with Johnny and tell me what to do with the problems he was having, not like I was a bad mom, but just suggestions.

Key point about what she wants and doesn't want.

THERAPIST: That was a very positive experience overall. Were there any times when you had less positive experiences with doctors or therapists?

A specific reflection could have highlighted the key point: not feeling blamed.

PATIENT: That's the only time I ever talked to anyone outside of friends or family. I always felt like I could handle it myself. My girlfriend went to see someone, and they put her on this medicine, and she just wasn't herself anymore. I'd rather feel like myself than be on the medication and change like she did. I tried to talk to my doctor once, and he wanted to put me on medicine.

Revealing a barrier: negative treatment expectations.

THERAPIST: And that was not something you felt comfortable with at all.

Reflection of feeling.

PATIENT: Yeah, he gave me a prescription, but I didn't have it filled. My friend, she was never the same.

THERAPIST: It was kind of scary for you to see the change in her. (*Patient nods.*) There are two different kinds of help that you've seen people get. One is medication, which you are really not comfortable with. It wasn't helpful when your doctor gave you medication, because you didn't feel it was right for you. On the other hand, having somebody to talk to, who understands you and seems to care and want to help—somebody you don't have to worry about taking care of— that feels like it could be a helpful thing. At least that was a helpful thing before.

Reflection of feeling.

Linking summary and reframe.

PATIENT: Yes, it seems like a very helpful thing.

Adherence talk.

THERAPIST: Well, what we offer is called "interpersonal therapy." It's a talking therapy that focuses on dealing with relationship problems to help relieve depression. The therapist will be in your corner, listening to you and helping you figure out what you can do to make things better.

Introducing the treatment.

PATIENT: That sounds good. Those are the kinds of problems I have.

Adherence talk.

THERAPIST: Looking down the road months from now, if the therapy works and is really helpful for you, how will things be different?

Looking forward.

PATIENT: What I would really like to be different is the situation with Johnny, but right now I don't see how that could change because it takes everything I have to keep my cool at work and get through the day and take care of him.

Expressing her wish and her pessimism—i.e., her ambivalence.

THERAPIST: A change with Johnny is one thing that you would really like, yet you can't quite see how that would happen.

Double-sided reflection.

PATIENT: Well, maybe if I could get a break or have a little time for myself, I wouldn't be so short with him and I could try some of the things his therapist suggests. Right now I spend my whole day working, and then I have to come home in the evenings and take care of everything there and fight with Johnny, and I never get a break.

Change talk: thinking about possible solutions.

THERAPIST: So, if you could wave a magic wand and everything with Johnny would be OK, that's what you would do. That may not be possible, but it sounds like if things could go really well with the therapy, one change would be that you would somehow find a way to get some help with Johnny so that you could have a break to focus more on yourself and take care of yourself instead of just taking care of everyone else.

Acknowledging her pessimism about a total solution . . .

. . . and highlighting a source of hope through reflection.

PATIENT: And I would like to have the energy to do that. I can barely drag myself out of bed to go to work and take care of Johnny.

More change talk.

THERAPIST: The way you are feeling now, it doesn't seem like there is any way you could do this, but if things went well and you had the energy again, you could figure out how to get some additional help or handle situations with Johnny more constructively or get a break to take care of yourself. Those would be some really positive changes.

Reframing in terms of the model of depression, from pessimism to hope.

PATIENT: Yeah. It would be really great if therapy could help with that.

Envisioning help.

Problem Solving Practical, Psychological, and Cultural Treatment Barriers

The goal in this phase is to draw out, explore, and problem-solve unaddressed barriers that could keep the patient from engaging in treatment. When the therapist encourages the patient to voice why it will be hard to come for treatment, practical barriers are usually the first ones offered; they are safe—socially appropriate and not too revealing. The therapist takes these at face value and works to resolve them; if they are the only barriers, that will soon become apparent, and if there are other underlying concerns, these will emerge once the practical barriers are dealt with.

In some cases the patient will not spontaneously offer any barriers; she may even initially deny that any exist. This may be true, but to ensure that important barriers are not going unspoken the therapist should suggest some:

> "Some people have told me that, even though they wanted to come for therapy, it might be hard to find the time or the money. Others have worried about what therapy would be like, or felt guilty about taking time for themselves instead of putting all their effort into taking care of their families, or had other concerns. It wouldn't be unusual if you had some doubts like these . . ."

This is also another part of the session where racially or culturally related concerns may emerge, either spontaneously or elicited by the therapist. Patients may harbor doubts as to whether someone who is of a different race, gender, ethnicity, religion, or social status can really understand their lives, or they may anticipate that they will be judged negatively for their differences. Alternatively, some patients from small minority communities may fear recognition and stigmatization by another member of the same community and prefer a therapist from a different ethnic or religious background. Trying to elicit the direct expression of these potential unspoken barriers, remaining nondefensive and open to patients' worries, and placing the patient in the role of teacher can often diffuse such concerns.

THERAPIST: If you decide to come in for treatment, what could make it hard to follow through with it?

Open-ended question to elicit barriers.

PATIENT: I don't know. I don't have much energy, and that makes it hard to do anything, but other than that I'm not sure.

A psychological barrier.

THERAPIST: Not having the energy to get here. . . . Tell me your how you think that could make it tougher for you.

Reflecting and asking for elaboration.

PATIENT: It takes all the energy I have to take care of Johnny and make it to work every day. I even had trouble getting here today, but I had to get Johnny here for his appointment and because I really needed to do that I made it here.

THERAPIST: So, it takes energy to get the help you might need so that you can have more energy.

Acknowledging the apparent dilemma.

PATIENT: And then there is Johnny and work. If I could see someone on Monday, I could probably come. That's my early afternoon off, and Johnny has his appointment that day. The rest of the week I have to be at work and take care of Johnny.

A potential practical barrier.

THERAPIST: The last thing we want to do is to put one more thing on you that's going to make your life more complicated and difficult. I'm certain we'll be able to work out the schedule so that you can come on your afternoon off. It sounds like, if we can do that, then it will clear one potential hurdle out of the way. That doesn't necessarily solve the energy problem, though. When you imagine yourself coming to the next session, what kinds of thoughts go through your mind?

Reflection of meaning.

Problem solving the practical barrier first . . .

. . . then returning to the psychological barrier, asking for specifics.

PATIENT: I know it will be hard to get here—I'll just want to go home and shut myself in my room. If I come, someone might try to tell me how to feel better, but I don't know if it's going to work. They might try to tell me that I should do this and that to feel better, but it's hard for me to do anything right now.

Specifying the "low energy" barrier and hinting again at worry about being blamed.

THERAPIST: You are imagining yourself getting ready to come in, and part of you will be wondering, "How is this going to go?"

A bit too general.

PATIENT: Yes, and I may not be able to do the things that they are going to tell me to do. If I didn't have the energy to do those things and someone didn't understand that, then I would be worried it wouldn't help anyway.

Tries again to get the therapist to understand her concern about blame or failure.

THERAPIST: I'm *sure* it wouldn't help. One of the things that would be really important is that your therapist understands how hard it is for you right now to get yourself to do the things you need to do, and not have unrealistic expectations. If you felt the therapist was going to be critical and give you things to do that you couldn't handle, it would be very discouraging for you.

Empathizing, and subtly reframing.

Implying the counterfactual: "If this were to happen... (but it won't happen here)."

PATIENT: Yeah, or things I didn't want to do, like "Take this pill."

An underlying concern.

THERAPIST: So, you're wondering if the therapist might tell you to do things that didn't feel right to you.

PATIENT: Yeah. I just want to make sure that they would understand certain things about my life. I need them to not be telling me things

She really wants this therapist to understand.

about work or Johnny or his father
that I can't do.

THERAPIST: What would not be helpful
would be for someone to come in
and say, "Just tell your boss you need
time off, and tell your son's father
that he has to help you"—things like
that.

The therapist "gets it" concretely.

PATIENT: Because that would just make
things worse—create problems at work
and more arguments with Johnny and
his dad.

THERAPIST: Right. You're in this delicate
situation. The therapist needs to
understand and respect that. I'm
wondering if you have any thoughts
about how you could make sure the
therapist understands that?

Eliciting her ideas for solving the problem.

PATIENT: I guess I need someone who
will listen to me. Someone to talk
to who understands my situation.
My mom doesn't even understand.
She doesn't know what it's like
to have no one who is really
there just for you, to listen to
you.

The patient says what she wants, but not how to get it.

THERAPIST: So, imagine a therapist who
is first going to sit down and
listen to you and really try to
understand your situation, not
start offering advice or suggestions
right away, but first really taking
the time to understand how difficult
things are for you and the delicate
situation you are in. If you knew
you were going to be coming to
see a therapist like that, would
that make it easier, do you think,
to make it here?

The therapist implicitly offers her what she is asking for . . .

. . . and then asks if this resolves the barrier.

PATIENT: Yeah, because I don't know how to get the energy to come to see someone if it isn't going to help. My situation is difficult. I'm not just making a big deal out of nothing.

Again, implicitly expressing her worry about blame or criticism.

THERAPIST: Absolutely. It is a bad situation and a very delicate one. You sort of feel like you're right at the edge and if you're not careful you could fall right off the edge.

Validates her perspective . . . but could have articulated her fear of being blamed.

PATIENT: Yeah, and I've got to do something to keep from doing that because I have to take care of Johnny.

Stronger adherence talk.

THERAPIST: I'm hearing both things: it really does feel important to you to get help with this, to find something that is going to help you feel better; and, if there is something that you really believe is going to help you feel better, you'll probably be able to find the energy you need to get there.

Reframing summary, with the implication that "energy" is a proxy for whether or not she wants to do something.

PATIENT: I have to because Johnny is difficult enough to handle when I am feeling good, and I'm afraid of what I might do if I don't start to get some relief.

Adherence talk.

THERAPIST: And the thing that would take your energy away would be if you felt like you were coming to someone who wasn't going to get your situation and understand how difficult it is.

Speaking her language.

PATIENT: Yes, like that doctor who tried to give me pills.

A potent potential barrier to adherence.

THERAPIST: You probably didn't feel like going back to see him at all.

PATIENT: No, I haven't gone back to him.

THERAPIST: What else can you think of that might make it tough or keep you from coming in?

Asking for more barriers.

PATIENT: Nothing, really.

THERAPIST: Some other mothers that we have worked with have identified some things that make it difficult for them to make it in to talk to someone. Would it be all right if I mention these things just to see if they apply to you? (*Patient nods.*) One thing that sometimes comes up is concern about whether a therapist *can* understand you, because of differences between you and the therapist or between the therapist's life and your life. Has that thought crossed your mind at all?

Asking permission to explore other possible barriers.

Probing for cultural barriers (which the patient has not raised spontaneously).

PATIENT: No. I just need somebody who will listen. As long as they are willing to listen, I think they could understand.

THERAPIST: It's not so important who the therapist is, their background, if they're a man or woman, white or black, rich or poor. What matters is how interested and willing they are to hear you and understand your situation and not impose their ideas on you.

Reflecting meaning . . .

. . . though still not being specific about her concern about being blamed.

PATIENT: Yeah, like the pediatrician Johnny had. She didn't have a life like mine. Well, I guess. We didn't really talk about her life. She would just listen to me.

Making clear just how important this is to her.

THERAPIST: It didn't look like you had similar lives. But that didn't matter because of how she cared and how willing she was to listen.

PATIENT: Yeah, and I guess I didn't really think about the rest of it.

Eliciting Commitment or Leaving the Door Open

The therapist's final goal is to elicit commitment to treatment. This begins with a recapitulation: the patient's perceived dilemma and change talk; the strengths she has shown in coping with this and other challenges; objective evidence of "no-fault" depression and expressed ambivalence about seeing herself as depressed or coming for treatment; what the patient most wants from treatment and the therapist and anything she does not want; and identified barriers to treatment participation and potential solutions. After providing information about the next steps in the treatment process, the therapist asks a "key question"— "How does this sound to you? Is this what you want to do?"—and listens for the opportunity to highlight the commitment talk that should emerge.

If the patient expresses commitment to treatment, the therapist makes the referral; if the patient remains ambivalent, the therapist reflects both sides of the ambivalence; if the patient offers resistance, the therapist rolls with it nondefensively. In all cases the therapist seeks to end the session on a positive note: communicating a nonpunitive message about "imperfect" treatment participation; taking a positive and inviting stance regarding the patient's ability to participate in and gain benefits from treatment, should she choose to participate; and offering hope by affirming the patient's participation, reiterating the view of depression as a treatable condition, and expressing the belief that the patient has already taken a first step toward feeling and functioning better.

THERAPIST: [Summary of the patient's *Recapitulation.*
story, dilemma, and strengths,
expressed need for change,
feedback on depression, perceived disadvantages and barriers for treatment,
perceived positives of treatment,
and resolution of ambivalence toward
treatment engagement] Is that a fair
summary?

PATIENT: Yeah, I think it is. (*Pause*)
I would be taking a chance,
I guess.   *Not quite a commitment.*

THERAPIST: How are you feeling about   *Key question.*
taking that chance right now?

PATIENT: Well, I need to find a way to cope with some of the problems I'm having. If it gets any worse, I might do something I'd regret. It's at least worth trying therapy to see if it will help.

Commitment talk.

THERAPIST: There's a part of you that feels "I'm taking a chance here," and at the same time it feels like not taking that chance might be even more risky for you.

Double-sided reflection, ending with a gentle reframe.

PATIENT: Right. I can't afford not to do something, so it's worth taking a chance.

THERAPIST: Great. Then, if you're ready, I can schedule an appointment for you to begin the therapy. Is that what you want to do?

Asking for commitment . . .

PATIENT: Yeah, I do. I think it would be good.

. . . and getting it.

THERAPIST: OK. I have you on the schedule for the next time you bring Johnny in. I'd like to mention a couple of things before we end. If you can't keep the appointment, we'd like you to call to let us know so that we can reschedule. At the same time, we also know that sometimes things come up at the last minute and you might not be able to call. We understand that when people's lives are as stressful as yours, these things can be unavoidable. I don't want you to feel like you can't call later to reschedule.

Recalling a barrier and its solution.

Emphasizing the nonpunitive stance.

PATIENT: That's good because I do have a very busy, hectic life and things do change at the last minute.

She appreciates this stance.

THERAPIST: I guess this seems especially important, because there is every reason to think that we will be able to

Expressing optimism about treatment success.

help you. We have had a lot of success in helping moms like you in the past. And as you said, our therapy tackles just the kinds of problems you're having. And you're already working hard to make things better. So, we don't want you to miss this chance. (*Patient nods, smiles.*) Is there anything else you'd like to ask about before we stop?

Affirming her efforts.

Eliciting questions/ reactions.

PATIENT: No. I think I've got it.

THERAPIST: I'm glad you came in today. It's not always easy talking with a stranger about such personal things. I think that this went well today, and that's a good sign for what's to come.

Ending with affirmation and optimism.

PROBLEMS AND POTENTIAL SOLUTIONS

Semistructured Intervention

A challenge in conducting semistructured interventions is to find the balance between adhering to the structure too rigidly or too loosely. The outline we provide represents an "ideal" form of the engagement session, and the structure is intended to ensure that the therapist accomplishes a set of tasks designed to enhance commitment to treatment. At the same time, the session should be delivered flexibly to meet the specific needs of each patient. If a particular area does not seem relevant to a given patient, it should be noted briefly and skipped; if the patient seems to be addressing topics in an order that differs from that specified here, therapists should follow the patient and not the outline. Being flexible may also mean that, in rare cases, the therapist may determine that the need for a given patient to tell her story and be heard is so great that the bulk of the session must be given over to simply listening empathically. Delivering the engagement session in a rigid or "cookbook" fashion is likely to undermine its purpose of meaningfully engaging the patient being interviewed.

Intervention Duration

The engagement session takes 45–60 minutes to complete. Factors that drive the duration of the interview include patient style (loquacious vs.

taciturn), mood disorder symptoms (psychomotor agitation vs. retardation), the number of treatment barriers, and the extent of patient ambivalence about treatment. If pressed for time, the therapist should focus primarily on those aspects of the session that seem most relevant for a given patient. For example, a patient may come for therapy already well educated about the nature of depression, making extended psychoeducation redundant; another may have had positive treatment experiences for another condition, yet may never have been depressed before, requiring more focus on understanding depression than on ambivalence about treatment. It is also important to explain the intervention duration to patients so that they allot enough time in their schedules to complete the interview.

Engagement Session versus Psychotherapy

Although the engagement session may be therapeutic for the patient, it is not intended as psychotherapy but as a "pretherapy" intervention. Therapists who are unaccustomed to starting this way may be tempted to revert to a more familiar initial agenda—for example, taking a thorough history, making a final diagnosis, and establishing a treatment plan. The rationale for conducting an engagement session is simple: patients who are ambivalent about treatment may be more likely to drop out; in such cases, history taking, diagnosis, and treatment planning are premature. Investing a session in engaging the patient prior to initiating the formal treatment process has the potential to get the treatment started on a more solid footing.

The Suicidal, Psychotic, or Agitated Patient

Good clinical judgment supersedes all protocols. If the therapist observes acute suicidal ideation, psychosis, uncontrollable agitation, or another critical condition, the intervention should be abandoned in favor of making arrangements for the patient's immediate safety and an appropriate level of care.

When the Engagement Session Therapist Is Not the Psychotherapist

In some settings, the individual conducting the engagement session may not become the patient's therapist. Although it is optimal to arrange for continuity of care, it may not always be practical. In these cases, the therapist conducting the interview should align him- or herself with the prospective therapist (e.g., "It will be very important for us to keep in mind that you felt intimidated by your last therapist") and emphasize that he or she will communicate the important aspects of the session. It goes without saying that ensuring that such communication occurs is essential.

When the Engagement Session Is Not the First Encounter with the Patient

In some settings, the first encounter with the patient must follow external guidelines promulgated by the facility or by regulatory agencies. In these cases, therapists who want to enhance engagement have two options. Therapists may choose to look for moments in the standard interview in which they can insert elements of the engagement session— for example, while inquiring about previous treatment episodes, the therapist could ask what the patient did and did not find helpful in each of those experiences. Alternatively, the therapist may conduct the initial visit in the standard way and then initiate an engagement session at the follow-up meeting. In these cases, the patient is likely to have already articulated key elements of her story, and the admitting diagnosis may have been discussed. Rather than repeating this material, the therapist can begin by summarizing what has already been discussed and then either ask for elaboration (if this seems likely to deepen the encounter) or move on to the next phase of the session.

Using the Engagement Session Prior to Other Forms of Treatment

Although developed as a prelude to IPT-B, the engagement session seems easily transferable to other contexts. Many of the issues the session is intended to address are found frequently in treatment of persons with anxiety, substance use, and other disorders. Similarly, we think it likely that therapists can adapt the intervention for use prior to CBT or other treatment modalities. The goal of helping patients to see how the help they want can be provided by a given treatment extends to multiple treatment approaches.

RESEARCH AND CONCLUSIONS

In an open prospective pilot study (Swartz et al., 2006), a group of depressed, nonsuicidal mothers of adolescents receiving mental health treatment were offered the engagement session and eight sessions of IPT-B. Of 13 mothers who met DSM-IV criteria for major depressive disorder and were not in treatment, 11 received an engagement session. Following the session, all completed the Client Satisfaction Questionnaire (CSQ), an eight-item instrument assessing subjective satisfaction with treatment, with possible scores ranging from 8 to 32 (Attkisson & Greenfield, 1994). The mean CSQ score for the engagement session was 27.2 (±4.0), indicating high levels of satisfaction. All 11 participants subsequently scheduled an initial treatment appointment, and all but 1 completed a full course of therapy. The one noncompleter, who was withdrawn after attending seven of the eight sessions, had also clearly "engaged."

In a randomized pilot study in the public care obstetrics clinic of a large urban women's hospital (Grote, Zuckoff, Swartz, Bledsoe, & Geibel, in press), 64 depressed economically disadvantaged pregnant women (63% of them African American) who were not seeking depression treatment were offered either the engagement session and eight sessions of IPT-B provided in the prenatal clinic or a referral for standard depression treatment by a community mental health provider in the prenatal clinic or in their neighborhood. Of 31 women assigned to "Engagement and IPT-B," 25 entered the study and received an engagement session; 24 women (96%) attended an initial treatment session, and 17 (68%) completed a full course of IPT-B. Of 33 women assigned to "standard referral and treatment," 28 entered the study, 10 (36%) attended an initial treatment session, and 2 (7%) completed a course of standard depression treatment. Extent of engagement and retention were both significantly superior in "Engagement and IPT-B" as compared to the "standard referral and treatment" (Fisher's Exact Test [FET], $p < .001$).

Research on the effects of the engagement session is currently in its preliminary stages. Our pilot work has demonstrated the feasibility of providing the intervention, and the rates of treatment initiation and attendance compare favorably to those found in typical practice, as reviewed earlier. A randomized pilot study comparing the engagement session with standard referral to treatment in depressed mothers and in depressed economically disadvantaged pregnant women is under way, and we have begun to evaluate the feasibility of training community therapists to conduct the engagement session in routine treatment settings.

Our work thus far has led us to view the engagement session with promise. At face value, the MI, ethnographic interviewing, and psychoeducational strategies work well together to address common barriers to treatment seeking. Anecdotally, women who have completed the session have consistently expressed the sense that it had helped them to clarify their treatment needs and goals and facilitated their participation in treatment. We have also trained numerous therapists from a variety of disciplines to conduct the intervention, with good results. We have thus concluded that the engagement session is worthy of further investigation to determine the extent to which the addition of an MI-based integrative engagement intervention can help to address the pressing problem of limited treatment engagement and participation among depressed individuals.

REFERENCES

American Psychiatric Association. (1994). *Diagnostic and statistical manual of mental disorders* (4th ed.). Washington, DC: Author.

Arkowitz, H., & Westra, H. A. (2004). Integrating motivational interviewing and cognitive-behavioral therapy in the treatment of depression and anxiety. *Journal of Cognitive Psychotherapy, 18,* 337–350.

Attkisson, C. C., & Greenfield, T. K. (1994). The client satisfaction questionnaire-8 and the service satisfaction questionnaire-30. In M. Maruish (Ed.), *The use of psychological testing for treatment planning and outcome assessment.* Hillsdale, NJ: Earlbaum.

Burke, B. L., Arkowitz, H., & Menchola, M. (2003). The efficacy of motivational interviewing: A meta-analysis of controlled clinical trials. *Journal of Consulting and Clinical Psychology, 71,* 843–861.

Daley, D. C., Salloum, I. M., Zuckoff, A., Kirisci, L., & Thase, M. E. (1998). Increasing treatment compliance among outpatients with comorbid depression and cocaine dependence: Results of a pilot study. *American Journal of Psychiatry, 155,* 1611–1613.

Daley, D. C., & Zuckoff, A. (1998). Improving compliance with the initial outpatient session among discharged inpatient dual diagnosis patients. *Social Work, 43,* 470–473.

Daley, D. C., & Zuckoff, A. (1999). A motivational approach to improving compliance. In D. C. Daley & A. Zuckoff, *Improving treatment compliance: Counseling and systems strategies for substance abuse and dual disorders* (pp. 105–123). Center City, MN: Hazelden.

Garcia, J. A., & Weisz, J. R. (2002). When youth mental health care stops: Therapeutic relationship problems and other reasons for ending youth outpatient treatment. *Journal of Consulting and Clinical Psychology, 70,* 439–443.

Grote, N. K., Bledsoe, S. E., Swartz, H. A., & Frank, E. (2004). Feasibility of providing culturally relevant, brief interpersonal psychotherapy for antenatal depression in an obstetrics clinic: A pilot study. *Research on Social Work Practice, 14,* 397–407.

Grote, N. K., Zuckoff, A., Swartz, H. A., Bledsoe, S. E., & Geibel, S. L. (in press). Engaging women who are depressed and economically disadvantaged in mental health treatment. *Social Work.*

Hettema, J., Steele, J., & Miller, W. R. (2005). Motivational interviewing. *Annual Review of Clinical Psychology, 1*, 91–111.

Mackenzie, C. S., Knox, V. J., Gekoski, W. L., & Macaulay, H. L. (2004). An adaptation and extension of the Attitudes Toward Seeking Professional Psychological Help scale. *Journal of Applied Social Psychology, 34*, 2410–2435.

McCarthy, K. S., Iacoviello, B., Barrett, M., Rynn, M., Gallop, R., & Barber J. P. (2005, June). *Treatment preferences impact the development of the therapeutic alliance.* Paper presented at the annual meeting of the Society for Psychotherapy Research, Montreal, Canada.

McKay, M. M., & Bannon, W. M. (2004). Engaging families in child mental health services. *Child and Adolescent Psychiatric Clinics of North America, 13*, 905–921.

McKay, M. M., McCadam, K., & Gonzales, J. J. (1996). Addressing the barriers to mental health services for inner city children and their caretakers. *Community Mental Health Journal, 32*, 353–361.

Miller, W. R., & Rollnick, S. (2002). *Motivational interviewing: Preparing people for change* (2nd ed.). New York: Guilford Press.

Miranda, J., Azocar, F., Komaromy, M., & Golding, J. M. (1998). Unmet mental health needs of women in public-sector gynecologic clinics. *American Journal of Obstetrics and Gynecology, 17*, 212–217.

Miranda, J., Azocar, F., Organista, K. C., Dwyer, E., & Areane, P. (2003). Treatment of depression among impoverished primary care patients from ethnic minority groups. *Psychiatric Services, 54*, 219–225.

Miranda, J., Azocar, F., Organista, K., Munoz, R., & Lieberman, A. (1996). Recruiting and retaining low-income Latinos in psychotherapy research. *Journal of Consulting and Clinical Psychology, 64*, 868–874.

Nock, M. K., & Kazdin, A. E. (2005). Randomized controlled trial of a brief intervention for increasing participation in parent management training. *Journal of Consulting and Clinical Psychology, 73*, 872–879.

Schensul, S. L., Schensul, J. J., & LeCompte, M. D. (1999). *Essential ethnographic methods: Observations, interviews, and questionnaires.* Walnut Creek, CA: AltaMira Press.

Scholle, S. H., Hasket, R. F., Hanusa, B. H., Pincus, H. A., & Kupfer, D. J. (2003). Addressing depression in obstetrics/gynecology practice. *General Hospital Psychiatry, 25*, 83–90.

Simon, G. E., Ludman, E. J., Tutty, S., Operskalski, B., & Von Korff, M. (2004). Telephone psychotherapy and telephone care management for primary care patients starting antidepressant treatment: A randomized controlled trial. *Journal of the American Medical Association, 292*, 935–942.

Swartz, H. A., Frank, E., Shear, M. K., Thase, M. E., Fleming, M. A. D., & Scott, J. (2004). A pilot study of brief interpersonal psychotherapy for depression in women. *Psychiatric Services, 55*, 448–450.

Swartz, H. A., Shear, M. K., Wren, F. J., Greeno, C., Sales, E., Sullivan, B. K., et al. (2005). Depression and anxiety among mothers who bring their children to a pediatric mental health clinic. *Psychiatric Services, 56*, 1077–1083.

Swartz, H. A., Zuckoff, A., Frank, E., Spielvogle, H. N., Shear, M. K., Fleming, M. A. D., et al. (2006). An open-label trial of enhanced brief interpersonal psychotherapy in depressed mothers whose children are receiving psychiatric treatment. *Depression and Anxiety, 23*, 398–404.

Walitzer, K. S., Derman, K. H., & Connors, G. J. (1999). Strategies for preparing clients for treatment—a review. *Behavior Modification, 23*, 129–151.

Westra, H. A., & Dozois, D. J. A. (2006). Preparing clients for cognitive behavioural therapy: A randomized pilot study of motivational interviewing for anxiety. *Cognitive Therapy and Research, 30*, 481–498.

Young, A. S., Klap, R., Sherbourne, C. D., & Wells, K. B. (2001). The quality of care for depressive and anxiety disorders in the United States. *Archives of General Psychiatry, 58*, 55–61.

Zuckoff, A., & Daley, D. C. (2001). Engagement and adherence issues in treating persons with non-psychosis dual disorders. *Psychiatric Rehabilitation Skills, 5*, 131–162.

Zweben, A., & Zuckoff, A. (2002). Motivational interviewing and treatment adherence. In W. R. Miller & S. Rollnick, *Motivational interviewing: Preparing people for change* (2nd ed., pp. 299–319). New York: Guilford Press.

CHAPTER 6

Motivational Interviewing as an Integrative Framework for the Treatment of Depression

Hal Arkowitz
Brian L. Burke

Upon seeing the title of this chapter, some readers may think: "Another therapy for depression?" We already have a number of treatments that have proven somewhat efficacious, including cognitive-behavioral (e.g., Westen & Morrison, 2001), psychoanalytic (Leichsenring, Rabung, & Leibling, 2004), humanistic (Elliott, Greenberg, & Lietaer, 2004), and drug therapies (Nemeroff & Schatzberg, 2002). Nevertheless, a significant percentage of clients who receive these therapies show improvement but not remission as well as high relapse rates. Many others are not helped at all. Motivational interviewing (MI) may be one way to enhance the effectiveness of psychotherapy and drug therapy for depression, because it emphasizes two issues that are highly relevant to depression—increasing intrinsic motivation and resolving ambivalence about change. In addition, meta-analyses (e.g., Burke, Arkowitz, & Menchola, 2003; Hettema, Steele, & Miller, 2005) have found that MI can be used in combination with other therapies and increases client retention in and adherence to other treatments. Many of these other treatments have been cognitive-behavioral in nature. Currently, there appears to be a great deal of interest in combining or integrating MI and cognitive-behavioral therapy (CBT). In this chapter, we will address the integration of these two therapies. However, our discussion will be broader and discuss MI not as another "school" of therapy but as a method that can be flexibly used to enhance treatment outcomes for depression. We propose that MI can be employed as an integrative framework that can incorporate other therapies and that can flexibly be used to enhance treatment outcome in depression.

THE CLINICAL POPULATION AND USUAL TREATMENTS

Depression is one of the most prevalent disorders of our time. Symptoms of major depression include five of the following nine: depressed mood; loss of interest or pleasure in the activities of life; weight loss or weight gain; insomnia or excessive sleeping; psychomotor agitation or retardation; fatigue or loss of energy; feelings of excessive worthlessness or guilt; problems with thinking, concentration, and decision making; and suicide thoughts or attempts. If the person displays milder depressive symptoms for a period of at least 2 years, he or she may be diagnosed with dysthymic disorder (American Psychiatric Association, 2000), which is more chronic but less intense than major depression.

In addition to major depressive and dysthymic disorders, there are other less common categories of mood disorders, including seasonal affective disorder, mood disorder due to a general medical condition, and substance-induced mood disorder.

Bipolar disorders, which are defined by the presence of manic or hypomanic episodes with or without depression, are also included under the category of mood disorders. In this chapter, our focus will be on unipolar depression, in which such episodes are absent.

Some 16% of the U.S. population have met the criteria for major depression at some point in their lives, while an additional 10% have met the criteria for minor depression, involving fewer but equally intense symptoms (Kessler, 2002). Many additional people experience less intense depression that still impairs their quality of life. Tragically, 10–15% of individuals with a diagnosis of depression eventually commit suicide (Clark & Fawcett, 1992). Clearly, depression is a serious problem in need of the most effective treatments we can find.

In recent years, there have been significant developments in both psychological (Craighead, Hart, Craighead, & Ilardi, 2002) and biological (Nemeroff & Schatzberg, 2002) treatments of depression. The two psychotherapies that have received the most research attention in randomized controlled trials are cognitive-behavioral therapy (CBT) and interpersonal psychotherapy (IPT; Weissman, Markowitz, & Klerman, 2000), while fewer studies have been done on psychoanalytic and humanistic therapies. The efficacy of various antidepressant drug therapies has also been evaluated in numerous studies.

A meta-analysis by Westen and Morrison (2001) of psychotherapy outcome studies through 1998 found that 54% of those depressed subjects who completed treatment improved significantly. However, at the end of treatment, a large percentage of participants still had some degree of depressive symptoms. This is problematic because the presence of residual depressive symptoms is a significant risk factor for relapse (Lewinsohn, Hoberman, & Rosenbaum, 1988). In addition, a high percentage of depressed clients were rejected from the studies on various grounds including comorbid substance abuse, psychoticism, and suicide risk, limiting the range of depressed persons to whom these results can be generalized. When analyses included not just completers but also those who began but did not complete treatment, improvement rates dropped to 37%. Furthermore, those studies that included follow-up found that relapse rates were disturbingly high.

While antidepressant drug therapies are helpful for many depressed people, (Nemeroff & Schatzberg, 2002), they also have many drawbacks. They can have troubling side effects such as sexual dysfunction and weight gain, are less cost-effective than psychotherapy (Barrett, Byford, & Knapp, 2005), and lead to greater relapse after treatment has ended (Hollon et al., 2005). Outcomes can be improved by trying a different antidepressant drug or augmenting it with another medication if the initial one is not tolerated well or doesn't have sufficient therapeutic effects (McGrath et al., 2006). However, Olfson, Marcus, Tedeschi, and Wan (2006) found that 42% discontinue antidepressant drug therapy within 30 days and 72% by 90 days. While there may be many reasons for discontinuation (e.g., lack of therapeutic effects or intolerable side effects), many people discontinue an otherwise tolerable and helpful medication. Potentially, MI can be helpful in increasing adherence to antidepressant medication when appropriate.

The outcomes of psychotherapy and antidepressant drug therapy are equivalent at the end of therapy, but when treatments are terminated, relapse rates are lower in psychotherapy (Hollon et al., 2005). There is a great deal of room for improvement in how many people are helped and how much they are helped, treatment adherence, and relapse rates in both drug therapy and psychotherapy. We hope to demonstrate that MI holds promise for improving the outcomes of both psychotherapy and drug therapy for depression.

RATIONALE FOR USING MI
IN THE TREATMENT OF DEPRESSION

There are several reasons that point to the potential utility in using MI in psychotherapy for all disorders and specifically for depression. First, MI can be integrated or combined with other treatments, enhancing client retention in and adherence to those therapies, thereby improving treatment outcomes. In addition, there are several more specific reasons that we discuss below.

MI Fits the Symptoms of Depression

Loss of interest and pleasure in most or all usual activities is a core symptom of depression and can easily be recast as low motivation. Burns and Nolen-Hoeksma (1991) found that motivation—as measured by "willingness" to participate actively in CBT treatment, to explore one's problems, and to make changes and sacrifices in order to improve— significantly predicted improvement in depression. The specific focus of MI on increasing motivation may therefore be a good fit to the motivational deficit shown by depressed people.

Depressed clients are often seen by therapists as "resistant." Both Miller and Rollnick (2002) and Engle and Arkowitz (2006) have reconceptualized resistance as ambivalence. Most clinicians who work with depressed clients are aware of how often such ambivalence arises, as in phrases beginning with "yes, but . . ." More than most other therapies, MI specifically addresses the ambivalence that is so prevalent in depression.

Finally, irritability and anger are present in about 25% of depressed clients (Pasquini, Picardi, Biondi, Gaetano, & Morisini, 2004) and the Project MATCH Research Group (1997, 1998) found that the presence of anger was a significant predictor of positive outcome in MI for alcoholism. This finding raises the possibility that MI might be particularly effective for people whose depression is associated with anger.

MI Can Help Depressed Persons Increase
Their Activity Levels

Increasing physical and social activities can decrease depressive symptoms (e.g., Burns & Spangler, 2000; Lewinsohn, 1974). Therapists of all persuasions often suggest to depressed clients that they increase their activity levels; yet, the manner in which these suggestions are made can have a significant influence on whether or not clients will act upon them. The supportive style that is characteristic of MI has been shown to generate less resistance than a more directive therapist style (Miller, Benefield, & Tonigan, 1993; Patterson & Chamberlain, 1994). As a result, when therapeutic suggestions are made in MI style, they are more likely to be carried out.

A Therapeutic Relationship Characterized by Empathy Reduces Depression

There are good data demonstrating that a therapeutic relationship characterized by empathy is a powerful agent of change in therapy (Bohart, Elliot, Greenberg, & Watson, 2002). Lambert and Barley (2002) concluded that therapeutic relationship variables including empathy were more highly correlated with therapy outcome than the specific techniques of the different therapies. They also concluded that therapists who were warmer and more empathic, understanding, accepting, and supportive were also more effective than therapists who were rated lower on these variables. Burns and Nolen-Hoeksma (1992) found that therapeutic empathy had a substantial causal effect on recovery from depression in clients receiving CBT. These studies suggest that MI, with its strong emphasis on an empathic therapeutic relationship, has the potential to enhance therapeutic outcomes in depression.

APPLYING MI IN THE TREATMENT OF DEPRESSION

Studies in the area of substance use disorders have shown that a few sessions of MI as a pretreatment enhance the outcome of subsequent therapies, including more directive ones (Connors, Walitzer, & Dermen, 2002; see also meta-analyses by Burke et al., 2003; Hettema et al., 2005). The use of MI as a pretreatment is more fully discussed in Arkowitz and Westra (2004), Westra and Dozois (Chapter 2, this volume), and Zuckoff, Swartz, and Grote (Chapter 5, this volume). MI as a pretreatment holds a great deal of promise for the treatment of depression and other disorders and warrants research scrutiny. However, our work has focused on MI as a treatment framework for the entire course of therapy.

Miller (1983) stated that MI was not originally intended as a standalone therapy but rather to be used in conjunction with other therapies. Consistent with this position, we consider MI to be *an integrative framework into which almost any therapy methods or theories can be incorporated.* However, in applying MI to depression in this integrative manner, we have found it necessary to address several issues that are discussed below.

The Healing Relationship

We have observed that in some instances the therapeutic relationship described by Carl Rogers (1951) and fostered by MI may be both necessary *and* sufficient for successful treatment outcome in depression. According to Carl Rogers, the therapeutic relationship is both necessary and sufficient for change. He argued that a particular type of therapy relationship containing certain conditions was needed to accomplish change. Three of the most central of these conditions are therapist genuineness, empathy, and unconditional positive regard or acceptance.

These attitudes are central to MI and are variously referred to as part of the "MI spirit" or "MI style." The very close relationship between Rogers's conditions for change and the MI spirit can be seen in several ways. Miller and Rollnick (2002, p. 25) state that

> First, motivational interviewing is client-centered or person-centered in its focus on the concerns and perspectives of the individual, as well as in our heavy reliance on and indebtedness to the work of Carl Rogers and his colleagues. In this sense, motivational interviewing is an evolution of the client-centered approach that Rogers developed.

However, MI differs from Rogers's approach in its emphasis on increasing intrinsic motivation to change, resolving ambivalence about change, and increasing change talk through selective responding. Miller and Rollnick (2002, p. 25) view the "MI spirit" or "MI style" as essential to achieving change, suggesting that MI methods used to accomplish these goals would lose most or all of their effectiveness without this spirit.

Further support for our view comes from the content of a major coding system that has been used in MI research (e.g., Moyers, Miller, & Hendrickson, 2005) that includes ratings of the specific core clinician skills for conducting MI. These are acceptance, empathy, genuineness, warmth, and egalitarianism. While there may be some differences in the meanings of these conditions between Miller and Rollnick's views and Rogers's views, the overlap is unmistakable.

Rogers's client-centered therapy, built on providing the same or similar conditions that are present in MI, has been shown to be efficacious in a number of studies (see, e.g., Elliot et al., 2004; Goldman, Greenberg, & Angus, 2006). These and other studies are discussed in more detail at the end of this chapter.

Given the substantial similarities between Rogers's conditions for change and the efficacy of his client-centered therapy on the one hand and the centrality of MI spirit to MI on the other, it is possible that the MI spirit may account for change in at least some clients, with the specific MI methods directed toward increasing change motivation and change talk and resolving ambivalence playing little or no role in the change process.

Many clients come to therapy with low self-esteem and self-acceptance as a central part of their problems. This is especially true in depression. By the therapist's providing unconditional positive regard, genuineness, and empathy to the depressed client, the client may come to internalize these attitudes, countering the usual depressive attitudes of conditional positive regard and lack of empathy.

Research has not yet clarified the relative contributions of MI spirit, resolving ambivalence, and increasing intrinsic motivation, respectively, in the change process. Such research would shed light on how MI works and the speculations proposed in this section. Research by Amrhein, Miller, Yahne, Palmer, and Fulcher (2003) has shown that change-commitment talk predicts outcome, but the question still remains as to what aspect or aspects of MI are necessary to accomplish such an increase.

Levels of Therapeutic Focus

Therapists who work with depression need to address not only the presenting symptoms of depression and other associated distress but also causal issues and ways of dealing with them. Unless there is some way to guide the therapist in developing the foci of therapy for depression, treatment may go in too many directions without making sufficient progress on any one, especially in short-term therapy. In our approach, we have developed a simple and useful method of thinking about foci of treatment for depression that could potentially be applied to other disorders as well.

We have defined three levels of foci: the overall symptoms of depression and other distress; the problems that contribute to the depression and distress; and what the client needs to do to change these problems. Working to increase motivation and resolve ambivalence about change are addressed at each level.

Level 1: Reducing Major Symptoms of Depression and Distress

The initial focus of therapy must be to reduce the overall symptoms of depression and associated distress. In addition to such frequently used MI methods as increasing change-commitment talk and working with value–behavior discrepancies, we have found decisional balance strategies to resolve ambivalence about depressive symptoms to be extremely helpful with depressed clients.

Differentially eliciting and reinforcing change-commitment talk is central to MI. Client talk that reflects maintenance of the status quo or reasons not to change is relatively deemphasized. For example, Miller and Rollnick (2002) even suggest shifting the focus of the conversation when such "no-change" talk arises. By contrast, we spend considerable time and emphasis in eliciting and reflecting reasons not to change, especially in the early stages of therapy that are aimed at building motivation to change. Our clinical observations suggest that focusing on *reasons not to change* as much as *reasons to change* early in treatment can help deepen the client's understanding and appreciation of that side of their ambivalence as well as bring out emotions associated with those reasons. In fact, the evocation and identification of painful emotions associated with not changing can add strength to the reasons to change by the client's realization that this distress will be reduced if change does occur. In addition our sense is that to resolve ambivalence, which we see as an inner conflict (Engle & Arkowitz, 2006), it is important to get "all the cards on the table." Otherwise, the client may have reasons not to change that have either not been sufficiently elicited and discussed or not sufficiently well appreciated. If this is the case, such reasons may continue to be obstacles to change. By evoking and examining these reasons in decisional balance work and focusing on them as much as we focus on reasons to change, we should thereby *increase* the likelihood of resolving the ambivalence and increase change-commitment talk.

Encouraging the client to discuss the obstacles or disadvantages to change can be a unique experience that may enhance a positive therapeutic relationship. This is due to the fact that the therapist listens nonjudgmentally and responds empathically to the client's discussion of thoughts and feelings that significant others may find incomprehensible or unacceptable. It is possible that after clients have experienced the therapist listening nonjudgmentally to their reasons not to change, they may be able to discuss their reasons *for* change more openly and genuinely rather than giving socially desirable responses and repeating what others have said to them about the need for change. We believe that the importance of focusing on reasons not to change as much as on reasons to change applies to the three levels of therapeutic focus discussed in this chapter.

As an example, consider a depressed man for whom one important reason not to change is the fear that if he is no longer depressed he will have to deal with the family problems that contributed to his becoming depressed in the first place. We would elicit his thoughts and fears about his ability to deal with these problems in some depth. Having done so, we can explore the advantages of dealing with this issue, and through open-ended questions and other MI methods we can examine how realistic that reason is. For example, we might explore and seek to elicit times in the past when he has dealt successfully with other family problems. Our ultimate goal is to help him resolve his ambivalence about remaining depressed and to increase his change-commitment talk in order to decrease his depression. We believe that exploring reasons not to change in depth is a means to this end. These speculations are based on our clinical experiences and remain to be examined in empirical studies.

The case of Brad illustrates work with ambivalence at this overall level of symptoms. Brad became seriously depressed and anxious during the year following his college graduation, fitting a diagnosis of major depression. During the course of the first three sessions, Brad was given a rationale and description of work on decisional balance and was asked to think of reasons not to change his depression. After much discussion, Brad came to focus on two related themes. First, if his depression and anxiety improved, he would have to deal with the difficult question of what to do with his life. He stated that this was one of the issues that may have precipitated his depression. Furthermore, if his symptoms improved, he expected that his parents "would be more on my case to get a job or do something or go back to school, and I still don't know what I want to do." He also listed several reasons to change, including how awful it was to feel sad, uninterested, and to take little pleasure from anything, as well as the negative impact his depression was having on his relationship with his girlfriend.

Level 2: Identifying Problems That Contribute to the Major Symptoms of Depression and Associated Distress

This is often a difficult area to assess, requiring considerable skill from the therapist. In addition, therapists of different orientations may conceptualize problems at this level differently. For example, a psychoanalytic view may see depression as related to anger turned inward or certain internalized mental representations, while a CBT approach may see it as due to distorted and negative thinking, beliefs, and underlying schemas. In our work, we look both to present and past determinants.

Consistent with MI, we consider the client as the expert and the therapist as a consultant to the change process. We start by asking the client what problems he or she believes may contribute to his or her depression. Sometimes, clients are readily able to identify these problems. When they do, the therapist helps define them more clearly through reflection and feedback offered tentatively. When they cannot, the therapist asks permission to offer some ideas about the causes of their depression and describes some possibilities, including repressed anger, social isolation and low levels of reinforcement, unresolved grief, and negative thought patterns. If the client chooses one or more of these that might apply, the therapist and client work together to develop the formulation(s) as they apply to the client.

William R. Miller (personal communication, December 7, 2006) has employed a very similar procedure with depressed clients, suggesting that their depression can be caused by a variety of factors and offering a menu of different options for the client to choose as possibly applicable to the circumstances. He reports that clients respond very well to this menu procedure, which takes advantage not only of the client's own wisdom and hunches but also of the fact that people tend to be more intrinsically motivated to do something they have freely chosen from among options.

Ricardo, a middle-aged man, described the main problem underlying his depression as "always seeing the half-empty part of the glass without being able to see the part that's half-full." In discussing the matter further, he attributed his depression primarily to his negative and pessimistic thinking. After exploring various options with him about how we might approach changing his thinking, he chose a cognitive therapy approach.

In exploring Level 2, we look to present not only factors that may be contributing to the depression but also patterns that may be carried forward from the past as well. The case of John provides an example of the latter. John became depressed after he was fired from his job. He stated that all he needed was a job with a "good" boss to eliminate his depression. However, exploration revealed that he had serious problems with authority dating back to his early childhood with a violent and authoritarian father. After a few sessions, he began to consider the possibility that his problem was more than situational and might reflect a more long-standing problem with authority figures. In this case, the therapy was more of a psychoanalytically oriented therapy done in the MI spirit and based on more modern conceptions of psychoanalytic approaches including object relations, self psychology, and the relational paradigm (see Wachtel, 1997, ch. 15, for a summary of these). It included interpretations relating to how patterns based on early attachments may carry forward into the present, where they are no longer appropriate. Interpretations also included those relating to transference, in which John treated the therapist as another authority figure with whom he had trouble. Working with the carryover from the past and pointing out the manifestations of this pattern in the therapy relationship were quite helpful. As we discuss later, however, interpretations were offered as tentative possibilities for understanding, and the client's thoughts about the interpretations often led to modification, rejection, or acceptance of them. It was psychodynamic therapy conducted in the MI spirit rather than from a more authoritative therapist stance.

Sarah, a 55-year-old woman, had been sexually abused as a child and manifested a great deal of shame because of it, leading her to become reclusive, lonely, and depressed. We defined the shame that she had been carrying around for so many years as an important problem contributing to her depression as well as other residual feelings about the abuse.

Charles, a middle-aged man, sought therapy with one of us (Hal Arkowitz) for depression associated with marital distress. His wife was increasingly upset with his inability to communicate his thoughts and feelings and was threatening to separate from him. I asked him if he could recall any early instances of difficulties in communicating with loved ones. He proceeded to describe that his parents had been unhappily married and that when he was a child his mother related to him more as though he were a counselor, sharing her intimate problems with him and getting upset if he tried to talk about his own concerns. As a result, he learned to be a good listener but a poor communicator. What had served him as a way of being close to his mother in the past had the effect of distancing himself from his wife in the present. This insight increased his motivation to explore being more open with his wife.

Level 2 is essentially a case formulation level. Input from any reasonable theoretical orientation is appropriate. In part, this is what makes MI an integrative framework into which different ways of conceptualizing the problem from diverse theoretical orientations can be incorporated.

Level 3: Changing the Problems that Contribute to the Major
Symptoms of Distress: Using MI in the Action Stage

Once the problems contributing to the depression are defined, they become the focus of treatment. As with Level 2, change strategies may
come from any bona fide psychotherapy approach. We have found that
working with MI in the action stage can be done in the context of the
MI spirit and may employ the methods of MI as well as those of other
therapy approaches. The procedures employed in the COMBINE study
also illustrate this clearly (Miller, 2004).

Therapy in Level 3 is directed toward behavior change, which is the
primary goal of MI. Sometimes, such change can be accomplished
through more action-oriented therapies such as CBT and in other cases
with therapies oriented more toward awareness, as in humanistic therapies, or insight, as in psychoanalytic therapies. But insight and awareness, while valuable for self-understanding, are not the end points of
such therapies. They are means to accomplish behavior change in the
problems concerning the client.

Consistent with MI, the therapist begins by asking the client what he
or she thinks can be done in order to change the Level 2 problems. Clients'
responses have included "get back to exercising," "stop beating up on myself," "stop seeing only the negative side of things," "be more open with
my wife," and "I don't know." When the client makes a concrete suggestion for a change plan, the therapist assists in its development if the plan
seems reasonable. We have found that clients often have a good sense of
what needs to be done. However, at times the plan may be problematic, or
the client may not know what to do to change the problem. In such cases,
the therapist asks permission to make suggestions and may offer a menu
of change strategies for the client to consider. The therapist's preferred
way of working with depression will be reflected by these suggestions. We
believe that it is most helpful if the therapy strategies that are employed
are conducted in the context of the MI spirit. However, as discussed
above, MI as a pretreatment has facilitated outcome even with more directive subsequent therapies. Nonetheless, even in this stage, waning of motivation and ambivalence may appear, and we believe that MI can be useful in addressing these problems as they arise.

A way of introducing this therapist input that we have found useful
is to say:

> "There are some ways of working on this problem that have been
> helpful for other people I've worked with who have had similar
> problems. Would you be interested in hearing about them?"

The therapist's relationship stance can vary within and across therapies, ranging from more directive[1] and authoritative at one end of the spectrum to more empathic and client-centered at the other. For example, the cognitive therapist can be more like an authoritative teacher in a psychoeducational enterprise or more client-centered and supportive. The psychoanalytic therapist can offer interpretations authoritatively or as tentative guesses for the client's consideration. The therapist style in the humanistic therapies is quite similar to the nondirective MI style because both were significantly influenced by the work of Carl Rogers (1951). However, methods from some humanistic therapies—for example, the two-chair approach originated by Perls, Hefferline, and Goodman (1951)—can be done either empathically and supportively or directively and authoritatively. For example, Hal Arkowitz was in a yearlong group with Fritz Perls, one of the founders of Gestalt therapy. In this group, Perls took the stance of "expert," who had ways of helping people to become aware of and to express feelings that had been suppressed or repressed. He was quite directive and authoritative in telling people what to do during the two-chair procedures, and he was not very supportive when people were dealing with painful emotions. By contrast, Leslie Greenberg uses the same two-chair procedure in a very empathic, supportive, and client-centered manner (Greenberg, Rice, & Elliott, 1993; Greenberg & Watson, 1998). Carl Rogers's client-centered therapy is always done in an empathic and supportive manner.

Even though people with high motivation and low resistance may respond well to a more directive style, we believe there are still advantages to carrying forward the MI spirit into the action stage. For one, ambivalence and motivation are not static—the client may reach a state of low ambivalence and high motivation at one point but regress at a later point. Continuing with the MI style ensures that these instances will be noted and that the therapist has the tools to work with them. Another advantage of continuing with the MI style pertains to maintenance of change after therapy. As Davison and Valins (1969) demonstrated, change that is attributed to internal sources (client's self and abilities) is more likely to endure than changes attributed to external sources (e.g., the therapist's expertise or a drug).

Consider how CBT might be conducted in an MI context. There are two major components of most cognitive-behavior therapies: (1) providing new experiences such as increasing activity levels or trying out new behaviors to test the accuracy of dysfunctional thoughts (e.g., "If I express my anger, my spouse will abandon me"); and (2) correcting overly negative thoughts and beliefs. New experiences (e.g., acting more assertively) may be discussed and even role-played during the session and then may be given as between-sessions homework assignments. Ideally, these assignments are developed collaboratively. However, the CBT therapist's attitude is often more didactic and authoritative. Even the phrase "homework assignments" conveys this attitude. CBT therapists also talk about "compliance" with homework assignments, again emphasizing the directive and completion-oriented characteristics of how these are used. The term "homework" is associated with a teacher giving assignments to students. The teacher is pleased when the student completes the assignment and displeased when the student does not.

Providing new experiences in between sessions can also be achieved in a more supportive and egalitarian manner in which the client is in charge and the therapist acts as consultant to the change plan. Arkowitz (2002) has suggested the use of the term "experiment" rather than "homework." Interestingly, in the seminal work of Beck, Rush, Shaw, and Emery (1979), the authors used the term "experiment" as well as "homework," but most subsequent cognitive-behavioral therapists have since employed the term "homework" for between-sessions activities. In using between-sessions experiments in an MI style, the therapist may raise the possibility that such experiences might be helpful and ask the client if they would like to hear more about this way of approaching their problem. If the client shows interest, the therapist might give some examples and then try to elicit from the client what specific activities they think might be helpful. The therapist may give input, but the client is in the driver's seat in this therapy. Then, if the client agrees that a particular activity might be worth trying (e.g., being more assertive with a significant other), the therapist and client agree that the client will try the experiment during the week. Arkowitz has described these experiments as discovery-oriented rather than completion- or validation-oriented. In presenting the experiment to the client, the therapist may say that the client's agreement to try the experiment is the experiment. All the rest are data that can be informative, no matter the outcome. If the client does not engage in the activity, this is an opportunity to learn about thoughts and feelings that came up when the client considered trying the activity, providing potentially valuable information to understand the obstacles to change. If he or she does complete the activity, the therapist and client also discuss what was learned from doing so. Contrast this to a completion-oriented homework assignment in which lack of completion is seen as a failure. Even when between-sessions activities in CBT are used to test hypotheses relating to dysfunctional beliefs that emerged in the session, the therapist can take a supportive rather than directive role in helping the client to implement them.

In one between-sessions experiment, a client with a writer's block agreed to try an experiment that involved sitting down at his desk for an hour a day in order to try to write. This "agreement to try" completed the experiment and, in effect, served as the independent variable. During the week, the client only sat down at his desk once, and even then he was still unable to write. However, his agreement to try led him to experience anxiety and to become more aware of the thoughts associated with his writer's block, which became useful to work with in subsequent therapy. With Charles, the client discussed above who feared expressing his thoughts and feelings to his wife, we agreed on an experiment in which he would try to tell his wife what he liked about the meals she prepared and what he did not like. He was mostly able to do this, and to his surprise (based on past experiences with his mother) she took it quite well and was actually pleased to hear him be more expressive. Thus, "experiments to try" can yield potentially useful data whether or not they are completed.

Another major component of CBT for depression is changing the negative thinking associated with depressed mood (Beck et al., 1979). In employing this approach in an MI context, the therapist asks if the client is interested in hearing about a strategy that has been useful with other depressed clients. If the client agrees, the therapist then proceeds to describe the procedures of identifying the thoughts most associated with depression, then examining evidence for and against these negative thoughts, and then revising the thoughts to fit the evidence. After this, the client is asked if he or she might want to try it to get an idea what it would be like. Beck's cognitive therapy actually employs a way of proceeding quite consistent with MI in emphasizing that the therapist only facilitates examination of the thoughts and evidence. Furthermore, unlike the procedure in other cognitive therapy approaches such as Ellis's rational emotive therapy (1994), Beck and colleagues' (1979) methodology does not align with the more positive-thinking approach, but rather takes a more Socratic role, allowing the client to examine the evidence and draw his or her own conclusions about whether the thought is overly negative or not. To emphasize self-efficacy, we often recommend the workbook *Mind over Mood* (Greenberger & Padesky, 1995), which encourages self-efficacy by taking the client through cognitive therapy step by step and providing a framework that makes it easy for clients to follow on their own.

If clients have significant reservations about cognitive therapy, they are encouraged to discuss them with the therapist. Client ambivalence can be examined and worked with, using the basic methods of MI. If clients persist in their objections to the cognitive approach, the client and therapist work to develop other ways to approach the depression.

Ambivalence about Antidepressant Medication

Various types of antidepressant medication have proven helpful for depression (Nemeroff & Schatzberg, 2002), with effects at the end of treatment generally equivalent to those found in psychotherapy. However, adherence rates to medication are very poor, with one large-scale study finding a discontinuation rate of 42% after 30 days and 72% after 90 days (Olfson et al., 2006). In addition, after treatment is terminated, the improvements from psychotherapy maintain better than those from medication (Hollon et al., 2005).

Nonetheless, there is a role for medication for some depressed clients, such as those who may resist seeking psychotherapy but who are willing to consider medication, those for whom psychotherapy is not available because of geographic or economic factors, and others who may be so depressed that they are unable to function in their work, family, and social environments.

When the therapist believes that medication may be helpful, the topic is introduced in MI style by asking if the client would like to hear about this possibility. If the client desires more information, the therapist can share his or her observations and knowledge about antidepressant medication, but more importantly the therapist should refer the client to sources of accurate information such as books or Internet sites or a consultation with a psychiatrist or family doctor. Good decisional balance work about whether or not to try antidepressants cannot be done without accurate information about the effects of these medications.

Length of Treatment

Most published work on MI has been relatively short-term. In fact, the *maximum* duration of treatment found in the meta-analysis by Burke, Arkowitz, and Menchola (2003) was only 4 sessions! Kopta, Howard, Lowry, and Beutler (1994) studied a wide range of outpatients receiving psychotherapy and found that, in 5 sessions, 50% showed improvement in acute distress (not necessarily remission), while longer durations of treatment yielded considerably better outcomes. For chronic distress, it took 14 sessions to reach the 50% improvement level, and 104 sessions to reach that level for characterological symptoms. Since depression often involves both chronic distress and a high prevalence of comorbid personality disorders (Shea, Widiger, & Klein, 1992), longer MI treatments may yield more powerful effects. Another rationale supporting longer treatments is that depression is not a homogeneous disorder, and there may be many problems to address at Levels 2 and 3 that cannot easily be dealt with effectively in short-term therapy.

PROBLEMS AND SUGGESTED SOLUTIONS IN USING MI WITH DEPRESSED CLIENTS

The three main problems we have encountered in using MI with depressed clients are multiple foci, shifting foci, and the perceptions of some clients that MI is not sufficiently action oriented.

Multiple Foci

At Level 1, there is often more than a single problem of depression. People with a diagnosis of depression are very likely to be diagnosed with other disorders as well. In fact, Kessler (1995) found that approximately 75% of clients with lifetime major depressive disorder met the criteria for at least one other DSM disorder, especially anxiety or substance use disorders. Fortunately, researchers have begun to address the treatment of clients with more than one diagnosis (e.g., Borkovec, Abel, & Newman, 1995; Daley, Sallhoum, Zuckoff, Kikrisci, & Thase, 1998).

The issue of multiple problems at Level 1 carries forward to Levels 2 (the issues underlying the major symptoms of distress) and 3 (working to change those issues) as well. In our use of MI, we ask the client which problem or problems they would find it most beneficial to focus on initially in the therapy. We approach this discussion in MI style, adding our input as appropriate and with the client's permission. Many times, what initially may seem like a plethora of diverse problems can be reduced to a few core problems at Level 2. For example, a client's problems with depression, generalized anxiety, and substance abuse at Level 1 may all be due to one or two core issues at Level 2, such as unresolved feelings about divorce or separation or the loss of significant sources of self-esteem, like a highly valued job. Identifying the core problems from the many that depressed clients initially present requires a longer course of therapy than the usual 12–16 sessions employed in most randomized controlled trials.

Our experience has been that working on the symptoms of depression is often the best place to start in people with multiple problems. As we discussed earlier in this chapter, depressed people generally show low levels of motivation to engage in the activities of life, and find efforts to change (at Level 3) difficult because of their ambivalence, fatigue, and/or pessimism. Once the symptoms of depression improve through either therapy or medication or both, the client is in a better position to tackle the underlying issues.

Shifting Foci over the Course of Treatment

Psychotherapy is a dynamic and emergent process. What seems to be a focus in the initial sessions can and often does shift over the course of subsequent sessions as the therapist gets to know the client better, as the client comes to understand his or her problems better, and as the client feels more comfortable disclosing things to the therapist that he or she fears the therapist will find unacceptable. In most cases, it is important for the therapist to be flexible and willing to follow the client as the foci change rather than being overly attached to the initial foci. Whenever the therapist thinks that the focus is shifting or changing entirely, it is important to mention this to the client and discuss what the appropriate focus should be at that point.

The case of Rachel illustrates this shifting of focus. Rachel, a 38-year-old nursing student, sought therapy (with Hal Arkowitz) for depression and anxiety. In the first few sessions, she attributed these problems to her procrastination in writing a major paper that was required for graduation from her nursing program. She felt overwhelmed by the task and was making little headway. She stated that she was questioning her career choice and not looking forward to a career in nursing. It appeared that the Level 1 focus was her depression and anxiety, and Level 2 involved her difficulties in writing and ambivalence about her career choice. We explored the pros and cons of a career in nursing and of her working on her paper, using decisional balance strategies. This, along with value–behavior discrepancies and increasing commitment change talk, led to some improvement in her depression and anxiety, and also to some progress on her paper. She decided that it was "silly" not to finish her degree, and that once she had the degree she could decide if she wanted to stay in the field or not. She realized that having the nursing degree would give her some financial security and that even if she decided to pursue other endeavors she could always earn some money through nursing.

In each of our first few sessions, Rachel alluded to sexual abuse that she had experienced as a teenager, saying that she thought it might help to talk about it, but was not sure if she could. A new focus had emerged. At Level 1, there was obviously still distress associated with memories of the abuse. At Level 2, the focus was the need to express and process some of the emotions relating to the abuse. However, it was clear she was not ready to do this. Over the course of the next four sessions, we examined her ambivalence about talking about the abuse. The "pros" of discussing the sexual abuse were "I'd probably feel better," "my sex life might improve," "I wouldn't feel so burdened by it," and "I know I should." The "cons" were "I don't want to make a bigger issue out of it than it is," "I don't want to dwell on it," "I'm afraid that I'll put a lot of effort into working out my feelings about the abuse, and my sex life still won't improve," and "maybe nothing will change if I do talk about it."

Over the course of these sessions, the balance began to tip toward her talking about the abuse, and during one session she began to talk about the events nervously and hesitantly. She continued to talk about the abuse over the next few sessions, each time showing more emotion as she did so. What had occurred was that when she was a young teenager and a virgin, she had met a considerably older man and fell in love with him. Unfortunately, he treated her poorly, used her for sex for 2 years, and then abandoned her. Rachel described how she thought that experience was still affecting her. She said that she was still angry and often used sex to get men to love her and to get power over them. Once she succeeded, however, she would lose interest in sex and in the man.

After several sessions of talking about the abuse, she reported that she did not feel as emotional about it as she had before. This session was in early December, just before the school winter break; after which Rachel went home to her family for a month. We met a few weeks after she returned. At that session, she reported that her depression had improved, and this was confirmed by her greatly improved scores on the Beck Depression Inventory. She also stated that she was feeling better about her relationship with her boyfriend and her feelings about sex. Finally, Rachel said that she was making slow but steady progress on her paper.

Client Perceptions That MI Is Not Sufficiently Action Oriented

There is no one therapy style or type that fits all clients. Some clients may do better with more active and directive approaches, while others may do better with more nondirective and client-centered approaches (Shoham-Salomon, Avner, & Neeman, 1989). Beutler and Harwood (2000) showed that when therapy was chosen to fit the person and problem, outcomes were better than if one approach was applied to all. So, it is quite possible that some clients respond best to an MI approach and others to more directive approaches.

Some depressed clients are highly passive (Miller & Seligman, 1975) and look for the therapist to direct them, whereas the MI therapist may be trying to elicit ideas for change from them in an MI style. This issue may be profitably explored via skilled reflective listening to identify the reasons for such passivity, which may in itself be a critical component of client progress. In addition, the therapist can actively provide advice and suggestions in the MI style without taking the change advocate position and thereby feeding into the passivity.

OBSERVATIONS ON TEACHING MI TO ADVANCED CLINICAL PSYCHOLOGY GRADUATE STUDENTS

One of us (Hal Arkowitz) has taught a year-long MI clinical practicum at the University of Arizona to advanced clinical psychology graduate students.[2] In addition to the usual graduate seminars, they had all completed at least 1 year of supervised clinical experience emphasizing CBT.

Most of the first semester was devoted to training and demonstrations, and the second to seeing clients under supervision. Each student saw 1–2 clients for a maximum of 10 sessions, limited largely by the length of the semester. In the three times I taught the practicum, the students and I saw a total of 26 clients. These clients had a range of presenting problems, including depression, anxiety disorders, procrastination, and relationship problems. For many, depression was the primary problem, while for others it was a secondary problem, and still others had problems that did not involve depression. Clients were given a short battery of self-report tests before and after treatment that included the Beck Depression Inventory. Results for all clients with primary or secondary depression will be discussed in the research section.

At the first class, I typically surveyed what the reasons were for the students' interest in MI, and although they used different words, one theme voiced by the majority was that, while they found their CBT training valuable, they were drawn to the *values* implicit in MI, or what we call the "MI spirit." They were clearly very enthusiastic and open to learning during the first semester of training.

By the end of the first semester, the students had received 45 hours of MI training, which included fairly extensive readings on MI, numerous role-playing exercises, and demonstrations of MI from training tapes prepared by Miller and Rollnick. In addition, the instructor saw a client and showed tapes of these sessions. We spent considerable time on interviewing based on open-ended questions and reflections. While the students needed to learn to shift therapy styles from a more directive one to MI, typically they learned this new style well and found it useful.

A frequent question that arose was how much clients could be helped by an approach that was not as directive or technique-driven as CBT. My chief response was to suggest: "Let's see how helpful it is in our work with clients next semester." So, throughout the first semester, many of the students discussed their (pardon the expression) ambivalence. On the one hand, they had read the outcome literature on MI and were impressed as well as drawn to the MI spirit. On the other hand, their previous training in CBT had emphasized the efficacy of more directive types of therapy, and they struggled to reconcile these two perspectives. Several mentioned that they had felt somewhat lost when clients were not cooperating with the CBT, and they thought that MI might have been helpful in such instances.

For most students, the first few sessions of therapy of doing MI with real clients were difficult despite their extensive training. The concern most often expressed was that they felt like they were not "doing" enough to help the client. Despite their interest in MI, it seemed that, without taking a more directive stance, they felt like they were not "doing their job." Once again, I counseled patience and a "let's see" attitude.

The majority of cases showed at least some degree of positive change, and, as the instructor, it was a pleasure to see the students' surprise and delight that their clients were showing improvements without the therapist taking a directive stance. I believe that one of the things that the students learned through their clinical experiences was the power of the therapeutic relationship in psychotherapy. In addition, we explored using active techniques like CBT, but delivered in the MI style, which some saw as a combination of the best of both approaches.

Given the strong emphasis in most clinical psychology graduate programs on CBT, I think that teaching MI in such programs will often encounter initial interest and then a subsequent feeling of "not doing anything." The best antidote for this feeling was the positive results that many saw in their cases. The practicum has been extremely well received by students and received very high ratings. I believe that they learned that MI and other therapies are not incompatible and that combining MI with other therapies, as we have described above, might be a very effective treatment indeed.

RESEARCH

As yet, there are no controlled studies of the efficacy of MI with depression. In this section, we will briefly review research that indirectly bears on this issue.

In the MI practicum described above, 17 of the 26 cases scored in the depressed range of the BDI at pretreatment, with scores ranging from 12 to 27. For some of these clients, depression was the primary problem, and for others it was secondary. Five clients terminated before the 10 sessions, three of whom were depressed. For some, this may have been due to the fact that they started therapy just before the lengthy winter break and may not have formed a sufficient alliance to return after it. Fourteen clients who scored in the depressed range on the BDI completed treatment. Of these, 11 no longer scored in the depressed range after treatment. Many also reported behavior changes in related areas.

This practicum data should best be considered a series of case studies rather than a single group design, since the way in which we used MI evolved over the course of the practicum, with later ones putting greater emphasis on integrating CBT and other therapies into work in the action stage, as described in this chapter. Nonetheless, the results of these cases tentatively suggest that MI has potential utility with populations of depressed people.

Some studies have examined the effect of an initial MI-style session for depressed clients on treatment seeking and adherence in subsequent non-MI treatments. For example, Swartz and colleagues (2006) evaluated a single-group intervention consisting of an engagement session that incorporated MI, followed by eight sessions of interpersonal therapy for depressed mothers of psychiatrically ill children. These mothers were originally not seeking treatment for themselves, although they did need it. Thirteen of these mothers who met the criteria for major depressive disorder and were not in treatment received an engagement session, following which they were offered brief interpersonal therapy for depression. The engagement session is described by Zuckoff, Swartz, and Grote (Chapter 5, this volume) and consists of MI along with methods to help the interviewer understand people from another culture without bias. All who participated in the engagement session attended at least one psychotherapy session, and the majority completed the full eight-session course of therapy.

In a randomized pilot study (Grote et al., in press), subjects were depressed economically disadvantaged pregnant women who were not initially seeking treatment. Some were assigned to a condition where they received an engagement session followed by eight sessions of interpersonal therapy (IPT) or a referral for standard depression treatment by a therapist in the community. Some 71% of the engagement session–IPT subjects completed a full course of IPT, while only 25% of the treatment-as-usual subjects attended an initial therapy session. None of the latter completed a course of therapy. These are very encouraging results that warrant further controlled studies.

In a different variation of the use of MI in affecting treatment adherence, Daley, Salloum, Zuckoff, Kikrisci, and Thase (1998) studied inpatients with depression and comorbid cocaine dependence. Upon discharge, subjects were randomly assigned to either an outpatient MI-based motivational therapy or outpatient treatment as usual. Those who received the motivational intervention were more likely to complete 90 days of outpatient treatment, attend more treatment sessions, report continuous sobriety, and were rehospitalized less often than the subjects who received treatment as usual. Subjects in the motivational group showed large reductions in Beck Depression Inventory scores at the end of the first 30 days of outpatient treatment.

Another piece of indirect support for the integrative approach described here comes from the COMBINE study (Anton et al., 2006). The Combined Behavioral Intervention was an integrative treatment that has similarities to what we have described in this chapter (see Miller, 2004, for details of this treatment). It integrated aspects of CBT, 12-step treatment, MI, and support system involvement, and yielded positive outcomes for alcoholism.

Research on Rogers's client-centered therapy for depression also bears indirectly on the efficacy of MI for depression. In many respects, client-centered therapy is the foundation of MI. The "MI spirit" is almost identical to the therapeutic attitudes described by Rogers as critical to therapy (Rogers, 1951), as was noted earlier.

MI differs from client-centered therapy in its explicit focus on increasing intrinsic motivation and resolving ambivalence. However, because of the considerable overlap, research on client-centered therapy for depression is of some relevance to the efficacy of MI for depression. Elliot and colleagues (2004) reviewed the literature on the efficacy of experiential therapies. Their review included five studies evaluating client-centered therapy for depression, wherein pre–post effect sizes averaged 1.40, with a range of 0.85–2.26. Because the effect sizes were pre–post and computed without data from a control group, they are higher than they would have been using a control group. Nonetheless, they are substantial and compare favorably to such effect sizes found in studies of other therapies for depression.

Greenberg and his associates have conducted two studies (Goldman et al., 2006; Greenberg & Watson, 1998) comparing client-centered therapy and an emotion-focused therapy (EFT) for major depression. EFT consisted of integrating client-centered therapy with emotion-focused experiential and Gestalt techniques to resolve affective–cognitive problems. Both studies supported the efficacy of client-centered therapy for depression. Interestingly, Goldman and colleagues (2006) found that EFT did significantly better than CCT on measures of depression, general distress, and interpersonal functioning.

The results of the studies reviewed above tentatively suggest that MI might be efficacious for depression. However, we clearly need well-controlled studies directly testing the efficacy of MI for depression before any conclusions can be drawn. Two types of studies that would be valuable in this regard involve the evaluation of MI as a pretreatment for CBT or other therapies as well as the evaluation of MI as an integrative framework throughout therapy, as described in this chapter. In addition, the results of the studies reviewed above also suggest that it would be useful to compare MI to CCT to determine if in fact the specific MI components add to the effectiveness of the CCT on which MI is based. They also raise questions about whether a greater emotional focus might enhance the efficacy of MI. Hopefully, researchers will begin to study various questions relating to MI and depression in the near future.

CONCLUSIONS

Our focus has been on the use of MI as an integrative framework into which other therapies can be incorporated for the treatment of depression. Although we have made only brief reference to the use of MI as a pretreatment to other therapies, we believe that this is a particularly promising direction for research and practice. We hope that the future will see clinical and research experimentation into MI with a variety of uses for depression including as a pretreatment and as an integrative framework for psychotherapy.

NOTES

1. By a directive stance, we refer to one in which the therapist is seen as the expert, often introducing new information and therapeutic strategies and "leading the way." This differs from the directive aspect of MI, which refers to the fact that the therapist has specific goals for the client (increasing intrinsic motivation and decreasing ambivalence) while not taking the role of change advocate or expert.
2. Copies of the syllabus for the MI practicum are available from Hal Arkowitz.

REFERENCES

Amrhein, P. C., Miller, W. R., Yahne, C. E., Palmer, M., & Fulcher, L. (2003). Client commitment language during motivational interviewing predicts drug use outcome. *Journal of Consulting and Clinical Psychology, 71*, 862–878.

American Psychiatric Association. (2000). *Diagnostic and statistical manual of mental disorders* (4th ed., text rev.). Washington, DC: Author.

Anton, R. F., O'Malley, S. S., Ciraulo, D. A., Cisler, R. A., Couper, D., Donovan, D. M., et al. (2006). Combined pharmacotherapies and behavioral interventions for alcohol dependence. The COMBINE study: A randomized controlled trial. *Journal of the American Medical Association, 295*, 2003–2017.

Arkowitz, H. (2002). An integrative approach to psychotherapy based on common processes of change. In F. Kaslow (Ed.) & J. Lebow (Vol. Ed.), *Comprehensive handbook of psychotherapy: Vol. 4, Integrative and eclectic therapies* (pp. 317–337). New York: Wiley.

Arkowitz, H., & Westra, H. (2004). Integrating motivational interviewing and cognitive behavioral therapy in the treatment of depression and anxiety. *Journal of Cognitive Psychotherapy, 18*, 337–350.

Barrett, B., Byford, S., & Knapp, M. (2005). Evidence of cost-effective treatments for depression: A systematic review. *Journal of Affective Disorders, 84*, 1–13.

Beck, A. T., Rush, A. J., Shaw, B. F., & Emery, G. (1979). *Cognitive therapy of depression.* New York: Guilford Press.

Beutler, L. E., & Harwood, M. T. (2000). *Prescriptive psychotherapy: A practical guide to systematic treatment selection.* New York: Oxford University Press.

Beutler, L. E. , Moleiro, C., Malik, M., & Harwood, T. M. (2000, June). *The UC Santa Barbara study of fitting patients to therapists: First results.* Paper presented at the annual meeting of the Society for Psychotherapy Research, Chicago.

Bohart, A. C., Elliot, R., Greenberg, L. S., & Watson, J. C. (2002). Empathy. In J. C.

Norcross (Ed.), *Psychotherapy relationships that work* (pp. 89–108). New York: Oxford University Press.

Borkovec, T. D., Abel, J. L., & Newman, H. (1995). Effects of psychotherapy on comorbid conditions in generalized anxiety disorder. *Journal of Consulting and Clinical Psychology, 63,* 479–483.

Burke, B., Arkowitz, H., & Menchola, M. (2003). The efficacy of motivational interviewing: A meta-analysis of controlled clinical trials. *Journal of Consulting and Clinical Psychology, 71,* 843–861.

Burns, D. D., & Nolen-Hoeksema, S. (1991). Coping styles, homework compliance, and the effectiveness of cognitive-behavioral therapy. *Journal of Consulting and Clinical Psychology, 59,* 305–311.

Burns, D., & Nolen-Hoeksma, S. (1992). Therapeutic empathy and recovery from depression: A structural equation model. *Journal of Consulting and Clinical Psychology, 92,* 441–449.

Burns, D. D., & Spangler, D. L. (2002). Does psychotherapy homework lead to improvements in depression in cognitive-behavioral therapy or does improvement lead to increased homework compliance? *Journal of Consulting and Clinical Psychology, 68,* 46–56.

Clark, D. C., & Fawcett, J. (1992). Review of empirical risk factors for evaluation of the suicidal patient. In B. M. Bongar (Ed.), *Suicide: Guidelines for assessment, management, and treatment* (pp. 16–48). London: Oxford University Press.

Connors, G. J., Walitzer, K. S., & Dermen, K. H. (2002). Preparing clients for alcoholism treatment: Effects on treatment participation and outcomes. *Journal of Consulting and Clinical Psychology, 70,* 1161–1169.

Craighead, W. E., Hart, A. S., Craighead, L. W., & Ilardi, S. S. (2002). Psychosocial treatments for major depressive disorder. In P. E. Nathan & J. M. Gorman (Eds.), *A guide to treatments that work* (2nd ed., pp. 245–262). New York: Oxford University Press.

Daley, D. C., Sallhoum, I. M., Zuckoff, A., Kikrisci, L., & Thase, M. E. (1998). Increasing treatment adherence among outpatients with depression and cocaine dependence: A pilot study. *American Journal of Psychiatry, 155,* 1611–1613.

Davison, G. C., & Valins, S. (1969). Maintenance of self-attributed and drug-attributed behavior change. *Journal of Personality and Social Psychology, 11,* 25–33.

Elliott, R., Greenberg, L. S., & Lietaer, G. (2004). Research on experiential psychotherapies. In C. R. Snyder & R. E. Ingram (Eds.), *Handbook of psychological change: Psychotherapy processes and practices for the 21st century* (pp. 493–539). New York: Wiley.

Ellis, A. (1994). *Reason and emotion in psychotherapy* (2nd ed.). New York: Birch Lane Press.

Engle, D. E., & Arkowitz, H. (2006). *Ambivalence in psychotherapy: Facilitating readiness to change.* New York: Guilford Press.

Goldman, R. N., Greenberg, L. S., & Angus, L. (2006). The effects of adding emotion-focused interventions to the client-centered relationship conditions in the treatment of depression. *Psychotherapy Research, 16,* 536–546.

Greenberg, L. S., Rice, L. N., & Elliott, R. (1993). *Facilitating emotional change: The moment-by-moment process.* New York: Guilford Press.

Greenberg, L. S., & Watson, J. C. (1998). Experiential therapy of depression: Differential effects of client centered relationship conditions and process experiential interventions. *Psychotherapy Research, 8,* 210–214.

Greenberger, D., & Padesky, C. A. (1995). *Mind over mood: Change how you feel by changing the way you think.* New York: Guilford Press.

Grote, N. K., Zuckoff, A., Swartz, H. A., Bledsoe, S. E., & Geibel, S. L. (in press). Engaging women who are depressed and economically disadvantaged in mental health treatment. *Social Work.*

Hettema, J., Steele, J., & Miller, W. R. (2005). Motivational interviewing. *Annual Review of Clinical Psychology, 1,* 91–111.

Hollon, S. D., DeRubeis, R. J., Shelton, R. C., Amsterdam, J. D., Salomon, R. M., O'Reardon, J. P., et al. (2005). Prevention of relapse following cognitive therapy vs. medications in moderate to severe depression. *Archives of General Psychiatry, 62,* 417–422.

Kessler, R. C. (2002). Epidemiology of depression. In I. H. Gotlib & C. L. Hammen (Eds.), *Handbook of depression* (pp. 23–42). New York: Guilford Press.

Kessler, R. C. (1995). The epidemiology of psychiatric comorbidity. In M. T. Tsaung, M. Tohen, & G. E. P. Zahner, (Eds.), *Textbook in psychiatric epidemiology* (pp. 179–197). New York: Wiley.

Kopta, S. M., Howard, K. I., Lowry, J. L., & Beutler, L. E. (1994). Patterns of symptomatic recovery in psychotherapy. *Journal of Consulting and Clinical Psychology, 62,* 1009–1016.

Lambert, M., & Barley, D. E. (2002). Research summary on the therapeutic relationship and psychotherapy. In J. Norcross (Ed.), *Psychotherapy relationships that work* (pp. 17–36). New York: Oxford University Press.

Leichsenring, F., Rabung, S., & Leibling, E. (2004). The efficacy of short-term psychodynamic psychotherapy in specific psychiatric disorders: A meta-analysis. *Archives of General Psychiatry, 61,* 1208–1215.

Lewinsohn, P. M. (1974). A behavioral approach to depression. In R. J. Friedman & M. Katz (Eds.), *The psychology of depression: Contemporary theory and research* (pp. 157–178). New York: Wiley.

Lewinsohn, P. M., Hoberman, H. M., & Rosenbaum, M. (1988). A prospective study of risk factors for unipolar depression. *Journal of Abnormal Psychology, 97,* 251–264.

McGrath, P. J., Stewart, J. W., Fava, M., Trivedi, M. H., Wisniewski, S. R., Nierenberg, A. A., et al. (2006). Tranylcypromine versus venlafaxine plus pirtazapine following three failed antidepressant medication trials for depression: A STAR*D report. *American Journal of Psychiatry, 163,* 1531–1541.

Miller, W. R. (1983). Motivational interviewing with problem drinkers. *Behavioural Psychotherapy, 11,* 147–172.

Miller, W. R. (Ed.). (2004). *Combined behavioral intervention manual: A clinical research guide for therapists treating people with alcohol abuse and dependence* (COMBINE Monograph Series, Vol. 1; DHHS No. 04-5288). Bethesda, MD: National Institute on Alcohol Abuse and Alcoholism.

Miller, W. R., Benefield, R. G., & Tonigan, J. S. (1993). Enhancing motivation for change in problem drinking: A controlled comparison of two therapist styles. *Journal of Consulting and Clinical Psychology, 61,* 455–461.

Miller, W. R., & Rollnick, S. (2002). *Motivational interviewing: Preparing people to change* (2nd ed.). New York: Guilford Press.

Miller, W. R., & Seligman, M. E. (1995). Depression and learned helplessness in man. *Journal of Abnormal Psychology, 84,* 228–238.

Moyers, T. B., Miller, W. R., & Hendrickson, S. R. (2005). How does motivational interviewing work?: Therapist interpersonal skill predicts client involvement within motivational interviewing sessions. *Journal of Consulting and Clinical Psychology, 73,* 590–598.

Nemeroff, C. B., & Schatzberg, A. R. (2002). Pharmacological treatments for unipolar depression. In P. E. Nathan & J. M. Gorman (Eds.), *A guide to treatments that work* (2nd ed., pp. 229–244). New York: Oxford University Press.

Olfson, M., Marcus, S. C., Tedeschi, M., & Wan, G. J. (2006). Continuity of antidepressant treatment for adults with depression in the United States. *American Journal of Psychiatry, 163,* 101–108.

Pasquini, M., Picardi, A., Biondi, M., Gaetano, P., & Morisini, P. (2004). Relevance of anger and irritability in outpatients with major depressive disorder. *Psychopathology, 3,* 155–160.

Patterson, G., & Chamberlain, P. (1994). A functional analysis of resistance during parent training. *Clinical Psychology: Research and Practice, 1,* 53–70.

Perls, F., Hefferline, R., & Goodman, P. (1951). *Gestalt therapy.* New York: Julian Press.

Project MATCH Research Group. (1997). Matching alcoholism treatments to client heterogeneity: Project MATCH post-treatment drinking outcomes. *Journal of Studies on Alcohol, 58,* 7–29.

Project MATCH Research Group. (1998). Matching alcoholism treatments to client heterogeneity: Project MATCH three-year drinking outcomes. *Alcoholism: Clinical and Experimental Research, 23,* 1300–1311.

Rogers, C. R. (1951). *Client-centered therapy.* Boston: Houghton Mifflin.

Shea, T. M., Widiger, T. A., & Klein, M. H. ((1992). Comorbidity of personality disorders and depression: Implications for treatment. *Journal of Consulting and Clinical Psychology, 60,* 857–868.

Shoham-Salomon, V., Avner, R., & Neeman, R. (1989). You're changed if you do and changed if you don't: Mechanisms underlying paradoxical interventions. *Journal of Consulting and Clinical Psychology, 57,* 590–598.

Swartz, H. A., Zuckoff, A., Frank, E., Spielvogle, H. N., Shear, M. K., Fleming, M. A. D., et al. (2006). An open-label trial of enhanced brief interpersonal psychotherapy in depressed mothers whose children are receiving psychiatric treatment. *Depression and Anxiety, 23,* 398–404.

Wachtel, P. L. (1997). *Psychoanalysis, behavior therapy, and the relational world.* Washington, DC: American Psychological Association.

Weissman, M. M., Markowitz, J. C., & Klerman, G. L. (2000). *Comprehensive guide to interpersonal psychotherapy.* New York: Basic Books.

Westen, D., & Morrison, K. (2001). A multidimensional meta-analysis of treatments for depression, panic, and generalized anxiety disorder: An empirical examination of the status of empirically supported therapies. *Journal of Consulting and Clinical Psychology, 69*(6), 875–899.

CHAPTER 7

Motivational Interviewing and Suicidality

Harry Zerler

Suicidality, related acts of deliberate self-harm, and suicide itself (see "Definitions," below) are among the most challenging subjects
for researchers and clinicians. The associated legal and ethical obligations of caregivers to act to attempt to maintain the safety of those at
risk of harm usually lead to highly structured assessments, and linkages
to further care. The insight, judgment, and emotional stability of suicidal clients are typically assumed to be so inadequate as to justify im-
position of intervention not only with minimal regard for the client's
free choice but also, if necessary, on an involuntary and legally mandatory basis. These constricted circumstances paradoxically present an excellent opportunity for the application of motivational interviewing
(MI) because of the significant value of MI in promoting autonomy, enhancing the therapeutic alliance, and examining ambivalence.

Like start-of-life issues (e.g., contraception, abortion, genetic manipulation) or end-of-life issues (e.g., euthanasia, assisted dying, or cap-
ital punishment), suicide evokes a range of controversy and argument
that often appears to overshadow efforts to find simple, effective ways to
help people in need or at risk while also upholding important community values. Readers who may be less familiar or experienced with the
care of suicidal clients are encouraged to explore the references and resources identified below with a special awareness that there are many

important conceptual, methodological, and ethical problems that impact empirical research and clinical study of this complex topic.

Suicidality and related acts of deliberate self-harm are best understood as existing along a continuum and as occurring within a process rather than as isolated events or transient behaviors. As a caregiver, your interaction with a client is part of that process, whether before, during, or after an "instance" of suicidality. In many encounters, caregivers seek specifically to screen out suicidal clients as a matter of risk management. Suicidal clients are often referred to designated mental health "screening centers" or "crisis counseling" services for specialized evaluation and linkage to further care. Your skill and sensitivity in managing those referrals may strengthen the therapeutic alliance and help to support such clients in coping positively with their next phase of care or, conversely, may destroy the therapeutic alliance and exacerbate the problems of the next phase of care. Your knowledge of that client will be an important resource for your colleagues who provide specialized screening and crisis counseling services. Your continuing *relationship* with that client can be an important consideration in establishing an appropriate plan for further care after crisis evaluation. You are likely to see that client again.

"So ubiquitous is the impulse to commit suicide that one of every two Americans has at some time considered, threatened or actually attempted suicide" (Lester, 1997). Acute or chronic suicidality or related acts of deliberate self-harm often "fly beneath the radar" and evade detection until or unless an "unanticipated" incident exposes the client to "crisis" management. Clients may frequently veil or distort information that could trigger detection. Viewed retrospectively, in the light of adequate information, many cases appear not only unsurprising but possibly predictable and preventable. Listening for change talk can be challenging in encounters with clients "in crisis." The drama of potential or actual suicidality, in the context of chronic illness, family conflict, or sudden destabilizing events, often includes many layers of information and communication that may obscure the client's actual desire, ability, reason, or need to engage in self-harm, or alternatively, to maintain safety. Exploring ambivalence, in the respectful and supportive spirit of MI, is a key to discerning appropriate further steps in the client's care while simultaneously supporting a therapeutic alliance and respecting the client's autonomy or, at a minimum, the right to receive treatment in the least restrictive setting possible. This chapter will describe the use of MI in crisis evaluation of clients who have just attempted suicide or who are believed to be threatening or contemplating suicide, or otherwise believed to be acutely at risk of suicide.

DEFINITIONS

"Deliberate self-harm" is "an acute non-fatal act of self harm carried out deliberately in the form of an acute episode of behavior by an individual with variable motivation. Other terms used to describe this phenomenon are 'attempted suicide' and 'parasuicide' " (Gelder, Mayou, & Cowen, 2001). For the purpose of this chapter, the term "deliberate self-harm" will be used throughout.

"Suicide" is defined as "an act with a fatal outcome that is deliberately initiated and performed by the person with the knowledge or expectation of its fatal outcome" (Gelder et al., 2001).

"Suicidality" is a condition that may be acute or chronic in which a person gives prominent consideration to whether they want, intend, or choose to live or want, intend, or choose to die; suicidality is characterized by an ambivalence that is influenced by many dynamic interpersonal and intrapersonal factors. Suicidality, as a cognitive or emotional state, can occur with or without deliberate self-harm or other acts of suicide.

THE CLINICAL POPULATION
AND USUAL TREATMENTS

The overall suicide rate in the United States is 10.9 per 100,000 persons annually, ranking as the 11th leading cause of death overall, but is the 3rd leading cause of death among young adults (ages 15–24). Suicide causes the premature death of more than 30,000 people a year in the United States. Age-specific rates of suicide have consistently been highest in the elderly (ages 65+), although the rate of suicide among adolescents and young adults has tripled since 1955 (American Association of Suicidology, 2004). Although 80% of persons who commit suicide are men, the majority of those who make nonfatal suicide attempts are women between 25 and 44 years of age. It is estimated that there are an average of 50–100 suicide attempts for every completed suicide, and the actual numbers are assertedly much higher than the officially documented ones, because many suicide attempts are never reported and many completed suicides are misrepresented as fatalities attributable to other causes.

Suicidality is a symptom or complex feature of other disorders, not a disorder in itself. Thorough assessment and optimal case management require comprehensive information gathering and integration with age-appropriate and culturally sensitive risk management models (American Psychiatric Association, 2003; Risk Management Foundation of the Harvard Medical Institutions, 1996, 2000). The MI approach in working with these clients may be seen as contrasting with the often overtly coercive processes initiated in response to the disclosure, discovery, or suspicion of suicidal ideation or behavior that constitute the "usual treatments" in the United States. These "usual-treatment" interventions often are triggered by requirements of compliance with clinical or institutional liability protocols, and also may be in compliance with statutory requirements in state law for mental health screening, evaluation, and care for those who appear to be imminently a danger to self or others. These requirements vary considerably in different jurisdictions, but they generally provide, at a minimum, for mandatory (that is, involuntary, if necessary) assessment by a designated mental health professional, usually in a hospital emergency department setting. Assessment and treatment are largely predicated on the identification of known *risk factors*—circumstances that are associated with an increased probability of self-harm—and also on the identification of known *safety factors*, which are associated with a decreased probability of self-harm.

The outcome of such assessment will generally determine referral and linkage to appropriate care and may vary widely, from declining referral for any further services, to accepting voluntary referral for further outpatient or inpatient mental health care, to being subjected to involuntary civil commitment for inpatient mental health care. Further treatments for suicidality or suicidal acts or deliberate self-harm may be situated within any of the many orientations of psychotherapy or combinations thereof. Typical interventions combine pharmacotherapy (e.g., antidepressant, anxiolytic, or mood-stabilizing agents), educational and recreational group therapy, and close observation (often as a component of a "patient safety plan" or "contract for safety"[1]). The combination of pharmacotherapy with structured activities in a controlled environment (i.e., inpatient mental health unit) monitored for safety is commonly called *milieu* therapy. Unless caregivers are persuaded of the client's relative ability to maintain safety, the indicated level of care of a client who is contemplating or has committed a serious act of deliberate self-harm will usually be an inpatient mental health setting or "acute partial hospitalization" (typically a daily part-day outpatient program). In the United States, these choices are also subject to the influence of managed-care gatekeepers, who control the healthcare benefits of many clients.

It is important to recognize that the evaluation and management of suicidal clients frequently occurs in an atmosphere of high anxiety: for the client, their family, significant others, their attending caregivers, and for others who may be involved, including teachers, employers, or police. If you first *attend to your client* and then respond also to the system, the protocols, the family, colleagues, and collaterals, you increase the probability of optimal outcomes. If a caregiver gets caught up in his or her own emotional responses, or those of the client's family or significant others, one may end up treating primarily the anxieties of these others and not the client.

RATIONALE FOR USING MI
WITH SUICIDAL CLIENTS

In caring for suicidal clients the use of MI promotes greater *autonomy* in the context of what may likely be limited choices for further treatment. Moreover, the benefits of using MI in this population may also be seen in the development of an enhanced therapeutic *alliance*. With the positive alignment of autonomy and alliance, clients may further benefit from actively identifying and adopting alternatives to passive compliance or to noncompliance, both of which are common problems in the usual clinical management and treatment of suicidality. Finally, the presence of marked and often complex *ambivalence* in this population offers ample potential for developing discrepancy to help promote readiness for life-affirming change.

MI can be particularly valuable for the importance it places on supporting and preserving client autonomy. As a counterbalance to the tendency of treatment systems to infantilize such clients, to limit their treatment choices to "voluntary" acceptance of or involuntary commitment to imposed psychiatric care, an MI stance in crisis evaluation seeks to recognize and nourish the client's innate capacity to make "good choices" to deal with "bad feelings." It is proposed that recognizing that capacity, however limited, in the client's own schema of their illness and needs may have a potentially critical positive influence on the course of care and on outcome. Because the client must ultimately survive by his or her own agency, adopting a posture that preserves and nourishes self-efficacy may be more prudent and potentially more effective than a stance that presumes the client is helpless in the face of imminent harm and assumes the role of rescuer; *the more that safety is imposed from without, the less there may be from within.* Moreover, encouraging and supporting the client in making his or her own appropriate choices may have associated benefits of increasing positive expectations, which seems especially critical in working with suicidal clients who identify themselves as hopeless and helpless.

Clinicians may be understandably concerned about adopting such a posture of equipoise. If the client commits an act of self-harm or actually completes suicide, will the clinician be considered responsible or held liable? Does simplified risk management (e.g., "just commit them, and sort the rest out later") impinge on the client's right to receive appropriate care in the least restrictive setting possible? If one chooses the often easier and apparently "safer" route of imposing involuntary psychiatric care in a controlled environment as a response to mitigate any level of risk, what are the consequences for the client? Will the client lose any slender vestige of self-efficacy and autonomy? What will be the impact on the therapeutic alliance with the client going forward? "Suicide and suicidal behaviors are statistically rare, even in populations at risk. For example, even though suicidal ideation and attempts are associated with increased suicidal risk, most individuals with suicidal thoughts or attempts will never die by suicide" (American Psychiatric Association, 2003). There are certainly cases in which the weight of risk factors and the limitations of a reasonable patient safety plan cannot support any other choice than hospitalization, and if the client will not accept a voluntary referral then involuntary commitment is a necessity. However, cases requiring hospitalization account for approximately only one-third of those I evaluate annually for suicidality, and in those cases the application of MI appears to minimize the rate of involuntary commitment. Expedient referrals for voluntary or involuntary hospitalization certainly shift the burdens of risk management and take less time than careful comprehensive assessments that allow and encourage the client to recognize resources and make choices, but they may undermine the further progress of the client. Clients may readily agree with proffered "safety" plans and agree to enter additional levels of further care, but these explicit choices may be processed with more or less recognition by a client (or caregivers) of the underlying, implicit, and ongoing complex ambivalence of the suicidal client. A common consequence is that inadequate attention to ambivalence may lead to limited progress in treatment beyond passive compliance and may contribute to a quick reversal, culminating in renewed attempts and success in self-harm. Many who successfully completed suicide had recently been discharged from an inpatient mental health unit. In the absence of adequate research, the implications of this association remain perplexing. Some think that these outwardly calm and cooperative clients, while compliant with their *milieu* therapy and seemingly well enough to leave a controlled environment, have during the course of their stay unfavorably resolved their ambivalence about life and death and then promptly take advantage of their newfound emotional peace and restored energy to effectively complete suicide. Wouldn't it be prudent to make effective exploration of ambivalence a focus not only of crisis assessment but also, on an ongoing basis, of inpatient treatment, discharge planning, and further care?

MI provides the clinician with an empathic but socially neutral relationship to ethically approach many types of ambivalence that constitute key existential dimensions of suicidality. Rather than solely adopting a clinical posture based exclusively on the medico-legal and prevailing sociopolitical assumptions that the client "must live" or "must not die," the MI stance recognizes that these are not necessarily "givens" from the perspective of the suicidal client, regardless of how important these assumptions may be to others or how much coercion may be brought to bear on the client. MI provides both an effective technique and the optimal spirit for reconciling many dilemmas attendant to the care of suicidal clients.

CLINICAL APPLICATION OF MI
WITH SUICIDAL CLIENTS

This application of MI is functionally integrated with crisis evaluation, which, in effect, allows crisis evaluation to also comprise brief therapy. This integrated approach also specifically looks forward, and is a prelude, to the subsequent care to which each suicidal client must be effectively linked. The objects of the use of MI in this context are to minimize coercion, to promote autonomy, and to promote self-efficacy. The measurable goal of the intervention is to promote change, specifically from a state of ambivalence or uncertainty to a state of reasonable readiness to maintain a patient safety plan. The near-term measurable outcome is the client's not taking any action to harm him- or herself or others in any way. Other measurable immediate outcomes include realizing the client's cooperation in facilitating the interview, gaining cooperation with medical clearance procedures and compliance with medication, optimizing the client's participation in and agreement to immediate and longer-term treatment planning, accomplishing the linkage of the client to further care in the least restrictive setting possible, and securing the client's agreement to and adherence with interventions arranged for the client's continuing care as part of the patient safety plan.

There are two related and significant modifications of MI in this application. The first is that, irrespective of the client's priorities, the encounter must necessarily touch all the key areas of a structured comprehensive risk and safety assessment, and consequently the therapist will ask many more direct questions, steer the dialogue, and occupy considerably more talk time than one would do otherwise in an MI session. The second is that the selective focus and the ultimate disposition of the session may be unavoidably coercive, in keeping with fundamental ethical and legal obligations of the caregiver to protect the safety of the client and the community. As in other applications of MI, the less coercive the circumstances, the less likely that "resistance" may be engendered or encountered. It is not uncommon in crisis evaluation to encounter suicidal clients who are either decidedly uncooperative toward their care or entirely passive or apathetic. Given these constraints, there is a corresponding need to evince superadherence to the *spirit* of MI, that is, to express and demonstrate genuine empathy, to listen and attend to what is said and not said, to be authentic and honest in a gentle and nonthreatening manner, and to discern, respect, reflect, affirm, and support every glimmer of positive energy. Regardless of how "cooperative" the client appears to be, there can be great divergence between the client's agenda and the necessities of competently assuring safety and further care—all the more reason and opportunity to put into practice the applicable principles of MI. In practice, there is ample room and compatibility for the integration of MI, with modifications, in the crisis management of suicidal clients.

This integrated process may be summarized as including each of the following elements in a dynamic mix that shifts emphasis in response to the unfolding presentation of the client:

Promote effective autonomy: *Collaboration—roll with resistance.*
Promote effective alliance: *Honesty–empathy–authenticity.*
Examine ambivalence: *Evocation—explore discrepancy.*
Support self-efficacy: *Reflect change talk.*

I emphasize courtesy, sensitivity, and asking permission at all times in the encounter. I put special effort into listening, reflection, and expressing genuine empathy, because that facilitates my relationship with the person for whom I'm caring, and in many cases that alone—establishing a meaningful sense that someone hears them, listens, and cares—is enough to enable clients to make "good choices" to deal with "bad feelings." In my experience, many that have long histories of poor outcomes, or have completed suicide, have had a lot of direction and coerced care and perhaps not nearly enough *relationship*. Within the structured framework of the crisis assessment, I allow the client to respond at his or her own pace and direction so that together we can build mutual trust and enable the client to maintain some sense of self-control. With greater ease in communications, it's possible to elicit and recognize the critical elements of ambivalence, being careful to avoid assumptions based on prior case history or presenting circumstances. As in other applications of MI, ambivalence may be operatively expressed as a choice of behaviors, and these normally inform the codetermination of further steps in care.

As in other applications of MI, decisional balance plays an important part in exploring or resolving ambivalence. There is no more authentic issue in existential terms than the question of life itself as a choice. In my work with suicidal clients I find that this is often experienced as not one choice but two: *Do I want to live?* and *Do I want to die?* In a reductionist view these may be seen as two sides of the same coin, but my clients have taught me that they are usually two distinct questions, parallel but not always congruent. Just as one might explore the good things and the less good things about abstinence, and also the good things and the less good things about continuing alcohol use with a problem drinker, so one may explore the good things and the less good things about continuing to live, and the good things and the less good things about choosing to die, with a suicidal client. In many instances this exploration promotes a realization that clients actually do not want to be dead but that they are so emotionally overwhelmed and so lacking in self-efficacy that they feel they have no other options. Suicidal clients may be at one place of readiness to deal with choices about the next steps in their care and be in an entirely different state of readiness to deal with existential choices about living or dying. It is important to understand that a client's agreement to a "safety plan" or to further care does not necessarily indicate a robust or stable resolution of ambivalence about either living *or* dying. There may be cases in which the client's expression of the good things about being dead is so powerful for them that there may be no better option than to seek the highest level of care. The deeper ambivalence surrounding how much one wants to live and how much one wants to die may take much more time in therapy and/or self-exploration to resolve. Yet, brief MI intervention in the acute stages of crisis seems to help clients often struggling with chronic depression and severe stressors to gain purchase on their own capacity to shed another tear and take another step without engaging in self-harm.

CLINICAL ILLUSTRATION

The following illustrative case example is a composite drawn from typical cases seen by the author in his practice as a crisis counselor at a busy suburban hospital emergency department. Space considerations allow only a very brief version here of what is typically an hour-long encounter in which I employ several MI tools to explore both problem acceptance and treatment acceptance.

James was a 29-year-old male who was referred by the local police and rescue squad after he called 911 and stated, "I'm dying, don't try to stop me." James had been seen in the emergency department twice in the preceding 12 months, both times after intentionally taking overdoses of prescribed and over-the-counter medications. On both occasions he was also intoxicated on alcohol and cocaine. He was a high school graduate, self-taught as a skilled mechanic but unemployed for several months. James reported no close family relationships and that his father was an alcoholic, and that for several months during their childhood he and a younger sister were sexually abused by his mother. At that time, his sister was 8 years old and he was 10 years old, and the abuse was never discussed or acknowledged in the family. He was divorced from a woman he married when he was 19 (their marriage, with no children, ended after 2 years, amid reports of mutual domestic violence). At the time of the assessment James was estranged from a current girlfriend who had recently obtained a restraining order against him because of threats he made to "get" her when she insisted that he move out of her apartment; James had a court date pending for allegedly violating the restraining order by repeatedly calling this woman at her home, at work, and on her cell phone. James had been in therapy on and off since his first suicide attempt a year previously. On the first occasion he was hospitalized voluntarily for 8 days and then attended a partial-hospital (half-day) program for 2 weeks. Subsequently he was referred for individual psychotherapy but stopped attending after his second appointment. His primary care physician prescribed medications 2 years earlier, but James acknowledged his poor compliance (saying "I don't like to take pills because I use alcohol—and I don't think they do anything for me but fog me out"). He similarly failed to continue taking other medications prescribed in the course of his hospitalizations. James minimized the importance of his cocaine abuse, saying, "I just do a little blow if it's around, like anybody. It's not like I'm a crack-head." On the earlier occasion of his second overdose, which he took in front of his girlfriend during an argument, he was brought to the emergency department, refused referral for voluntary inpatient psychiatric care, and was involuntarily committed to a state hospital, where he remained for 6 weeks. The current suicide attempt was more serious than the two previous ones (this time he took a large quantity of acetaminophen, with his blood alcohol level over .24), and he spent 2 days in an intensive care unit before becoming medically stable enough to be evaluated for further care. Based on this presentation, James was clearly a high-risk low-safety client. He had a history of significant and escalating self-harm, significant co-occurring substance abuse, noncompliance with treatment recommendations, poor insight and judgment and high impulsivity, limited positive social support, and increasingly apparent borderline personality traits.

James was assessed at his bedside in the intensive care unit with both a "one-to-one" nurse observer and a security guard nearby, because he was regarded as an active risk for elopement and for intentional self-harm. He presented as cooperative but guarded during the assessment. In addition to reviewing his history as described above, the assessment was significant for his disclosure that he owned two firearms, a hunting rifle and a shotgun, that he said he kept "in a safe place," and also for his repeated requests for me to assist him in making a phone call to his estranged girlfriend ("I just want to talk to her. I want her to work this out"). After an initial information-gathering phase of the assessment, I suggested taking a break so that James could have his lunch; after about a half-hour I returned to sit at his bedside, and our dialogue continued:

HARRY: Hi, James, I'm back. How are you doing?

JAMES: You know, I *really* want to make that call. I *have* to talk to her . . .

He starts to weep and then cries openly. I am quiet but maintain eye contact, and my expression reflects the client's sadness and my own concern for him. I hand him some tissues. I do not speak, and patiently sit, inclined toward James, attentive, simply allowing us to share the moment. After a minute or two his tears stop, he wipes his eyes, and then looks at me and releases a great sigh, and looking at him, I sigh in return.

JAMES: I'm finished, I f__ed up everything, I want to die.

HARRY: You seem to be feeling worn out, hopeless . . .

JAMES: It would be different if she'd give it a chance—why can't I just talk to her?

HARRY: James, it seems the restraining order was placed because you threatened to hurt her, and you've had some past incidents of fights at home, and you've done some things before to hurt yourself.

JAMES: They always bring up that old stuff; I did those things when I was drunk! And I was provoked plenty, too.

HARRY: What do you think it would take for people to see you differently?

JAMES: Maybe just to see me sober, I'm a nice guy, maybe too nice, and I get hurt all the time. Why aren't they putting restraining orders on people that hurt *me*? I'm the one that ends up living in a car.

HARRY: It doesn't seem fair to you . . .

JAMES: Hell, no! (*Slumps down.*) I don't care anymore.

HARRY: It sounds like you feel you may do better if you're not using alcohol or drugs.

JAMES: Sure, I was doing great for a while. But if I party a little just like anybody else, she starts nagging me, and I don't need to be told what to do like a little kid.

HARRY: You don't like other people telling you what to do. How about choices you can make now?

JAMES: I'm not going back to the state hospital, I'll tell you that. I'd rather be dead. Do I get to choose?

HARRY: That depends a lot on you, and on how you feel about your safety issues. We can talk about that if you like . . .

JAMES: What safety issues?

HARRY: Well, one thing that definitely is a concern is your firearms, James. I know you told me you like to hunt . . .

JAMES: I never hurt anybody with a gun. If I wanted to do that to myself I would have done it.

HARRY: What do you think stopped you?

JAMES: I don't know, I just can't see myself doing that. Those guns cost me a lot of money. They're put away safe anyhow.

HARRY: Well, I appreciate that you don't want to use them except for hunting, and it's good that you're careful how you keep them, but you know people might have a lot more confidence in your ability to make choices if you would consider letting us make sure your guns are really in a safe place . . .

JAMES: I don't want the cops taking them . . .

HARRY: As long as they're legal hunting weapons you may be able to have a responsible family member or friend keep them for now.

JAMES: That's already done. I got them up at my friend Al's place, he was my foreman at work, and we go hunting every year. He keeps them in his gun safe.

HARRY: If I could call Al to verify that, and to let him know how you're doing, that would be great, James. . . . I will ask Al not to let you have them unless you guys are going hunting and he's sure you're sober and feeling OK.

JAMES: Well, that's OK with me.

At this point I completed a written consent form that James signed and I witnessed, and I expressed appreciation for his cooperation, and offered affirmation, saying "This really helps us to be able to talk about more choices for your care." I excused myself to immediately phone James's friend and was able to verify that the weapons were, in fact, in a gun safe to which James had no direct access. His friend Al told me that he was aware of James's history of emotional and behavioral problems and assured me that he would not allow any access to the weapons except for hunting together, and then only if he is assured that James is sober and appears stable. I thanked him, documented our conversation, and resumed the encounter with James:

HARRY: I spoke with your friend Al; he asked me to tell you he's sorry you're not doing too well right now, and he'll be responsible for your guns. He seems to like you and care about you a lot.

JAMES: Yeah, Al is really a great guy; he's like family to me. So, what happens now—when do I get out of here? I need to get my car back, all my stuff is in it.

HARRY: James, you did some real damage to your health this time. Have you talked with the doctor about that?

JAMES: Yeah, he showed me my liver tests. Do you think I'll be OK?

HARRY: I'm not a doctor, but I think that will mostly depend on how you choose to take care of yourself. The doctors will want you to stay in inpatient care on the mental health unit until everyone agrees that you're well enough to do partial hospital again. Are you OK with that?

JAMES: I really don't have much choice, do I?

HARRY: You have a choice between voluntary and involuntary mental health care, and you know from past experience what the difference is. . . . If you don't mind me saying so, we would like you to stay with us, as you have before, James. You know we care about you here. What do you think?

JAMES: OK, I guess I'll stay here.

The total face-to-face time spent in the MI-based assessment of "James," excerpted above, was 1 hour.

Does MI make a difference as compared to similar encounters without MI? For the sake of comparison, let's revisit the encounter with James as it might have occurred *without* an MI approach. In this contrasting example, the entire assessment and disposition took only 40 minutes, with no breaks. This dialogue, like the first, is based on a composite of actual encounters conducted with similar clients by interviewers without an MI stance, as observed in my practice. The interviewer pursues a disposition, as in the first example, after the initial assessment data has been established:

INTERVIEWER: James, we need to decide now what further care you will have.

JAMES: You know, I want to talk to her; I really want to make that call.

He starts to weep and then cries openly. The interviewer hands James some tissues and says, "That's why you're in trouble now, for not following a restraining order. I'll give you a minute" and leaves the room. About 3 minutes later, James is no longer tearful, and the interviewer returns.

INTERVIEWER: Are you ready for us to talk now?

JAMES: I'm finished, I f__ed up everything, I want to die.

INTERVIEWER: Well, you certainly have to stay in the hospital in that case.

JAMES: It would be different if she'd give it a chance—why can't I just talk to her?

INTERVIEWER: James, you have to take that up with the judge who issued the restraining order.

JAMES: They always bring up that old stuff; I did those things when I was drunk! And I was provoked plenty, too.

INTERVIEWER: We'll make sure you get detox and treatment for your alcohol and drug problems, too.

JAMES: Look, I'm no alcoholic and I'm not a drug addict. Why aren't they putting restraining orders on people that hurt *me*? I'm the one that ends up living in a car.

INTERVIEWER: Maybe you need to take a look at that . . .

JAMES: (*Slumps down.*) I just don't care anymore. I'm not going back to the state hospital, I'll tell you that. I'd rather be dead.

INTERVIEWER: Right now I don't feel that I could trust you to be safe outside a state hospital.

JAMES: Why not? You don't really know anything about me . . .

INTERVIEWER: Well, I have a big concern about your firearms, James. I know you told me you like to hunt . . .

JAMES: I never hurt anybody with a gun. If I wanted to do that to myself I would have done it.

INTERVIEWER: James, I'd like to know where those guns are now.

JAMES: I don't have 'em anymore. I sold them.

INTERVIEWER: Who did you sell them to and when?

JAMES: It's none of your business, but I sold them at a gun show last year.

INTERVIEWER: Can you verify that?

JAMES: Look, I'm not comfortable talking about this anymore. I want to be discharged. When do I get out of here? I need to get my car back, all my stuff is in it.

INTERVIEWER: James, you're a risk to yourself and to others, and you have to remain hospitalized. You're uncooperative and I have no choice but to send you to the state hospital for further care.

JAMES: That's what you think. I'm leaving . . .

James stands up and pulls out his intravenous line and removes a cardiac monitor, and the interviewer loudly issues a stat call for physical restraints. Later that day James is transferred to a state hospital for involuntary inpatient psychiatric care.

This fictional composite case example is drawn from actual encounters with real clients and is intended to provide a representative comparison of how working with suicidal clients can be enhanced with the use of MI. This is not to suggest that MI is a panacea; in reality, there are limits to what may be achieved. As a cautionary postscript to the first, MI-based, dialogue with "James," an hour after that dialogue was completed, James broke a plastic spoon that he had saved from his lunch and, in the presence of a nurse and security guard, superficially lacerated his throat and one wrist. He was physically restrained and later transferred to a state hospital for involuntary inpatient psychiatric care. Three weeks later, when James was discharged from the state hospital, he called our community "crisis line" number and asked to speak to me:

HARRY: Hi, this is Harry.

JAMES: Hey, man, it's James. Do you remember me?

HARRY: James, how are you? Sure, I remember, I've been wondering how you were doing; where are you calling from?

JAMES: I'm at a group residence they sent me to from the state hospital. You know, I really need to get my act together now. I'm going to do things different this time. I thought maybe we could get together to talk.

HARRY: I'd be happy to see you again—what time is good for you?

PROBLEMS AND SUGGESTED SOLUTIONS

One problem that may be considered in light of the foregoing examples is the view of some colleagues that the MI intervention was "a waste of time. Look what he [James] did. We see these clients all the time, you can't do anything with them; you should have just sent him to involuntary long-term care right away." Understanding and acceptance of ambivalence regarding MI-based practice innovations among colleagues is no different than being sensitive to mixed feelings about change within clients. While we are not practicing MI with our colleagues in the same sense that we do with a client, the value of promoting change while avoiding argument, judgment, or persuasion has been evident in my practice. Some colleagues remain temperamentally or philosophically opposed to altering treatment as usual. Many, however, have shown genuine appreciation and interest in MI as an approach to enhancing our work with suicidal clients.

Skeptics ask, "What was the better outcome with MI in the case of James?" In both examples, he was involuntarily committed. However, I would argue that in the MI-based intervention his cooperation in safeguarding his weapons and his subsequent decision to reconnect with the counselor with whom he came to feel comfortable, and trust, are valuable dividends for the client and the community and are suggestive of a continuing opportunity to promote positive change over time. By contrast, one may consider the apparent mistrust, anger, and alienation that characterize the alternative example, which suggest continuing high-risk circumstances for the client and the community.

Colleagues without MI training or experience are often skeptical that this approach can be "practical" or "manageable" to accomplish the required procedures in the limited timeframe that is often a workplace reality of many healthcare settings. They typically employ a somewhat more distanced and more rigidly structured linear method of completing the evaluation. Though not supported by experimental data, my observations and experience suggest that the time taken for an MI-based intervention is generally only moderately longer than other approaches; moreover, the qualitative differences appear to be quite meaningful and include supporting completeness and accuracy of information essential to a thorough assessment, establishing a positive therapeutic alliance in support of further care, and identifying and minimizing barriers to further positive engagement. Once required data gathering is completed, I will literally reset the process for the next scene: suggesting and providing a brief intermission for everyone's comfort and personal needs, and again asking clients for permission to talk with them about "what happens next." It is surprising how easily basic considerations of comfort and common courtesy are eclipsed by the exigencies of crisis management of suicidality, and this deliberate attention to personal needs—a concrete expression of MI spirit—helps to moderate anxieties, to reduce conflicts, and to not exacerbate ambivalence that will impact critical decision making regarding further care. At that point the client, other caregivers, participating family, significant others or collaterals, and I in the role of facilitator are positioned to build on our alignment, to agree on what the problems are, and to seek agreement on what happens next. Appreciating that there may often be differences among these many stakeholders, my MI stance places respect for the client's autonomy and personal responsibility as the paramount objective while maintaining a congruent respect for the risk factors and safety factors that must also influence the client's disposition and plan for further care.

The value of providing an MI basis for the crisis examination of these dilemmas can be critical, in part because (considering the rarity of skilled MI therapists) it is very exceptional and contrasts greatly with the more directive or coercive approaches commonly associated with "treatment as usual." One of the most challenging aspects of using MI with clients in such difficult circumstances is to do so in a way that prepares them for the likelihood of their subsequently having to encounter many people using more directive and decidedly non-MI approaches. After voluntary or involuntary admission to a secure mental health unit, many clients will be discharged to a lower level of care within a relatively short time, and the dilemma of ambivalence is unlikely to be so quickly resolved. Yet, the client's response to the assault on his or her personal autonomy may well have reduced "readiness" for change. I encourage clients to express their feelings about being enmeshed in circumstances very different from what they would have chosen or planned, most often by saying, "Tell me about how you might cope with what's happening now and with what happens next in your care." There are still relatively few clinical settings where MI is routinely practiced; at this time I am the sole MI practitioner in my community. My solution is to do what I call "seeding" MI: I use MI with clients as much as I can whenever I can; I gently promote awareness of the method among colleagues, family, police, and other collaterals; and for anyone who expresses interest in further MI education or training, I connect them with accessible resources.

Another way I approach this problem is the exploration with clients of what I call "autono-MI," a take-some-with-you, do-it-yourself extension of our MI encounter, in which the client acquires some MI spirit that they can use in a time of need, when they are in situations where there may not be any to be had. This product of conscious modeling on the part of the clinician during the MI encounter leads to an explicit mutual pact in parting that recognizes that there's more here than we can use right now—would you like to take some with you to have later? For most clients, their further care may be very unlike their brief MI encounters with me. All the more reason to seek to provision them with positive expectations, genuine affirmations, and an intrinsic awareness of some options they may employ in coping with other more inflexible, demanding, or distanced approaches to treatment. It is a simple matter to take a few extra minutes to rehearse possible choices to help support the client's sense of self-efficacy and capacity to tolerate further care that may be much less flexible or sensitive as compared to MI, being careful to reflect and summarize with attention to change talk.

Finally, it is important to be aware of the limitations of this application of MI. It is obvious that not all suicidal clients are responsive to MI—or to other approaches. The clinician must be observant of the context and climate in which each encounter with a suicidal client is embedded, as suicidality is rarely an uncomplicated function of solely intrapersonal conflict. A client's web of social relationships and conflicts, economic resources and stressors, chronic and persistent illness or behavioral dysfunction, and other negative circumstances often are well beyond the scope or power of any brief intervention. It is also important for any whose practice involves the care of suicidal clients to follow prudent recommendations for clinician wellness protections in undertaking this work.

RESEARCH

Empirical research on suicide has been quite limited, with very few randomized controlled trial (RCT) studies of any kind and many limitations affecting the interpretation of correlational studies (Gaynes et al., 2004; Soomro, 2005). Methodological problems for researchers begin with controversy over how to define the actual behavior; the difficulty of obtaining evidence from persons who have completed suicide; the use of substitute subjects, usually suicide attempters, to represent suicide completers; and the difficulty of adequately defining and matching control groups (Lester, 1997). There are currently no published research studies on the use of MI with suicidal clients. Some prominent researchers whose work on prevention of suicide and management of suicidality and deliberate self-harm appears quite consistent with the application of MI are Jobes (2006; Jobes & Drozd, 2004), Linehan (1993; Linehan & Bagge, 2000), Shaffer (Shaffer, Garland, Gould, Fisher, & Trautman, 1988; Mann et al., 2005), and Gould (Velting, Kleinman, Lucas, Thomas, & Chung, 2004; Gould et al., 2005).

CONCLUSIONS

There are many challenges to the clinical application of MI in working with suicidal clients; yet, the benefits of strengthening therapeutic alliance, of supporting autonomy, responsibility, and self-efficacy, and of opening up dichotomous thinking and exploring ambivalence seem likely to be as valuable in your practice as they have been in mine. I know that clients appreciate this application of MI, because they tell me so, often saying, "I've been to counselors before, but no one ever treated me the way you did," or words to that effect; they appear to be especially pleased that I take time to listen rather than having to feel that they've been rushed through a standardized assessment; and they appreciate that I offer them choices and options at every stage of the interview. A more objective indicator is that among crisis clients in my practice there is a comparatively low rate of involuntary commitment for inpatient psychiatric care—less than 7%—while some 33% accept voluntary referral for inpatient care. The application of MI in the evaluation and treatment of suicidality invites and deserves greater attention from researchers and caregivers.

NOTE

1. The use of an oral or written "contract for safety" in the management of suicidality has been demonstrated to have serious limitations and to lack sufficient evidential basis for having a protective impact on acts of deliberate self-harm (American Psychiatric Association, 2003, pp. 5, 41–42).

REFERENCES

American Association of Suicidology. (2004). *U.S.A. Suicide: 2002 Official Final Data.* Washington, DC: Author.

American Psychiatric Association. (2003). *Practice guideline for the assessment and treatment of patients with suicidal behaviors.* Arlington, VA: American Psychiatric Publishing.

Gaynes, B. N., West, S. L., Ford, C. A., Frame, P., Klein, J., & Lohr, K. N. (2004). Screening for suicide risk in adults: A summary of the evidence for the U.S. Preventive Services Task Force. *Annals of Internal Medicine, 140,* 822–835.

Gelder, M., Mayou, R., & Cowen, P. (2001). *Shorter Oxford textbook of psychiatry.* Oxford, UK: Oxford University Press.

Gould, M. S., Velting, D., Kleinman, M., Lucas, C., Thomas, J. G., & Chung, M. (2004). Teenagers' attitudes about coping strategies and help-seeking behavior for suicidality. *Journal of the American Academy of Child and Adolescent Psychiatry, 43,* 1124–1133

Gould, M. S., Marrocco, F. A., Kleinman, M., Thomas, J. G., Mostkoff, K., Cote, J., et al. (2005). Evaluating iatrogenic risk of suicide screening programs: A randomized controlled trial. *Journal of the American Medical Association, 293,* 1635–1643.

Jobes, D. A. (2006). *Managing suicidal risk: A collaborative approach.* New York: Guilford Press.

Jobes, D. A., & Drozd, J. F. (2004). The CAMS approach to working with suicidal patients. *Journal of Contemporary Psychotherapy, 34,* 73–85.

Lester, D. (1997). *Making sense of suicide: An in-depth look at why people kill themselves.* Philadelphia: Charles Press.

Linehan, M. M. (1993). *Cognitive-behavioral treatment of borderline personality disorder.* New York: Guilford Press.

Linehan, M. M. (2000). Behavioral treatments of suicidal behaviors: Definitional obfuscation and treatment outcomes. In R. W. Maris, S. S. Canetto, J. L. McIntosh, & M. M. Silverman (Eds.), *Review of suicidology* (pp. 84–111). New York: Guilford Press.

Linehan, M. M., & Bagge, C. L. (2000). Reasons for living versus reasons for dying, a letter to the Editor. *Suicide and Life-Threatening Behavior, 2,* 180–181.

Mann, J. J., Apter, A., Bertolote, J., Beautrais, A., Currier, D., Haas, A., et al. (2005). Suicide prevention strategies: A systematic review. *Journal of the American Medical Association, 294,* 2064–2074.

Risk Management Foundation of the Harvard Medical Institutions. (1996). *Guidelines for identification, assessment, and treatment planning for suicidality.* Cambridge, MA: Author.

Risk Management Foundation of the Harvard Medical Institutions. (2000). *Decision support outline: Emergency/crisis coverage of a suicidal patient.* Cambridge, MA: Author.

Shaffer, D., Garland, A., Gould, M., Fisher, P., & Trautman, P. (1988). Preventing teenage suicide: A critical review. *Journal of the American Academy of Child and Adolescent Psychiatry, 27,* 675–687.

Soomro, G. M. (2005). Deliberate self harm (and attempted suicide). *Clinical Evidence, 13,* 1–3.

ADDITIONAL RESOURCES

Some of the works referenced above are accessible in electronic form through the Internet. Readers will find additional valuable resource material and further links at any of these websites:

www.suicidology.org—American Association of Suicidology
www.afsp.org—American Foundation for Suicide Prevention
www.nimh.nih.gov/suicideprevention—National Institute of Mental Health
www.psych.org/psych_pract—American Psychiatric Association

CHAPTER 8

Motivational Interviewing in the Management of Eating Disorders

Janet Treasure
Ulrike Schmidt

The eating disorders—anorexia nervosa (AN), bulimia nervosa (BN), and related disorders (eating disorders not otherwise specified [EDNOS] and binge-eating disorder [BED])—are quite prevalent disorders that affect mainly young women. In a recent community survey, lifetime prevalence rates were 4.6% for AN, 7.7% for BN (including partial and subthreshold cases), and 0.6% for BED in young females (Favaro, Ferrara, & Santonastaso, 2003). These disorders typically have a chronic course with major psychiatric and medical comorbidities and sequelae (Fairburn & Brownell, 2001; Zipfel, Löwe, & Herzog, 2003). Anorexia nervosa has the highest mortality of any psychiatric disorder, with the risk of death three times higher than that of depression, schizophrenia, or alcoholism (Harris & Barraclough, 1998).

The etiology of eating disorders is complex (Jacobi, Hayward, de Zwaan, Kraemer, & Agras, 2004). BN is a Western culture-bound syndrome (Keel & Klump, 2004), with dieting being a major risk factor for this condition. In contrast, there are descriptions of AN from non-Western cultures and well-documented cases dating back to the Middle Ages. In these historical non-Western cases the psychopathology is not based on concerns about weight or shape; rather, those affected complain of lack of appetite and inability to eat or justify their food restriction in terms of ascetic or religious ideals. While the current diagnostic criteria of both AN and BN focus on weight and shape concerns as *the* central psychopathology of these disorders, we—along with others (Palmer, 2003)—believe that weight and shape concerns are central in BN but not in AN. Instead, the essence of AN appears to be eating restraint motivated by a range of factors, including weight/shape concerns (Palmer, 2003).

Some experts suggest that the diagnostic categories (such as AN, BN, BED) and subcategories (e.g., purging or nonpurging type) should be abandoned and all forms of eating disorders considered together (Fairburn & Bohn, 2005). However, we would argue that while there is some overlap among different eating disorders, the distinctions in etiology, clinical features, and maintaining factors among the disorders continue to have utility in planning treatment and management (Collier & Treasure, 2004; Jacobi et al., 2004; Schmidt & Treasure, 2006).

In this chapter, while we will consider the use of motivational techniques in the management of different eating disorders, the main emphasis will be on AN. We have chosen to focus on AN because people with this disorder are typically less ready to change than people with other eating disorders, such as BN or BED (Blake, Turnbull, & Treasure, 1997). People with BN or BED typically are distressed by their symptoms and seek help of their own accord, making it easier to form a treatment alliance and effect change. In contrast, one key feature that sets AN apart from all other psychiatric disorders is that it is highly valued by the person herself, even when faced with the prospect of death. This point is summarized by Bemis (1986) as follows: "When asked to characterize their reactions to weight loss, anorexics report that they feel delighted, inspired, triumphant, proud and powerful, . . . special, superior and deserving of the respect and admiration of others." Naive therapists may thus find themselves pleading or arguing with their patients to halt their "self-destructive path." As weight loss progresses and with increasing risk to the patient's life, therapists may become more controlling and coercive. Patients treated in this way tend to "fight the system" by cheating (e.g., carrying weights in their pockets or drinking lots of fluid before being weighed) or "eat their way out of the hospital" to get away from coercive treatment.

Motivational interviewing (MI) has been an instant "hit" with eating disorder therapists, as it has given them a framework for working *with* their patients rather than against them. However, as we discuss below, modifications of the standard MI model need to be made to make it useful for patients with AN. As we go along, we will also compare and contrast the treatment approach to AN with that applied to other eating disorders.

THE CLINICAL POPULATION AND USUAL TREATMENTS

The history of AN treatment stretches back over the last 150 years. In the past a medical model of treatment was applied whereby the person with AN was admitted to the hospital, given bed rest, and refed. Psychotherapeutic approaches have been developed during the past 20 years. The earliest psychological treatments of AN were behavioral, with an exclusive focus on achieving weight gain using strict operant conditioning (Schmidt, 1989); patients were being kept on bed rest and isolated from their families, with "privileges" being reintroduced upon the requisite weight gain. This was often experienced as coercive and unhelpful by patients and led to fierce resistance (Touyz, Beumont, Glaun, Phillips, & Cowie, 1984). More recently, treatment guidelines based on systematic reviews of the evidence have been compiled in the United Kingdom, Australia, and New Zealand (Beumont et al., 2004; National Collaborating Centre for Mental Health, 2004). These guide- lines suggest that the first line of treatment should be outpatient psy- chological treatment with an emphasis on psychological as well as nutritional change. The U.K. treatment guideline (National Collabo- rating Centre for Mental Health, 2004) explicitly states that strict oper- ant conditioning regimes should not be used in the treatment of AN.

AN commonly begins in the mid-teens. One of the classic features of this disorder is that the individual does not consider herself to have a problem and resists treatment (although this resistance may to some ex- tent be the product of coercive treatment). This stands in marked con- trast to the concerns of family, friends, and teachers, who are able to make a "spot diagnosis" and who are drawn to want to help. Given this disparity, it is not surprising that the most effective interventions for ad- olescents in the early stages of AN are family-based treatments (Na- tional Collaborating Centre for Mental Health, 2004). While in the early days of family therapy, treatment was very directive, with an emphasis on "restructuring the family system" and "putting the parents back in charge" and with little regard for the concerns of the young person (Minuchin, Rosman, & Baker, 1978), more modern family-based treat- ments are more flexible and compatible with a motivational approach. The emphasis now is on engaging all family members, respect for the family's unique style, teaching parents to find the right balance between setting appropriate boundaries and respecting adolescent autonomy, and giving adolescents more of a voice. Variants of family therapy such as parental counseling (where the parents are seen on their own and the child is seen separately) have been found to be as effective as conjoint family therapy (Eisler, Dare, Hodes, Russell, Dodge, & LeGrange, 2000).

Adults with AN usually have had a long history of the problem and have additional features indicative of a poor prognosis. In general, there is more certainty about what does *not* work rather than what does work for this group of patients. Dietetic treatment or nutritional counseling alone are associated with poor treatment adherence (Serfaty, 1999) and are less effective than psychological therapy (e.g., cognitive-behavioral therapy [CBT]) (Pike, Walsh, Vitousek, Wilson, & Bauer, 2003). Similarly, admission to the hospital for refeeding and weight restoration is not as acceptable to patients as outpatient care, as evidenced by low adherence rates (Crisp et al., 1991); nor is inpatient refeeding sufficient in itself to produce recovery. Relapse following inpatient care is common, and additional psychosocial treatments are necessary. Medication has not proven helpful in the treatment of AN (Claudino et al., 2006; Treasure & Schmidt, 2005).

In contrast to AN, bulimia nervosa is a relatively new disorder, first described in 1979 (Russell, 1979). While the typical onset is also in the teenage years, the disorder often goes unnoticed by others, and there are usually delays of several years before people with BN access treatment. By the time they do seek treatment, it is usually the person's own decision to ask for help rather than that of concerned close others. In BN there is a large body of high-quality evidence about what works in treatment. Cognitive-behavioral therapy for BN (CBT-BN) is currently the treatment of choice (Hay, Bacaltchuk, & Stefano, 2004; National Collaborating Centre for Mental Health, 2004). Nevertheless, there is still room for improvement, as less than 50% of patients treated with CBT-BN make a full recovery. New models of CBT are being developed that build on and refine existing approaches (Cooper, Wells, & Todd, 2004; Fairburn, Cooper, & Shafran, 2003). It is possible that those who respond poorly to CBT-BN do so because of low motivation.

RATIONALE FOR USING MI
IN EATING DISORDERS

The theme of anorexics' reluctance to change has been a recurring one in the eating disorders literature (Vitousek, Watson, & Wilson, 1998).

Different empirical models for conceptualizing and assessing motivation and readiness for change exist. One prominent framework for this is provided by the transtheoretical model of change (Prochaska, DiClemente, & Norcross, 1992). The key assumptions of this model are first that, to change a behavior, people move through a sequence of stages, from *precontemplation*, to *contemplation*, *preparation/action*, and finally *maintenance*. Studies in adults with AN found that about half of those presenting for treatment were either in the precontemplation phase (i.e., had no desire to change) or the contemplation phase (i.e., were very ambivalent about change) (Blake et al., 1997; Ward, Troop, Todd, & Treasure, 1996).

The mismatch in the desire for change between the person with anorexia nervosa and those around them, coupled with the sense of urgency of intervention resulting from the person's compromised medical state, makes the process of engaging people with AN into treatment a challenging task. In the past, AN treatments have often been directive or outright coercive, leading to a breakdown in trust between patients and their health care providers. MI offers a way of circumventing the hostility and resistance that so easily arise in this context.

People with BN more often present for treatment of their own accord (Blake et al., 1997), albeit often after a protracted period of time. They too may have mixed feelings about change. On the one hand, they are desperate to get control of their bingeing, but they are reluctant to let go of their weight- and shape-control measures. In addition, they are ambivalent about eliminating their extreme food restriction and compensatory behaviors such as vomiting. Thus, motivational approaches may be appropriate not just for AN but for other eating disorders as well.

CLINICAL APPLICATION OF MI
TO EATING DISORDERS

For most cases of AN, a simple motivational feedback session or a short course of motivational enhancement therapy is not sufficient to achieve weight restoration and psychological recovery. Rather, a mixture of additional techniques such as CBT or interpersonal interventions is needed—an approach akin to that used in Project COMBINE, a study combining MI with CBT in the treatment of addictions (COMBINE Study Research Group, 2003).

The Maudsley Model of Anorexia Treatment

We have developed a specific and evidence-based model of how AN is maintained (Schmidt & Treasure, 2006). Based on this, we have developed a treatment that combines MI with a cognitive-interpersonal approach (the Maudsley model of anorexia treatment) (Schmidt & Treasure, 2006). A full description of the model is beyond the scope of this chapter. In brief, we propose that the core psychopathology of AN is a need for the avoidance of intense negative emotions in people who have anxious/avoidant and perfectionist/rigid personality traits and who develop beliefs about the positive function of the anorexia in their life (pro-anorexia beliefs). These pro-anorexia beliefs about the utility of AN help them manage difficult emotions and the relationships that arouse them (e.g. "anorexia stifles emotions" or "anorexia helps me to express distress"). A further maintenance factor is the response of others, which is characterized by concern and worry, or criticism and hostility, which give rise to additional pro-anorexia beliefs (e.g., "anorexia makes me special," "anorexia makes others care for me"). If the benefits of AN are unacknowledged or unrecognized in therapy, treatment can be sabotaged or increased resistance to change can occur. The techniques of MI are very useful for helping clients question these valued functions of AN.

An outline of the stages of treatment for AN, based on the Maudsley model, is shown in Figure 8.1. The whole treatment is conducted in the MI spirit, that is, using a collaborative, empathic, and respectful stance throughout, as described by Miller and Rollnick (2002). There is however, one important difference. In the classical applications of MI (e.g., in the field of addictions), the patient's autonomy to accept or reject treatment at any stage is an integral part of the spirit of MI. In contrast, in the treatment of AN, the patient is not always an autonomous agent. Many cases begin in early adolescence or preadolescence.

Ongoing Risk Monitoring					
Engagement	Nutrition	Collaborative Case Conceptualization	Joint Treatment Plan	Working for Change	Relapse Prevention and Ending
Involve Close Others for Support					

FIGURE 8.1. Maudsley anorexia treatment.

The illness impedes and interrupts the process of maturation, and people remain dependent on their parents beyond the usual age. Moreover, the starvation itself has profound effects on cognitive function, in particular executive function. Thus, an individual's capacity to make autonomous decisions can be severely impaired. Indeed, in many countries this is recognized in the law. In the United Kingdom, for example, the Mental Health Act is used to treat some patients who suffer from life-threatening AN in the hospital involuntarily, including being fed against their will. At a more basic level, there is no choice as to whether food is eaten or not. All living beings have to eat. Thus, there are limits to individual freedom that both the practitioner and patient have to abide by.

Within these boundaries set by our biological makeup, the law, or by parental authority (in the case of children and adolescents), it is nonetheless possible to use a motivational approach offering choices to individuals. Thus, it is possible to give feedback about medical risk with a clear bottom line, which is that medical treatment for refeeding is to be recommended when certain risk parameters are met (see *www.eating research.com*). Yet, even at the point of life-threatening AN, patients still have some choices as to whether they would prefer to work on moderating their risk as an outpatient or within the confines of an inpatient setting. If they choose the former, there are choices about the kinds of nutritional steps to be taken to make the situation safer, for example, whether to start dietary supplements such as high-calorie drinks or whether to increase calorie intake by adding in greater amounts of normal food into the diet, how much and what kinds of support to enlist from which close others, and about the nature and frequency of medical monitoring.

It is important that when information about nonnegotiable matters is presented in the treatment of AN, the practitioner avoids presenting it as a threat and instead adopts an empathic "one-down position," pointing out that both the patient and practitioner are bound by the law and/ or societal rules.

Assessment and Engagement Phase

The aims of the first meeting with the patient are to have a conversation that explores her concerns, in the context of her eating disorder history and background, and to conduct an assessment of medical and psychosocial risk. Significant others are invited to attend the second part of the initial meeting to express their views and concerns. The person with AN often attends only because of family pressure. Thus, it is not uncommon in the initial meeting to be faced with a person who is stony-faced and silent and whose whole demeanor radiates protest. Below we illustrate how we use the principles and techniques of MI in the first few minutes of contact with the patient.

Clinical Illustration 1: Opening Moves

Emma, a 19-year-old student, was referred to the eating disorders unit by her general practitioner (GP). The referral letter noted that Emma has lost 22 pounds during her first term at college. Emma had been a top student in high school but found the transition to college life difficult, as she no longer was the brightest and best student. Her mother had told the GP that Emma seemed to be studying all the time, unable to relax, eating little, and responding very irritably when confronted with this.

THERAPIST: Thank you for coming to the appointment with me today. I wonder whether you could tell me how you came to be here?

PATIENT: I very nearly didn't come. I didn't want to come.

THERAPIST: I appreciate you're being so honest with me and letting me know that you really, really don't want to be here. [The therapist positively connotes the patient's frank communication and somewhat overstates the patient's reluctance to be there.]

PATIENT: I am really just here because of my mom—she made me come because she was worried. She had been on my case for quite a while, saying that I am not eating properly and that I am too thin. In the end I couldn't take her nagging any more, and I went to see our GP with her, and he wrote the referral to you. I know I have lost some weight, but I don't really think there is anything wrong with that. I am perfectly fine. I think I am wasting your time.

THERAPIST: So, what you are saying is that you just played along with the referral to keep your mom and GP happy and that you don't have a clue what all the fuss is about.

PATIENT: That's right.

THERAPIST: That must be confusing—other people around you are concerned, and you don't have any concerns whatsoever. [The therapist reflects by using undershooting, that is, minimizes more than the patient.]

PATIENT: Well, sometimes I am a bit worried, because since I started losing the weight I get tired quite easily now. [The patient now comes back for the first time with some concern of her own.]

THERAPIST: Can you tell me a bit more about that?

PATIENT: Well, I am supposed to study for my exams at college, but I can't really concentrate on my studies at all. I sit down for 15–20 minutes at a time and that's it. My brain just goes fuzzy.

THERAPIST: That sounds really tough, with you trying so hard to study and not managing to. Are there other changes that you have noticed since your weight has gone down?

PATIENT: Well, I do feel really cold all the time. At home it is all right—I can put the heater on full-blast—but in my dorm room at college I am never warm enough.

THERAPIST: That sounds rather miserable to feel so cold all the time. (*Patient nods vigorously.*) [The patient is gradually opening up a bit and seems quite willing now—with prompts from the therapist—to talk about some of her concerns.]

THERAPIST: Do you mind me asking about a couple of other things that people often say they notice when they have lost some weight?

PATIENT: That's fine.

THERAPIST: I wonder whether you have noticed any other changes in your physical health.

PATIENT: Like what?

THERAPIST: Some people we see notice that their skin becomes dry and flaky or their nails become brittle. Have you noticed anything like that since you started losing weight?

COMMENT

The therapeutic style of MI requires the therapist to take his or her cues from the patient—to ask open-ended questions and reflect on the answers. Patients with AN, who are often rather shy and inhibited young people, may find this approach somewhat alien, and the conversation may dry up quickly. We therefore tend to provide more structure early on and do not rely exclusively on open-ended questions. Instead, we go through a number of different life domains (see Table 8.1) and ask people whether they have noticed any changes in these areas, using some of the suggested prompts about the kinds of things that people often notice when they lose weight. It is important that the clinician not "rattle through this" like a checklist but rather use these prompts to give patients time to reflect on what is happening.

After exploring these different life domains, the therapist summarizes what has been discussed so far.

THERAPIST: So, if I have understood you, you mainly came today because your mom had been concerned about your health. You yourself have noticed that you get tired more easily. You feel cold all the time, and you haven't had your period for 6 months. You have also noticed that you have become more irritable with your family. You don't find pleasure in going out with friends like you used to, and it has been more difficult to concentrate on your studies.

PATIENT: (*sounding suddenly quite concerned*) Hmmm, I hadn't realized how much losing weight was affecting me. What can be done about it?

THERAPIST: In the first instance, it might be helpful if we talked a bit more about where you are at right now with your weight, eating, and other things in your life, how that fits in with what things were like before all of this started, and where you'd like to go with some of this in the future. I'd also like for you to have a physical checkup and get some blood tests done. And after that we can look at some of the options of what can be done. How does that sound?

This initial phase takes about 15–20 minutes and paves the way for a more in-depth exploration of the current situation, the person's per-

TABLE 8.1. Life Domains and How They May be Affected in AN

Physical Health	Periods stop, hair loss, sensitivity to cold, reduced stamina, dental problems, bladder dysfunction, poor sleep
Psychological Health	Low mood, irritability, obsessions, rituals, compulsions, poor concentration, and preoccupation with food
Social Life	Disinterest, difficulty in joining in with groups, fear of eating
Romantic Life	Disinterest, no libido
Family	Anger, anxiety, frustration
Work or Study	Poor concentration, lack of ambition, stigma
Legal	Shoplifting, for example, stealing food

sonal and family background, eating disorder history, and her hopes and plans for the future. A detailed physical risk assessment, including body mass index, degree of weight loss, physical examination, and laboratory tests are also conducted. In the next section we show how the empathic, reflective style of MI is used to feed back information about the person's risk in regard to nutritional health and safety and to set the scene for a dialogue about how to change.

Clinical Illustration 2: Giving Medical Feedback

The following scenario illustrates the use of a body mass index feedback chart (see *www.eatingresearch.com*), which delineates areas of increasing risk, in providing feedback about nutritional health. The patient is a 22-year-old college student with severe AN and high medical risk who is attending for her first outpatient therapy session. The therapist uses this opportunity to examine the patient's mixed feelings about the illness.

THERAPIST: If we take your height and weight and plot them on this body mass index chart, you can see that you fall into this navy blue area. Do you want to read what that means and what the risks are?

PATIENT: (*reading aloud*) Critical anorexia nervosa, inpatient treatment recommended, organs begin to fail, muscle, bone marrow, and heart. So, those organs begin to fail if people are in that zone?

THERAPIST: Yes, in the blue zone that's the general risk. Does it make sense to you that you are in that zone?

PATIENT: I didn't realize that I was in that area.

THERAPIST: Where did you think you may have been?

PATIENT: A part of me thinks that I am underweight. Sometimes I can see that I am underweight, but other times I just think that it's everybody else who is concerned about me and making a fuss. I didn't realize that I was in that section there. I am a bit shocked actually. I don't know why I didn't understand before.

THERAPIST: You look very puzzled.

PATIENT: I am. I just don't understand why people have said that I am low-weight, and I can't see it. I can look at myself and I see me. I look in the mirror and I don't see what other people are seeing. So, I can't believe it.

THERAPIST: So, the tricks that the anorexia plays are confusing to you. It sounds as though at times you get a glimmer of what other people see, but at most times the anorexia nervosa tricks you and puts all of that to the back of your mind.

PATIENT: When I am with other people and they express concern, I know I am underweight. I can tell by people's faces, and I can tell when they are making comments about me.

THERAPIST: So, on the one hand, you are pretty sensitive at using the mirror of other people. You read their concern and worry, and on the other hand it's difficult for you to truly believe because your anorexia nervosa tricks you into thinking that it's not true.

PATIENT: Yes, and because I spend a lot of time on my own, I don't really see many people apart from my family now. I just don't see my friends, so a lot of the time I am on my own. So, I believe myself. I trust what I see and I trust what I feel.

THERAPIST: So, that's another trick that the anorexia nervosa plays on you. It isolates you, which cuts you off from feedback and also must make you feel very lonely.

COMMENT

The therapist externalizes the AN and lightens the discussion of the typical psychopathology by using the word "tricks." The interpersonal impact of AN is clear from this transcript. The therapist then proceeds to give further feedback about medical risk. This includes markers of cardiovascular, metabolic, and muscular function. The therapist moves on to the use of a "nutritional ruler" to elicit thoughts about change.

THERAPIST: So, let's think about your nutritional safety on a scale of 0 to 10. 0 is where you are not able to ensure your nutritional safety, and 10 is where you are confident that you can care for your nutritional health. Before we started talking, where would you have said you are on that line?

PATIENT: I would have thought I was maybe 6, 6½. But since we've been talking and seeing this and how compromised I am, I have to believe what this is saying. I have to believe the results that you are giving me. I don't want to but it's saying that I am not able to feed myself, and I thought I was. If I am honest, I think I am maybe only a 2 or so.

THERAPIST: You would have given yourself a 6, meaning there was part of you that recognized a glimmer perhaps through other people's eyes that you were not healthy-looking. You saw people's fear about your nutritional health. Most of the time you were able to ignore that, and so you had given yourself a reasonably high mark. However, you have heard feedback from your health checkup that makes you give yourself a much lower mark.

PATIENT: Yes, it makes me feel really ashamed to think that I can't do this for myself. I can't do what other people do naturally.

THERAPIST: It is a challenge to start to get your head around how the anorexia nervosa was able to trick you, leaving your life in danger.

PATIENT: I think I am still shocked seeing these results.

THERAPIST: How do you think we can care for your nutritional safety?

PATIENT: I don't want to go to the hospital.

THERAPIST: That strength of determination is a tool to power you into being able to fight the anorexia nervosa. However, it isn't a question of just choosing. We both are having to work here within a legal and safe-practice context. In our mental health legal system it is recognized that anorexia nervosa does trick people and puts their health in jeopardy, so if someone has a very low score on the nutritional safety ruler, we may need that procedure. At the other end is where you can be totally independent of others. You are saying you don't want to come into the hospital. What is needed are signs that you can care for your nutritional health. What do you think you can do?

COMMENT

After further discussion the patient and therapist decide that they are going to try to work together on an outpatient basis, which is the patient's preferred option. However, given the severity of her condition and her own recognition that she is finding it hard to look after her nutritional needs, she has agreed to temporarily move back home and let her mother help her at mealtimes.

At the end of the assessment session a personalized feedback letter is sent to the patient. The letter is written using nontechnical language incorporating verbatim statements of the patient wherever appropriate. The tone of the letter is empathic and nonjudgmental. The letter usually starts with a description of the presenting problem and the impact of the problem on the patient's life, as perceived by the patient. The patient's hopes and fears vis-à-vis a positive or negative outcome are identified. Obstacles to change are listed, as are factors that might increase hope for recovery. This is followed by a summary of the patient's life story, with an emphasis on areas of difficulty and strengths. Where appropriate, a diagnosis is given and the treatment options are outlined. Feedback on the patient's physical status (e.g., from the physical examination and blood tests) is also included. The length of the feedback letter typically is between two to three typed pages. The first page of the letter to the patient (Emma) discussed earlier, in clinical illustration 1, might read as follows:

Dear Emma,

I enjoyed meeting with you in my clinic today, and in what follows I will attempt to summarize what we talked about. This is so that you can check whether I have understood what you told me. If I have left out anything important or gotten anything wrong, I would be grateful if you could let me know.

You were referred to us by your general practitioner, Dr. Taylor. You had gone to see him mainly to keep your mom happy, who had become quite concerned about your recent weight loss. You felt quite strongly that there was nothing wrong with you and that perhaps you were wasting my time.

As we talked a bit more, it emerged that you yourself have some concerns about your health and relationships since you started to lose weight. You get tired more easily, you feel cold all the time, and you haven't had your period for 6 months. You have also noticed that you have become much more irritable with your family and feel rather guilty about this. You don't find pleasure in going out with friends like you used to, and it has been more difficult for you to concentrate on your studies.

In addition, you have noticed a number of positives about your weight loss. Especially when you started losing weight, you felt much more in control of your life than before, you felt energized, able to focus on your work, and much less vulnerable to feeling upset or distressed. You also had a number of positive comments from your peers who admired your willpower in eating little.

You have recently begun to wonder whether at times the negatives of losing the weight outweigh the positives, but when concerned others like your mom "go on and on and on" at you about the dangers of losing weight, you have very much felt like wanting to defend your position . . .

The next few sessions focus on building motivation for change. This is done using standard MI techniques such as exploring readiness and confidence to change, examining the pros and cons of change, and looking forward and backward and considering values and value–behavior congruence. An important part of this is an exploration of the valued function of the anorexia in the person's life together with the identification of relevant pro-anorexia beliefs, which are usually closely linked to the reasons the person has for not wanting to change. These beliefs are most simply explored by asking people about what is good about their anorexia and what they value about it. An additional technique for identifying positive and negative beliefs about AN is through asking the patient to write two letters to anorexia, first as a friend and then as an enemy. We give this as a homework task early on in treatment, introducing this as a task that the patient might want to try and might find helpful in clarifying her position vis-à-vis her AN. An example of one such letter is given below.

> *Dear anorexia,*
>
> *You are always there for me even when others let me down or turn away. You are faithful to me and have been my salvation. Others think that you are bad for me, but in truth it is your support that has carried me through. Without you I'd be aimless and lost. You have given me something to focus on when my world fell apart and have given me back some of the control I lost.*

In this letter it appears that the dependable nature of the anorexia, as well as the focus and sense of control it has given her, is valued by the patient. Other people's letters focus more on how AN helps to elicit care or concern from close others or approval from slim peers (see Lavender & Schmidt, 2006).[1]

A conversation about the good things that the AN provides for the person sheds light on key interpersonal relationships and yet the deficits in them and provides important pointers about underlying beliefs the person may have about herself, others, and the world at large, as well as personal values and rules. For example, a person who believes that the anorexia makes her special and makes others notice and admire her may have core beliefs about being boring and unlovable. As treatment progresses, the focus of the discussion should shift to look at how—other than through the AN—the person may be able to achieve her legitimate goals of, for example, feeling safe and getting care and approval from others and how she can better care for herself.

Ongoing Risk Monitoring

This is an integral part of treatment. Risk is monitored regularly, with the timing and breadth of the examination depending on the level of risk. At a minimum this involves measurement of the patient's weight by the therapist at every session. This is presented to the patient as an essential requirement (enshrined in U.K. guidance on good practice), as without regular weighing an increase in medical risk may go unnoticed, potentially resulting in dangerous consequences. Patients' views about being weighed are carefully explored and reflected upon, and if they are reluctant to be weighed, options are explored to make weighing less anxiety-provoking. For example, some people find it easier not to know what exactly their weight is, and therefore they might prefer to be weighed with their back to the scales.

Weighing occurs at the beginning of the session, because if there are emotional and planning issues that arise contingent on the change in weight, it is important that they be addressed in the meeting. Weight gain is a primary sought outcome of all interventions with AN, and is an important marker of engagement and the success of therapy. If weight is falling, this indicates that the therapist needs to reflect on the process of engagement and the development of the therapeutic alliance. Weight loss or failure to gain weight in therapy are also discussed in terms of the function and importance of AN in the person's life and her readiness and confidence to change.

Clinical Illustration 3

A patient with AN who early in therapy was very motivated to change and made good progress in terms of weight gain has reached a plateau, and over the past five outpatient sessions her weight has remained stably in the AN range.

THERAPIST: Let's just plot today's weight on your chart. It looks like your weight has really leveled off a bit recently. What do you make of that?

PATIENT: I started out with all good intentions, but it is just too scary. I don't think I can go any further right now.

THERAPIST: It is all going a bit fast for you, and you are putting on the emergency brakes. I wonder whether it might be helpful to revisit our readiness and confidence ruler. When we looked at it a little while ago, your motivation to overcome AN was a 7 and your confidence a 6. Where do you think you are with this right now?

PATIENT: I don't know I guess I have lost the plot a bit; I think my motivation at best is at a 4 now, and confidence-wise I am not much higher. I find it really hard to remember why I wanted to make the changes. I guess I can mainly see the downside of giving up the anorexia now.

THERAPIST: You have lost touch with the reasons for change, it all seems scary and unfamiliar, and you don't feel ready to move further. Just for argument's sake—let us pretend it is 5 years from now and your anorexia hasn't changed. What would that be like for you?

PATIENT: I'd hate that—I'd be 30 by then, and I promised myself I would no longer have AN by then. My boyfriend would probably have given up on me. He is very keen to start a family, as am I, but we both agreed that I would need to be over the anorexia first. I guess starting a family then would still not be an option. I would have run out of goodwill from some of my friends, and it would break my parents' heart.

COMMENT

It is quite common that people with AN find it hard to keep up the momentum of change, especially if they have put on some weight rapidly. It is therefore often useful to revisit their original reasons for wanting to change with them.

Nutritional Health Phase

A focus on nutritional health is ongoing in therapy but is used flexibly. If, as in clinical illustration 2 earlier, a patient's nutritional health is poor and she is at high risk, motivating her to make some changes in her nutritional state and to reduce her overall risk will be a priority. However, if a patient is able to maintain her nutritional health at a level where the risk is only moderate, then there is less of a requirement for immediate change in the nutritional state. In such a situation, the patient and therapist can choose to move on to other areas of change. It may be appropriate to only come back to the issue of nutritional change after there is a greater understanding of the person's relationship with AN.

Once a person with AN becomes more open to the idea of improving her nutritional health, it can be helpful to go through what this implies in detail. Information is provided in the treatment manual on what a person who wants to recover from AN would need to eat and what a person with high medical risk would need to do to keep safely out of the hospital. Once again, the spirit and techniques of MI are employed in having a dialogue about this (as in the next clinical illustration, below). It maybe helpful to use the process of calculating the patient's typical daily energy expenditure as a means of monitoring personalized feedback. This straightforward and transparent process serves to build up trust, as the person with AN is able to see how the values are derived in a standardized way. The therapist then tries to elicit in detail a change plan relating to nutrition.

Clinical Illustration 4: Developing a Plan for Improving Nutritional Health

THERAPIST: Let's go back to think about what a day in your life would be if you were improving your nutritional safety. How do you see that rolling out?

PATIENT: I guess I'd need to eat a bit more and more regularly, like having meals and snacks. I find it very hard to remember that I have to eat when I am on my own. I am always so busy, and there are a thousand other things that I would rather do than eat. I get very frightened when I start eating—there is always that little voice in my head telling me I am too fat already and that I don't deserve to eat. It is very upsetting.

THERAPIST: Let me see whether I have understood this. At one level you know exactly what you need to do to improve your nutritional health. Yet, when you try to put that into practice, the anorexic voice gets very strong and stops you from going further. Focusing on other things rather than eating then helps you to reduce your distress.

PATIENT: (with sadness) When you say it like that, I can see I am really stuck.

THERAPIST: That makes you feel quite uncomfortable.

PATIENT: I just don't know how to get started.

THERAPIST: Would you like me to talk a bit about what other people in a similar situation to yours have found helpful when making a start in looking after their nutritional health?

PATIENT: (*Nods*).

COMMENT

The patient and therapist then brainstorm a number of different practical steps that may work for her in overcoming her impasse.

Involving Significant Others

Eating disorder symptoms strike at the core of family life, as the symptoms arise with each meal throughout the day. In addition to the core eating disorder symptoms, there are often additional symptoms such as compulsions, obsessions, self-harm, and violent verbal and physical outbursts. The interpersonal reactions to the illness within the family can be important in maintaining the illness. The anxiety about the illness frequently leads to an overprotective response from others, but this is interspersed with hostility engendered by the person's refusal to eat and deceit (e.g., pretending to have eaten when she hasn't) that develops. These responses of significant others are the core features of high expressed emotion, which may adversely affect the outcome of many psychiatric illnesses (Butzlaff & Hooley, 1998). As the average duration of AN is 6 years, the coping resources of significant others can easily become strained.

In our model, significant others—typically parents or partners—are invited to participate flexibly in sessions as required, to help them support the person with AN. On the whole, significant others of adults with AN are happy to be involved in the care of the patient—that is, to have health professionals share information with them and to have some input into the decisions for treatment. Patients, too, are generally happy to cooperate with some form of involvement from significant others. If the person with AN is at high medical risk, then it is considered good practice to involve close others, hopefully at a stage before there are legal imperatives to do so. The issue of confidentiality can be problematic. Patients should be made aware that only information essential to a patient's care will normally be disclosed to others. In the following example the patient discusses how she wants her parents to be involved.

Clinical Illustration 5

PATIENT: I need to be able to talk to somebody when I have had my breakfast or when I am having my breakfast.

THERAPIST: Talking to somebody will distract you from the anorexic voice. Who might be able to do that?

PATIENT: My parents will. It's going to be difficult because I haven't eaten with people for such a long time. So, to eat in front of them is going to be a real struggle. It's really scary.

This exchange would then be followed by the patient and therapist's developing a more detailed plan for how her parents might support her during and after mealtimes and how this would be discussed in a session with the parents. These joint therapy sessions are supplemented by optional separate MI-based skills workshops for significant others that have been developed to reduce conflict and criticism in the family.

Case Formulation and Working for Change

In the formulation phase a collaborative cognitive-behavioral case formulation is developed (Lavender & Schmidt, 2006). This is shared with the patient as a diagram and a letter. The practice of writing formulation letters is derived from cognitive analytical therapy (Ryle, 1995). A treatment plan is developed based on the formulation. Carefully chosen behavioral experiments focused on reducing emotional avoidance, perfectionism, and rigidity are also conducted. An example of a diagrammatic case formulation is given in Figure 8.2, together with an excerpt from the accompanying formulation letter outlining the patient's treatment plan.

Clinical Illustration 6: Case Formulation and Treatment Plan

Sarah was a 20-year-old woman who had a 6-year history of restricting anorexia and at the start of treatment had a body mass index of 15.5 kg/ m². Her daily food intake followed a rigid pattern of two small calorie-restricted meals during the day. Sarah lived at home with her parents and sister, Clare. Clare (age 23) had Down's syndrome and a number of associated medical difficulties. Sarah herself had been born prematurely

Early Experiences and Predisposing Factors

- Preterm birth, tendency to be anxious from early age
- Mom was anxious, always worried about us, protected us, especially Clare
- Clare was often ill and got a lot of attention as a result of this—I felt less important
- Dad was critical of me when I didn't achieve as well as he thought I could
- I never felt I fitted in that well—not one of the popular girls at school, always quite shy
- My family doesn't talk to each other about emotional issues—people keep things to themselves

Core Beliefs

- I'm weak, powerless, and vulnerable.
- I'm not good enough, different/defective.
- Others are likely to judge and criticize me.

Attitudes, Rules, and Assumptions

General:
- If I let people see I'm weak, or if they realize I'm different and not good enough, I'll be more vulnerable.
- I should keep my feelings to myself and others at a distance, so they don't find out I'm not good enough, weak, and different.
- I should be able to achieve the highest standards; if I don't, its proof I'm not good enough.
- If I work hard and keep focused, I might be able to reach the standards I need to.

Anorexia specific:
- If I can control my eating, I'm less weak and less vulnerable.
- Being able to control my eating means I'm good at something, and different in a good way rather than in a bad way.
- If I can control my eating, I can keep safe, focused, and clear.
- Keeping focused on my eating means I can keep others at a safe distance.
- If I'm ill, it hides the fact that I'm not good enough.

Triggers: Why Anorexia?

- Feeling stressed about schoolwork, my friends getting boyfriends; discovered losing weight and going to the gym made me feel better and initially others admired me for it

Functions of My Anorexia and My Beliefs About It

Intrapersonal (within me):
- Safety, keeps me in my "bubble"
- Control: everything is clear and simple
- Achievement: it's something I'm good at
- It makes me "good" different rather than "bad" different
- Avoidance: means I don't have to think about or feel bad about other things

(continued)

Interpersonal (with others):
- Avoidance: means I can keep others away, stay in my safe "bubble"
- Care: although I get annoyed with my parents for interfering, at least they notice me, and because it's an "illness" it's not so much my fault or because I'm not good enough

Behaviors

- Restrict my food, follow my rules exactly.
- Keep my emotions to myself, and don't get too near to people.
- Try really hard with everything—don't stop until its perfect.

Other Factors That Maintain My Anorexia

Starvation effects:
- I feel bloated if I eat anything at all
- I feel OK at this weight—its hard to believe that there's anything wrong when I feel well.

FIGURE 8.2. Example of a diagrammatic case formulation.

and had needed to spend a month in the hospital before being allowed to go home. Sarah described her family as generally close and caring, although they did not talk a great deal about their personal feelings, and there had been a lot of arguments over the past few years about her eating habits and weight. She said she and her mom got on well but that her father could be quite critical when she did not do as well as he thought she could, and sometimes was "a bit of a bully" as a result of this. Sarah said she loved Clare, but she felt that it had been hard growing up having an ill sister, as she had sometimes felt that Clare got all the attention. She added that she felt guilty for feeling like this, as she "shouldn't think selfish things like that."

As may be seen in this formulation, AN has important intra- and interpersonal functions for Sarah.

Below we provide an excerpt from the therapist's formulation letter for Sarah, taken from the end of the letter, where the jointly developed treatment goals are discussed.

> *Together we have decided on a plan for your further treatment. The key changes you would like to make in your life are (1) to be able to express your thoughts, feelings, and needs to other people openly and assertively and to say "no" to other people rather than to always please others and comply with their requests; (2) to learn to "be good enough" rather than always having to do things perfectly;*

(3) to relearn to eat healthily and maintain a healthy weight. Over the next 10 to 15 sessions we will be working together to help you develop new skills and new ways of approaching situations relevant to your goals, and I very much look forward to this.

Relapse Prevention and Ending

During the final phase of treatment there is a focus on relapse prevention and ending. This involves the client and the therapist taking stock of what has been achieved in treatment, what remains to be done, and their plan for the future, including a discussion of the pros and cons of further change. Both the therapist and the patient write each other a good-bye letter.

Additional Facets of Treatment: Narrative and Externalizing Approaches

We found that people with AN are often much more able to express their thoughts and feelings on paper than face to face, perhaps because it gives them more control over what is said. Thus, in addition to the usual strategies of MI and the tools to elicit change talk, such as the motivational ruler and the decisional balance sheet, we use narrative techniques in the form of written tasks throughout treatment. For example, the letters written to AN as a friend or enemy highlight the positive and negative aspects of AN in the person's life and help to explore the decisional balance. Moreover, these letters serve to introduce the concept of externalizing the disorder. There is a tendency for the person to take on the mantle of AN as an identity perhaps—because the illness strikes when adult identity is forming, and the two become entangled. Thus, many patients have no concept of a mature identity without AN (Tan, Hope, & Stewart, 2003). We use the term "anorexic voice" or more personalized epithets to refer to AN symptoms. Writing tasks set in a hypothetical future either with or without the eating disorder enable the individual to take a broader perspective on her illness and to think about other goals, values, and life directions she would like to take. Thus, many of these writing tasks are adaptations of standard MI procedures designed to increase discrepancy, and they include elements such as looking forward, looking backward, describing a typical day, looking at the best and worst aspects of continuing problematic behaviors, and so on.

Later in the therapy, writing tasks focused on the role of AN in the person's life or on key events or relationships are used to reduce emotional avoidance and foster the processing of emotionally salient material while giving the patient control over what and how much she feels able to divulge. Specifically constructed writing tasks are also used to aid perspective shifting and to help patients get away from an excessive focus on detail and instead to see the bigger picture "in life" and resolve ambivalence about change. Writing also allows coming to terms with upsetting things, finding new meanings, and finding new solutions to difficulties. These tasks are presented to patients as homework assignments but always in a motivational style, that is, offered as something that they may wish to try. Further details about the use of these writing tasks can be found in Schmidt, Bone, Hems, Lessem, and Treasure (2002).

Family Skills Workshops

Significant others have deficits in skills and knowledge about managing eating disorder symptoms (Whitney et al., 2005). We have developed a model of significant other coping and have designed a manualized collaborative care intervention (Treasure, Smith, & Crane, 2007; Treasure, Whitaker, Whitney, & Schmidt, 2005). The curriculum includes modules on coping, medical risk, understanding change, communication, emotion processing, problem solving, interpersonal relationships, and managing eating and other difficult behaviors. This is supplemented by skills-based workshops and teaching significant others the spirit and key skills of MI and CBT. Some of the elements of this treatment resemble those of community reinforcement family treatment (CRAFT; Smith, Meyers, & Miller, 2001), where families of people with addictions are taught how to increase the motivation of their close other for treatment.

Teaching significant others some of the skills of MI serves to open up communication with the patient. Significant others especially value the skills of reflective listening. The following comment from a parent illustrates the positive impact that being taught reflective listening had on his interaction with his anorectic daughter:

> "Yeah, [I] just like practicing reflective listening. I came out of that and went, wow, that's going to change how I'm going to talk to D. And when I've really tried to consciously use it, it has. And it's worked and I think, I mean, I think that's what it was. It wasn't like trying to be like an analyst or anything like that—it was just listening and not feeling like I had to solve D's problems in one conversa-

tion. And just kind of, it's OK that everything isn't OK, and just accepting. I think that's a lot of it—just accepting the situation as it is now and not constantly feeling guilty about it. That was quite a revelation."

We also use writing tasks with significant others, analogous to the work with our patients, as a way of processing emotions and repairing the relationship with the loved one, giving them such tasks as writing about "what my daughter means to me."

RESEARCH INTO MOTIVATIONAL INTERVENTIONS IN EATING DISORDERS

In contrast to the situation with BN, where there are many clinical trials available, conducting treatment research into AN is difficult. The relative rarity of the disorder makes it hard for any one center to have sufficient cases to mount well-powered large studies, and the life-threatening nature of the disorder makes it difficult to study "pure" interventions. As yet, only a handful of randomized controlled clinical trials (RCTs) exist, none of them on motivational interventions. However, there is some information on the impact of pretreatment motivation, readiness and confidence to change, and treatment outcomes.

In the treatment of AN, variables such as motivation, readiness or confidence to change, or "stage of change" have been found to predict whether people start treatment (Geller, 2002) or drop out (Gowers, Smyth, & Shore, 2004), whether they gain weight during treatment (Gowers et al., 2004; Rieger et al., 2000) and longer-term outcomes (Schubert, Landau, & Treasure, 2008), underscoring the importance of addressing these variables in treatment. In AN, individual case studies (Treasure & Ward, 1997) and two small uncontrolled studies (Feld, Woodside, Kaplan, Olmsted, & Carter, 2001; Gowers et al., 2004) have examined the effect of a motivational intervention on patient outcome. In one of these, an assessment that used an MI style was associated with an increase in motivation from before to after the assessment (Gowers et al., 2004). In the second study (Feld et al., 2001), a four-session motivational enhancement therapy (MET)[2] intervention was offered to people with eating disorders, mainly those with AN. Motivation and confidence to change increased significantly from session one to four.

In BN, motivational variables do not consistently predict outcomes. In one study "stage of change" failed to predict dropout but did predict outcome from interpersonal therapy, though not from CBT (Wolk & Devlin, 2001). In another study, "stage of change" predicted change in the expected direction in bingeing but not in weight-control measures (Katzman et al., 2007; Treasure et al., 1999). In yet another study, patient desire to stop bulimic behaviors and expected success of treatment did predict remission of bulimic symptoms (Mussell et al., 2000). Finally, poor motivation to change has been found to predict relapse from BN (Halmi et al., 2002). The transtheoretical model of change, on which concepts such as "stages of change" have been based, has recently come under criticism on conceptual and methodological grounds (Wilson & Schlam, 2004). Thus, the inconsistent results regarding "stage of change" may not be all that surprising.

Three RCTs have examined MI or MET in bulimic disorders. In one of these on 90 participants with BN or binge eating disorder, MI plus a CBT self-help manual achieved higher abstinence rates from bingeing at 6 months than the CBT self-help manual alone (Dunn, Neighbors, & Larimer, 2006). In another RCT, 225 participants with BN or eating disorder not otherwise specified were allocated to one of three groups to receive four sessions of individual MET either followed by eight sessions of group or individual CBT or four sessions of individual CBT followed by group CBT. (The obvious fourth group of four sessions of individual CBT followed by eight sessions of individual CBT was not included due to resource constraints.) MET demonstrated no advantage over CBT in terms of engaging participants in subsequent CBT or in terms of short-term (at 4 weeks) or longer-term (12 weeks, 1 year, and 2.5 years) eating disorder outcomes (Katzman et al., 2007; Treasure et al., 1999). In this study, all therapists conducted both MET and CBT treatments, with separate supervision and treatment manuals for both conditions. However, resource constraints did not allow for formal assessment of treatment fidelity and therapist competence. Thus, the possibility that treatment fidelity or therapist competence was suboptimal cannot be excluded. The majority of patients in this study were already in the contemplation stage, and none was in precontemplation at the start of treatment (Treasure et al., 1999). It is possible that MET might be more effective in improving adherence and subsequent outcome in a less motivated group.

A third RCT of 61 patients with BN examined the addition of repeated personalized motivational feedback, as is typically part of MET, to a cognitive- behavioral guided self-help treatment (Schmidt et al., 2006). Feedback on bulimic and other symptoms such as anxiety, depression, and interpersonal functioning was used to initiate motivational conversations with patients about their readiness and confidence to change and potential barriers to this. While added feedback did not have an effect on adherence to treatment, it did reduce self-induced vomiting and dietary restriction more effectively than guided self-care without added feedback.

CONCLUSIONS

MI and related approaches are highly relevant and applicable to the field of eating disorders. Although in this chapter we have focused mainly on anorexia nervosa, we wish to stress that we see MI as potentially relevant to all eating disorders. Miller himself cautioned that "the popularity of MI has largely preceded the availability of efficacy data" (Miller, 2001), and this is certainly true in eating disorders. Much more research into MI and MET in eating disorders is needed for us to be able to fully gauge what the place of these interventions is in our therapeutic armamentarium. So far, in eating disorders MI and MET have been mainly used as pretreatments prior to other interventions, in particular CBT. However, in milder or partial cases of eating disorders, MI or MET could be explored as a stand-alone treatment, as in those cases a formal case conceptualization and the skills building that is required in more complex cases may not be necessary. Finally, teaching those who care for people with eating disorders to use MI strategies to reduce conflict and help the AN patient move toward recovery seems a promising strategy to pursue.

NOTES

1. We studied the contents of these letters and extracted the themes that emerged (Serpell, Treasure, Teasdale, & Sullivan, 1999). These were then synthesized into a research instrument that measures the pros and cons of anorexia (Gale, Holliday, Troop, Serpell, & Treasure, 2006; Serpell, Neiderman, Haworth, Emmanueli, & Lask, 2003; Serpell, Teasdale, Troop, & Treasure, 2004). The most important pro-anorexia themes identified in studies using this instrument were that AN helps people to feel safe and in control and that it stifles emotions and communicates distress.

2. Motivational enhancement therapy is a brief treatment based on the stages-of-change model and motivational interviewing (Miller, Zweben, Di Clemente, & Rychtarik, 2002). The aims of this treatment are to increase people's intrinsic

motivation to change. Treatment includes giving feedback, MI techniques, discussion of obstacles and options for change, emphasis on personal choice and the patient's own problem-solving skills, and formulating a change plan.

REFERENCES

Bemis, K. M. (1986). *A comparison of the subjective experience of individuals with eating disorders and phobic disorders: The "weight-phobia" versus the "approach-avoidance" models of anorexia nervosa.* Unpublished doctoral dissertation, University of Minnesota, Minneapolis.

Beumont, P., Hay, P., Beumont, D., Birmingham, L., Derham, H., Jordan, A., et al. (2004). Australian and New Zealand clinical practice guidelines for the treatment of anorexia nervosa. *Australian and New Zealand Journal of Psychiatry, 38,* 659–670.

Blake, W., Turnbull, S., & Treasure, J. L. (1997). Stages and processes of change in eating disorders: Implications for therapy. *Clinical Psychology and Psychotherapy, 4,* 186–191.

Claudino, A., Hay, P., Lima, M., Bacaltchuk, J., Schmidt, U., & Treasure, J. (2006). Antidepressants for anorexia nervosa. *Cochrane Database of Systematic Reviews;* (1), CD004365.

Collier, D. A., & Treasure, J. L. (2004). The aetiology of eating disorders. *British Journal of Psychiatry, 185,* 363–365.

COMBINE Study Research Group. (2003). Testing combined pharmacotherapies and behavioral interventions in alcohol dependence: Rationale and methods. *Alcoholism: Clinical and Experimental Research, 27,* 1107–1122.

Cooper, M. J., Wells, A., & Todd, G. (2004) A cognitive model of BN. *British Journal of Clinical Psychology, 43,* 1–16.

Crisp, A. H., Norton, K., Gowers, S., Halek, C., Bowyer, C., Yeldham, D., et al. (1991). A controlled study of the effect of therapies aimed at adolescent and family psychopathology in anorexia nervosa. *British Journal of Psychiatry, 159,* 325–333.

Dunn, E. C., Neighbors, C., & Larimer, M. E. (2006). Motivational enhancement therapy and self-help treatment for binge eaters. *Psychology of Addictive Behaviors, 20,* 44–52.

Eisler, I., Dare, C., Hodes, M., Russell, G., Dodge, E., & Le Grange, D. (2000). Family therapy for adolescent anorexia nervosa: The results of a controlled comparison of two family interventions. *Journal of Child Psychology and Psychiatry, 41,* 727–736.

Fairburn, C. G., & Bohn, K. (2005). Eating disorder NOS (EDNOS): An example of the troublesome "not otherwise specified" (NOS) category in DSM-IV. *Behaviour Research and Therapy, 43,* 691–701.

Fairburn, C. G., & Brownell, K. D. (Eds.). (2001). *Eating disorders and obesity: A comprehensive handbook* (2nd ed.). New York: Guilford Press.

Fairburn, C. G., Cooper, Z., & Shafran, R. (2003). Cognitive behaviour therapy for eating disorders: A transdiagnostic theory and treatment. *Behaviour Research and Therapy, 41*, 509–528.

Favaro, A., Ferrara, S., & Santonastaso, P. (2003). The spectrum of eating disorders in young women: A prevalence study in a general population sample. *Psychosomatic Medicine, 65*, 701–708.

Feld, R., Woodside, D. B., Kaplan, A. S., Olmsted, M. P., & Carter, J. C. (2001). Pretreatment motivational enhancement therapy for eating disorders: A pilot study. *International Journal of Eating Disorders, 29*, 393–400.

Gale, C., Holliday, J., Troop, N. A., Serpell, L., & Treasure, J. (2006). The pros and cons of change in individuals with eating disorders: A broader perspective. *International Journal of Eating Disorders, 39*, 394–403.

Geller, J. (2002). Estimating readiness for change in anorexia nervosa: Comparing clients, clinicians, and research assessors. *International Journal of Eating Disorders, 31*, 251–260.

Gowers, S. G., Smyth, B., & Shore, A. (2004). The impact of a motivational assessment interview on initial response to treatment in adolescent anorexia nervosa. *European Eating Disorder Review, 12*, 87–93.

Halmi, K. A., Agras, W. S., Mitchell, J., Wilson, G. T., Crow, S., Bryson, S. W., et al. (2002). Relapse predictors of patients with BN who achieved abstinence through cognitive behavioral therapy. *Archives of General Psychiatry, 59*, 1105–1109.

Harris, E. C., & Barraclough, B. (1998). Excess mortality of mental disorder. *British Journal of Psychiatry, 173*, 11–53.

Hay, P. J., Bacaltchuk, J., & Stefano, S. (2004). Psychotherapy for bulimia nervosa and binging. *Cochrane Database of Systematic Reviews*; (3), CD000562.

Jacobi, C., Hayward, C., de Zwaan, M., Kraemer, H. C., & Agras, W. S. (2004). Coming to terms with risk factors for eating disorders: Application of risk terminology and suggestions for a general taxonomy. *Psychological Bulletin, 130*, 19–65.

Katzman, M. A., Bara-Carril, N., Rabe-Hesketh, S., Schmidt, U., deSilva, P., Troop, N., et al. (2007). *A randomized controlled two-stage trial in the treatment of bulimia nervosa, comparing CBT versus motivational enhancement in phase 1 followed by group versus individual CBT in phase 2.* Manuscript submitted for publication.

Keel P. K., & Klump, K. L. (2003). Are eating disorders culture-bound syndromes?: Implications for conceptualizing their etiology. *Psychological Bulletin, 129*, 747–769.

Lavender, A., & Schmidt, U. (2006). Cognitive-behavioral case formulation in complex eating disorders. In N. Tarrier (Ed.), *Case formulation in cognitive behaviour therapy: The treatment of challenging and complex cases* (pp. 238–262). East Sussex, UK: Routledge.

Miller, W. R. (2001). Comments on Dunn et al.'s "The use of brief interventions adapted from motivational interviewing across behavioral domains: A systematic review." When is it motivational interviewing? *Addiction, 96*, 1770–1772; discussion, 1774–1775.

Miller, W. R., & Rollnick, S. (2002). *Motivational interviewing: Preparing people for change* (2nd ed.). New York: Guilford Press.

Miller, W. R., Zweben, A., DiClemente, C. C., & Rychtarik, R. (2002). *Motivational enhancement manual: A clinical research guide for therapists treating individuals with alcohol abuse and dependence* (Project MATCH Monograph Series, Vol. 2). Rockville, MD: National Institute of Alcohol Abuse and Alcoholism.

Minuchin, S., Rosman, B. L., & Baker, L. (1978). *Psychosomatic families.* Cambridge, MA: Harvard University Press.

Mussell, M. P., Mitchell, J. E., Crosby, R. D., Fulkerson, J. A., Hoberman, H. M., & Romano, J. L. (2000). Commitment to treatment goals in prediction of group Cognitive-Behavioral Therapy treatment outcome for women with bulimia nervosa. *Journal of Consulting and Clinical Psychology, 68*, 432–437.

National Collaborating Centre for Mental Health. (2004). *National Clinical Practice Guideline: Eating disorders: Core interventions in the treatment and management of anorexia nervosa, bulimia nervosa, and related eating disorders.* London: National Institute for Health and Clinical Excellence.

Palmer, B. (2003). Concepts of eating disorders. In J. Treasure, U. Schmidt, & E. Van Furth (Eds.), *Handbook of eating disorders* (2nd ed.). Chichester, UK: Wiley.

Pike, K. M., Walsh, B. T., Vitousek, K., Wilson, G. T., & Bauer, J. (2003). Cognitive behavior therapy in the posthospitalization treatment of anorexia nervosa. *American Journal of Psychiatry, 160*, 2046–2049.

Prochaska, J. O., DiClemente, C. C., & Norcross, J. C. (1992). In search of how people change. *American Psychologist, 47*, 1102–1114.

Rieger, E., Touyz, S., Schotte, D., Beumont, P., Russell, J., Clarke, S., et al. (2000). Development of an instrument to assess readiness to recover in anorexia nervosa. *International Journal of Eating Disorders, 28*, 387–396.

Russell, G. (1979). Bulimia nervosa: An ominous variant of anorexia nervosa. *Psychological Medicine, 9*, 429–448.

Ryle, A. (1995). *Cognitive analytic therapy: Developments in theory and practice.* Chichester, UK: Wiley.

Schmidt, U. (1989). Behavioural psychotherapy for eating disorders. *International Review Journal of Psychiatry, 1*, 245–256.

Schmidt, U., Bone, G., Hems, S., Lessem, J., & Treasure, J. (2002). Structured therapeutic writing tasks as an adjunct to treatment in eating disorders. *European Eating Disorders Review, 10*, 1–17.

Schmidt, U., Landau, S., Pombo-Carril, M. G., Bara-Carril, N., Reid, Y., Murray, K., et al. (2006). Does feedback improve the outcome of guided self-care in bulimia nervosa?: A preliminary randomised controlled trial. *British Journal of Clinical Psychology, 45*, 111–121.

Schmidt, U., & Treasure, J. (2006). Anorexia nervosa: Valued and visible. A cognitive-interpersonal maintenance model and its implications for research and practice. *British Journal of Clinical Psychology, 45*, 3443–366.

Schubert, I., Landau, S., & Treasure, J. (2008). *The role of inpatient treatment in reducing medical risk in people with anorexia nervosa: A study of the predictors of the duration of treatment and short and long term body mass index in a series of cases with severe anorexia nervosa.* Manuscript in preparation.

Serfaty, M. A. (1999). Cognitive therapy versus dietary counselling in the outpatient treatment of anorexia nervosa: Effects of the treatment phase. *European Eating Disorders Review, 7*, 334–350.

Serpell, L., Neiderman, M., Haworth, E., Emmanueli, F., & Lask, B. (2003). The use of the Pros and Cons of Anorexia Nervosa (P-CAN) Scale with children and adolescents. *Journal of Psychosomatic Research, 54*, 567–571.

Serpell, L., Teasdale, J. D., Troop, N. A., & Treasure, J. (2004). The development of the P-CAN, a measure to operationalize the pros and cons of anorexia nervosa. *International Journal of Eating Disorders, 36*, 416–433.

Serpell, L., Treasure, J., Teasdale, J., & Sullivan, V. (1999). Anorexia nervosa: Friend or foe? *International Journal of Eating Disorders, 25*, 177–186.

Smith, J. E., Meyers, R. J., & Miller, W. R. (2001). The community reinforcement approach to the treatment of substance use disorders. *American Journal of Addictions, 10*(Suppl.), 51–59.

Tan, J. O., Hope, T., & Stewart, A. (2003). Anorexia nervosa and personal identity: The accounts of patients and their parents. *International Journal of Law in Psychiatry, 26*, 533–548.

Touyz, S. W., Beumont, P. J., Glaun, D., Phillips, T., & & Cowie, I. (1984). A comparison of lenient and strict operant conditioning programmes in refeeding patients with anorexia nervosa. *British Journal of Psychiatry, 144*, 517–520.

Treasure, J. L., Katzman, M., Schmidt, U., Troop, N., Todd, G., & De Silva, P. (1999). Engagement and outcome in the treatment of bulimia nervosa: First phase of a sequential design comparing motivation enhancement therapy and cognitive behavioural therapy. *Behaviour Research and Therapy, 3*(7), 405–418.

Treasure, J., & Schmidt, U. (2005). Anorexia nervosa. *Clinical Evidence, 14*, 1140–1148.

Treasure, J., Smith, G., & Crane, A. (2007). *Skills-based learning in caring for a loved one with an eating disorder: The new Maudsley method.* London: Routledge.

Treasure, J. L., & Ward, A. (1997). A practical guide to the use of motivational interviewing in anorexia nervosa. *European Eating Disorders Review, 5*, 102–114.

Treasure, J., Whitaker, W., Whitney, J., & Schmidt, U. (2005). Working with families of adults with anorexia nervosa. *Journal of Family Therapy, 27*, 101–103.

Vitousek, K., Watson, S., & Wilson, G. T. (1998). Enhancing motivation for change in treatment-resistant eating disorders. *Clinical Psychology Review, 18*, 391–420.

Ward, A., Troop, N., Todd, G., & Treasure, J. (1996). To change or not to change—"how" is the question? *British Journal of Medical Psychology, 69*, 139–146.

Whitney, J., Murray, J., Gavan, K., Todd, G., Whitaker, W., & Treasure, J. (2005). Experience of caring for someone with anorexia nervosa: Qualitative study. *British Journal of Psychiatry, 187*, 444–449.

Wilson, G. T., & Schlam, T. R. (2004). The transtheoretical model and motivational interviewing in the treatment of eating and weight disorders. *Clinical Psychology Review, 24*, 361–378.

Wolk, S. L., & Devlin, M. J. (2001). Stage of change as a predictor of response to psychotherapy for bulimia nervosa. *International Journal of Eating Disorders, 30*, 96–100.

Zipfel, S., Löwe, B., & Herzog, W. (2003). Medical complications in eating disorders and obesity. In J. Treasure, U. Schmidt, & E. van Furth (Eds.), *Handbook of eating disorders: Theory, treatment and research.* (2nd ed.). Chichester, UK: Wiley.

Motivational Interviewing in the Treatment of Problem and Pathological Gambling

David Hodgins
Katherine M. Diskin

THE CLINICAL POPULATION

Gambling is generally understood to incorporate the element of risk in an organized way, in which the individual risks something he or she has in the hope of acquiring more. Forms of gambling have existed across the ages and cultures of humanity. Primitive dice made from the knucklebones of sheep (astralagi) have been found in caves dating from 3,500 B.C. (Bernstein, 1996), while in 2006, 6.5 million Americans visited Internet gambling sites (American Gaming Association, 2007). Even when gambling has not been legally sanctioned, illegal gambling opportunities such as floating card and crap games, bookies, numbers, and illegal slot machines have been available. Some forms of gambling are legal in all provinces of Canada and every state in the United States except Utah and Hawaii, with local and regional governments participating in providing gambling opportunities and sharing in gambling revenue.

The majority of gamblers, like the majority of drinkers, do not experience adverse effects from their activities; however, excessive gambling has been a source of serious distress for centuries. Romans who could not pay their gambling debts were sold into slavery (National Research Council, 1999), while gambling-related suicide attempt rates for problem and pathological gamblers currently range from 7 to 26% (Hodgins, Mansley, & Thygesen, 2006).

Although "gambling mania" was identified as a form of "monomania" in the early 1800s, pathological gambling was included in the American Psychiatric Association's *Diagnostic and Statistical Manual of Mental Disorders* (DSM) for the first time in 1980 as a disorder of impulse control. The criteria for pathological gambling disorder have continued to be modified in subsequent editions of the manual. At present, according to DSM-IV-TR (American Psychiatric Association, 2000), "the essential feature of pathological gambling is persistent and recurrent maladaptive gambling behavior . . . that disrupts personal, family or vocational pursuits" (p. 671). The criteria for pathological gambling disorder combine criteria relating to the effects of gambling (for example, legal and relationship problems, hiding losses) with criteria similar to substance abuse (tolerance, withdrawal) and include the use of gambling as a means of escaping from problems or relieving a dysphoric mood (Cunningham-Williams & Cottler, 2001). Estimates of the prevalence of pathological gambling are about 1% in the past year (Gerstein et al., 1999; Shaffer & Hall, 2001; Welte, Barnes, Wieczorek, Tidwell, & Parker, 2004).

Unlike substance use disorders there is no "abuse" classification in DSM-IV to take into account subclinical but still problematic gambling behavior. Nonetheless, rates of problem gambling are typically estimated in prevalence surveys and fall in the range of 2–3% (Shaffer & Hall, 2001). These estimates suggest that in total about 4% of adult North Americans experienced negative consequences from gambling last year.

The effects of problem and pathological gambling are wide-ranging. Gamblers are at high risk for stress-related physical illnesses and comorbid psychiatric disorders. It is clear that problem gambling affects more that just the gambler. Family, friends, employers, and health and social welfare systems all feel the impact of problem gambling. Gamblers often face serious legal problems as a result of committing illegal acts to finance their gambling. More specifically, problem and pathological gamblers are more likely than recreational gamblers to be divorced, to have received welfare, to have experienced bankruptcy, to have been arrested, and to have physical and psychological health problems (Report to the National Gambling Impact Study Commission, cited in Volberg, 2001). The relative speed at which increased gambling opportunities have become available has made it difficult to accurately estimate the extent of the financial and social costs of gambling problems.

USUAL TREATMENT

Based on various understandings of the factors that cause and maintain problem gambling, modalities used in its treatment have included psychoanalysis, client-centered supportive therapy, various forms of group therapy, marital therapy, behavioral and cognitive therapies including self-help manuals, Gamblers Anonymous (GA) groups, and pharmacological treatments. Empirical research on treatment efficacy has not been extensive, with few randomized clinical trials in the literature. A recent review of gambling treatment noted that much gambling treatment research has involved case studies, small samples, and uncontrolled interventions (Toneatto & Ladouceur, 2003). Only 11 randomized clinical trials were identified, with numerous methodological limitations. These studies encompassed a number of behavioral interventions, including various combinations of imaginal desensitization, electric aversion, and *in vivo* exposure to gambling situations; cognitive behavioral interventions; two pharmacological studies using fluvoxamine and naltrexone; and two studies that used self-help workbooks with and without telephone support. The authors of the review concluded that "interventions that fall within the cognitive-behavioral spectrum, even when delivered via a manual and involving only minimal therapist contact, have the most empirical support. The limited evidence also suggests that the length or intensiveness of treatment may not be important variables in regard to outcome" (Toneatto & Ladouceur, 2003, pp. 13–15).

RATIONALE FOR USING MOTIVATIONAL INTERVIEWING WITH GAMBLING PROBLEMS

Motivational interviewing (MI) is a natural fit for the area of problem and pathological gambling for a number of reasons. First, it is clear that impairment of control and motivation are important features of the disorder. The conceptualization of pathological gambling is a matter of some debate, with some theorists focusing on its similarity to addictive disorders such as substance abuse. Some view pathological gambling as an impulse control disorder, and others consider it to fall on the obsessive–compulsive spectrum (National Research Council, 1999). The diagnostic criteria of the DSM-IV-TR reflect the lack of clear a consensus: the criteria are modeled after those of substance dependence, but the disorder is placed within the impulse disorders section of the manual

(American Psychiatric Association, 2000). Regardless, the various conceptualizations share the recognition that impairment of control over gambling is a central feature of the disorder and, as a result, a struggle with motivational factors is pivotal in outcome. It is common to use treatment approaches for pathological gambling that are adapted from substance abuse treatment models, such as cognitive-behavioral treatments.

Recently the idea of addiction as a "disorder of motivation" (Heather, 2005) has been suggested. It is based on the idea that the "addict" is choosing to behave in a way that is against his or her long-term interests. This definition includes more than the idea that the person is doing something that society finds unacceptable—this is something that the individual him- or herself (at least sometimes) wants to change, resulting in "a motivational conflict composed of the contrasting incentives and disincentives. . . . The resolution of such a conflict is, of course, at the heart of MI" (Heather, 2005, pp. 4–5).

A second reason that MI fits with pathological gambling is the observation that recovery from gambling problems without treatment (i.e., natural recovery) is common (Hodgins, Wynne, & Makarchuk, 1999). The existence of self-directed recovery is consistent with the notion that motivation is central in the change process. Interviews with recovered pathological gamblers confirm that cognitive-motivational factors are perceived to be primary in maintaining abstinence from gambling (Hodgins & el-Guebaly, 2000).

CLINICAL APPLICATION OF MI TO PROBLEM AND PATHOLOGICAL GAMBLING

As with many mental health disorders, rates of treatment seeking are low relative to the prevalence estimates of the number of people suffering from the disorder. Less than 10% of problem gamblers in the United States seek out the available treatments (Cunningham, 2005; National Gambling Impact Study Commission, 1999). To the extent that low treatment seeking is related to motivation and lack of access to treatment, two potential complementary solutions are to increase the motivation of individuals to seek formal treatment and to broaden the treatment options by offering more accessible types of treatment. We present examples of both these approaches that use MI principles. First, we present the use of a brief motivational intervention to increase the efficacy of a self-help workbook for pathological gambling. Second, we provide a description of a one-session motivational intervention to encourage reduction of gambling behavior.

A third application of MI to gambling treatment relates to treatment compliance. Dropout rates in both psychosocial and pharmacological clinical trials are unacceptably high (Grant, Kim, & Potenza, 2003; Hodgins & Petry, 2004; Toneatto & Ladouceur, 2003). An Australian study illustrated the value of a variety of compliance-improving interventions in increasing attendance in outpatient cognitive-behavioral therapy for problem gambling (Milton, Crino, Hunt, & Prosser, 2002). The compliance-improving interventions included providing written and verbal reinforcement for attendance, encouraging a sense of optimism and self-efficacy about the outcome, providing feedback on assessment results, the regular use of decisional balance exercises between sessions, and the discussion of barriers to treatment involvement. A number of these strategies were adapted from the MI literature. Together these compliance-improving interventions increased treatment completion rates to 65% from a baseline of 35% completion before the changes.

Promoting Self-Recovery in Pathological Gamblers Using Motivational Enhancement

To capitalize on the desire of some problem gamblers to recover without formal help (Hodgins & el-Guebaly, 2000), a self-help workbook was developed that incorporated the techniques that recovered gamblers identified in interviews as significant in the recovery process (Hodgins & Makarchuk, 2002). The content of the workbook includes sections on self-assessment, goal setting, cognitive-behavioral strategies, relapse prevention strategies, and information about more formal treatment resources.[1]

We assessed the efficacy of providing self-help materials to pathological gamblers who did not wish to enter formal treatment in a clinical trial. Media recruitment was used, and two alternative self-help protocols were compared to a 1-month waiting-list control (see Hodgins, Currie, & el-Guebaly, 2001, for details). The first approach involved simply providing a self-help workbook via the mail (workbook-only group); the second involved a telephone motivational interview prior to receiving the workbook (motivational group). The workbook was distributed as a bound booklet, with the instruction that the participant work through the exercises at his or her own pace.

The motivational interview took between 20 and 45 minutes and was conducted using MI principles (Miller & Rollnick, 2002). The general aim of the interview was to be supportive and empathic and to demonstrate interest in the client's problem. The interview had four goals in addition to collecting basic assessment information. The interviewer attempted to elicit the gamblers' concerns, including the difficulties they were experiencing. For example:

> "What worries have you had about your gambling? What makes you think you need to change your gambling?".

The interviewer queried effects on financial and legal status, relationships, and emotional functioning and elicited gamblers' thoughts about the advantages of quitting. The second and third goals of the interview were to explore the gambler's ambivalence about change and to promote self-efficacy:

> "What might make it difficult to accomplish a change in your gambling? How successful do you think you will be? Looking back, what makes you think you can accomplish it?"

Finally, the interviewer suggested specific strategies for the individual based on past successful change attempts. These strategies were tied to a section of the workbook. For example:

> "It sounds like starting exercising was helpful when you quit drinking. There is a section in the workbook that recommends taking on new activities—that might be helpful."

After the interview, the clinicians prepared a brief personalized note to the gambler that was sent in the mail along with the workbook.

Many U.S. states and Canadian provinces offer problem gambling help lines to provide treatment information and personal support to individuals. This motivational intervention protocol is ideally suited to be integrated into such a service, as has been done in the statewide gambling treatment system in Oregon. Our research experience is that it does successfully attract individuals not interested in formal treatment.

Description of a Typical Participant

Belinda is married and is in her late 40s. Her husband is in charge of their finances and has recently told her that if she doesn't get her slot machine gambling under control he will leave her. She has tried GA, but found that she didn't like the religious aspect of it and that listening to other people talk about gambling made her gambling urges even stronger. She also found it difficult to identify herself as the type of person who goes to GA. The idea of a treatment approach in which she can work at her own pace and speak with someone over the phone really appealed to her.

During the motivational interview, Belinda spoke a lot about her self-image and how she did not see herself as the type of person who would get addicted. She identified a sense of challenge and the pleasure of escaping the boredom of life for a while as significant positive aspects of playing the slots for her, although she recognized the negative impact on her marriage, finances, and self-esteem. Belinda described herself as being highly self-directed and having a reasonable amount of self-control. She was interested to hear that many people successfully recover from gambling. When asked about previous behavior changes, she described how she had lost a great deal of weight when she was a teen. The therapist linked the strategies that she had used to lose weight—setting short-term goals, exercising regularly with friends, and reminding herself of her long-term goals—to the contents of the workbook.

The telephone interview lasted about 40 minutes and ended with the therapist giving a summary statement, as recommended in MI. At the end of the interview, the therapist told Belinda:

> "I am impressed with how open you are to talking about your struggles. It sounds like you like the challenge of playing the slots and like the fact that it gives you time alone. On the other hand, it has caused you a number of problems—both you and your husband are upset with the financial cost, and you are starting to spend your savings, which will have implications for your long-term goal of retiring to the coast. As well, you are a strong person, so the gambling takes its toll on your self-esteem. You find it hard to believe that you would continue to gamble. You have tackled hard personal issues before—your weight—and it sounds like you might be ready to tackle this one."

Belinda did, in fact, set some short-term gambling goals, following the suggestions in the workbook. These goals included not gambling for 2 weeks as an evaluation period. She changed her behavior by arranging to go for daily walks with a friend right after work, which was when she typically would visit the casino. She decided to track her finances more closely to monitor her "savings" from not gambling. She also prepared herself for how she would handle the urges to gamble through distraction and reminding herself about her long-term goals.

Belinda gambled once after the 2-week period but immediately felt that she wanted to make it her last time. She recommitted herself to her goals and strategies and did not gamble again.

One-Session Motivational Intervention for Problem Gambling

The promoting self-recovery approach that was described above was focused on providing a telephone contact and written materials to individuals seeking to change their behavior. This next study involved comparing a face-to-face motivational intervention with a clinical interview that did not contain motivational components in order to determine whether the MI elements of the contact specifically accounted for the response. We advertised for participants who were experiencing some concerns about their gambling. They were invited to attend an interview and were given the self-help workbook described above.

In developing a brief interview that could be used with a wide range of individuals with varying levels of gambling problems and varying levels of concern about their gambling, our primary goal was to incorporate the spirit of MI into the intervention. The interview was intended as an opportunity for a collaborative encounter—a dialogue about gambling. We hoped to provide an opportunity for gamblers to explore their concerns and ambivalence about gambling in a nonjudgmental context. To this end it was necessary for the interviewers to sincerely commit to the idea that the impetus and responsibility for change must come from the gambler. We found that gamblers who received a motivational intervention reduced their gambling significantly more over a 12-month period following the interview than gamblers receiving the nonmotivational interview.

The Interview

The intervention included these basic components: a brief discussion about gambling habits; a discussion of the things people liked and disliked about gambling; a normative and personalized feedback section; a decisional balance exercise; an exploration of self-efficacy; a future-oriented imagination exercise; ratings of motivation to change and confidence; and, if appropriate, a discussion of the participant's thoughts about changing his or her gambling behavior. The discussion about potential changes was left to the discretion of the interviewer in order to tailor the interview to the client. Some participants were not ready to consider change or didn't feel they had a problem. Insisting on a discussion of possible change strategies may have alienated the participant and would have served to detract from the purpose of the interview, which was to allow the participant time to access and reflect on his or her thoughts and feelings about what he or she was doing. Although all of the components were expected to be included in the interview if possible, the order and emphasis was at the discretion of the interviewer, to promote flexibility. If, for example, a question about the "good things" about gambling evoked a litany of worries, we did not require that individuals stop expressing their concerns. Instead, we followed their lead and asked for more information. We would ask about the "good things" at a later point in the interview, perhaps framing the question historically, for example:

> "You've told me a lot about the problems you've been having with gambling, but I'm wondering what was it about gambling that attracted you when you started—what did you like about it?"

The intention was for the interviewer to retain control of the direction of the encounter while allowing the participant to discuss what was important to him or her. We often employed brief summaries of the discussion to shift to the next section of the interview.

HOW DID THE INTERVIEW PROCEED?

All the interviews began with a very general question about the participants' gambling. After describing their gambling preferences and the frequency of their gambling, gamblers often started to describe their current difficulties, which led smoothly to an initial discussion of current problems. For people who had some difficulty warming up to the interview, we asked what had prompted them to participate in the study. For people who seemed unconcerned or unsure about why they had volunteered, we asked if other people had "said anything" about their gambling. If others had voiced concerns, we would then ask if the gambler had any concerns or if he or she did not feel that the issues identified were a problem. For less talkative gamblers we sometimes asked for a description of a typical gambling day, which often generated a discussion about employment (or lack of it), situational factors that made gambling attractive on certain days, and their feelings before and after gambling.

The interviews typically started as follows:

"We advertised for people who have been wondering about their gambling. Can you tell me a bit about your gambling?"

- "Well, I started off going to Vegas for fun, but now it's not fun anymore."
- "I go to the bar and play the machines and spend money that I need for other things."
- "My wife and I separated about 2 years ago, and I'm lonely, so I want to go out; but I know I should be spending more time with the kids and not wasting my money."

GOOD AND NOT-SO-GOOD THINGS ABOUT GAMBLING

We next took time to explore what the gambler enjoyed about gambling. Often this line of questioning would generate mixed responses—gamblers would start out talking about some positive aspects of gambling but would begin to introduce negative elements. We tried to make sure that gamblers got the opportunity to explore their attraction to gambling—what drew them to it initially and what they still enjoyed.

"Tell me what you like [or liked] about gambling—what's the best part . . . what else . . . ?"

- "It gives me somewhere to go and meet people—I often see the same people there."
- "I like the rush, the feeling that I might win this time."
- "It's a really good feeling when I win. I get excited and imagine that I can get out of debt."
- "I get to forget what's going on at home."

We would then move into a discussion of the not-so-good things about gambling. For example:

"You already told me about some concerns you have had about your gambling [summarize]. What else is a concern? What else is not so good about your gambling?"

- "I get depressed when I lose, I feel stupid, I feel like a loser."
- "I think of the things I could have bought for the kids."

- "I'm going further into debt, don't know how I'm going to pay the bills."
- "I never have any extra money."
- "I'm afraid people will find out and think I'm stupid."

During this discussion of good and not-so-good things about gambling, the interviewers were encouraged to remain sensitive and attentive, using reflective listening to encourage exploration of emotional responses and multiple issues. During the discussion of the "not-so-good things," emotions were often quite close to the surface, and the interviewer could often use an initial statement to explore the effects of gambling. For example, in response to "I think of the things I could have bought for the kids," the interviewer could simply reflect perceived emotion— "It makes you sad to think that your kids are missing out because of gambling"—and allow the participant time to sit with this feeling. Alternatively, the interviewer could choose to delve further into the impact of gambling on the family. For example:

> "It sounds like gambling has impacted your ability to buy things for your kids. Has gambling affected your relationship with them in other ways?"

FEEDBACK

After giving the gamblers an opportunity to talk about gambling and explore ambivalence, they were asked if they were interested in receiving information about how their scores on a measure of gambling problems compared with others who had taken the survey. We used data from a recent local survey to provide comparisons with participants' scores on a measure of gambling severity. Such information is available in the majority of states and provinces and in many locations worldwide. The feedback section was the only component of the intervention that is not part of the "classic" motivational interview as described by Miller and Rollnick (2002), although it is described as a critical element of related brief intervention approaches (Miller & Rollnick, 1991). The approach to feedback delivery was consistent with the general MI approach. Participants were first asked if they were interested in finding out how their scores compared with other adult Albertans. After they were told how their scores compared to others and the risk category associated with their score, participants were asked for their reaction to the feedback.

None of the study participants declined the offer of comparing their scores to the general population. Some responded without surprise, and some were quite distressed. Some had difficulty believing that their level of gambling was as unusual as it appeared from the comparison. We did not argue with participants who felt this way or who suggested that other respondents must have minimized their own gambling habits. Instead, we reflected their responses—for example, "It seems to you that lots of people gamble about as much as you do," or "It's hard to believe some people don't gamble at all." Reflections rather than arguments allowed for further exploration of their perceptions of whether or not their level of gambling involvement was unusual as compared to others and allowed for a consideration of how and with whom they spent time. If participants indicated that the feedback confirmed their concerns, the interviewer would reinforce their concern and ask for more—for example, "This is something you have been thinking about for a while—have you thought about what you might want to do about it?" At the end of the 12-month follow-up we asked if gamblers remembered receiving the normative feedback. About two-thirds of the gamblers who had received normative feedback remembered it, and all but one felt it had been helpful.

NORMATIVE FEEDBACK

"When you called in response to the ad, the research assistant asked you some questions about your gambling—that was a questionnaire that has been given to thousands of people. Would you like to see how your score compares to others? You are in the group that is considered to be [either at moderate risk for developing gambling problems or having a substantial level of gambling-related problems]. Does that surprise you at all?"

- "It depresses me a little. . . ."
- "No, that's why I came in."
- "Wow! That's scary."
- "That confirms I have a problem."
- "People were lying when they answered this—I told the truth."
- "I know lots of people who gamble as much as I do."

Personalized Feedback

"We have another way to look at what's going on with you and your gambling if you're interested. We can look at how much you're spending as compared to how much you take home in a month. You told the research assistant that you take home about $ ____ per month. You also talked about how much you spent gambling in the last 2 months, which would average about $ ____. Does that sound about right? If we divide what you spend by the amount you make, we can see what percentage of your income goes to gambling each month. It looks like you are spending about ____ % of what you take home on gambling. What do you make of that?"

- "It makes me feel even worse, but committed to change."
- "It depresses me a little—I might cut out scratch cards, but I really like the casino."
- "I'm not sure why I do this, I'm an intelligent person."

DECISIONAL BALANCE

The decisional balance exercise was introduced. This was done in a paper-and-pencil format, and a copy was given to the gambler to take home. The decisional balance was done as a hypothetical cost–benefit exercise. Participants were asked to think about the costs to them if they chose to stay the same and continue gambling at the same level (a further exploration of the not-so-good things about gambling). They were then asked to think about the benefits if their gambling stayed the same (another chance to explore what was important to them about their gambling). We next asked them about the costs of changing—providing an exploration of what they would be giving up if they did make changes (this gave them an opportunity to express some of their fears and concerns about changing their gambling). And finally they were asked to consider the benefits of changing their gambling (giving them an opportunity to imagine a future without gambling). This discussion was framed in terms of the thought that that they might be entertaining the possibility of making some kind of change in their gambling—quitting or cutting down was not introduced unless the gambler brought it up. By maintaining the hypothetical nature of the discussion, participants were free to talk about what might be different without having to commit to any changes at all.

> "We have talked a bit about the good and not-so-good things about gambling for you—this is an exercise that is a little bit the same but gives us a different way to look at things. We can look at these questions even if you aren't sure you want to quit or cut down."

Costs of Staying the Same. We started with thinking about what life would be like if no changes were made in gambling—what the costs would be to the gambler if he or she made no changes at all in behavior, including some of the previously discussed problems.

- "I'm leading a double life—lying to family and friends."
- "Stealing."
- "Feeling guilty."
- "Growing debts."
- "I will go broke."
- "I worry about money all the time."
- "I could go bankrupt."

Benefits of Staying the Same. Next we talked about the benefits of not changing—what are the important things about maintaining their gambling? This is an opportunity to understand what people like about gambling, what purpose it serves in their lives.

- "I might win."
- "It's entertainment."
- "It's a chance to dream."
- "I like the excitement, rush."
- "Getting away from home, socializing."
- "It's an escape."

Many people could not think of anything that would be good about staying the same—often this question would generate a quick response—"there's nothing good about it." After reflecting the feeling we would proceed to the next quadrant. We often found that when people moved to thinking about the costs of changing their gambling (what they would be giving up) they were more able to identify their reasons for persisting with gambling, and these were discussed as perceived benefits when the thoughts were generated.

Costs of Making Changes. This was a very useful area to explore—it provoked a great deal of thought in terms of what the gambler would be giving up and what might be difficult about changing. It also was a springboard for the gamblers to generate alternatives to their current activities.

- "I would lose the chance to go out, boredom."
- "I would lose the chance to escape from stuff at home."

- "It's hard to change."
- "It's hard to be responsible."
- "I'd have to give up the chance of winning."

Benefits of Making Changes. What would he or she imagine would be different if a change were made? This was an opportunity to imagine a hypothetical future—an opportunity to think about the things besides gambling that are important. Again, some of the items raised from the previous discussion could be discussed and expanded.

- "I could trust myself more, not feel guilty."
- "I could do things with the money: eat healthier food, travel, give kids more, pay debts, buy a house."
- "I could have less stress, be healthier, spend time with kids, friends."
- "My spouse wouldn't divorce me."

ENCOURAGEMENT OF SELF-EFFICACY

This was an opportunity to talk about change more generally, to ask about how this individual makes changes in his or her life. People could usually think of something that they had had some success with, even if they hadn't been totally successful. Even if they had not succeeded in changing a behavior, they could often generate some thoughts about what had and hadn't worked. This was an opportunity to restate that the client is the best authority on him- or herself and is the person most likely to know what he or she is willing to undertake. Often people would start to generate ideas about how they could change their gambling if they wanted to by using previously successful strategies. If they had no personal experience or ideas around change, we might ask if they knew of any strategies other people had used. We also asked about situations where they had the opportunity to gamble but chose not to, exploring what they had done differently in those situations.

"We've been talking about the idea of making changes—have you ever made changes in other areas of your life? What works best for you?"

- "I need to do it cold turkey."
- "Telling people, being open with them, getting help."
- "Getting counseling."

- "Just deciding—made a decision I didn't want it."
- "I have to cut ties with people who were involved in same things (e.g., drinking, drugs)."

FUTURE-ORIENTED IMAGINATION EXERCISE

We asked people to think about their lives in 5 or 10 years. What did they imagine their lives would be like based on two scenarios—if they did make changes in their gambling and if they didn't?

"If you decided you don't want to change anything about your gambling, what do you imagine your life would be like in 5 or 10 years?"

- "The same, maybe worse."
- "I'd be homeless."
- "I would disappear, be lonely."
- "I would get more depressed."
- "I would lose my family."

"If you decide you want to make some changes in your gambling, what do you imagine your life would be like in 5 or 10 years?"

- "I could have a different house."
- "I would be healthy, less anxious."
- "Better marriage."
- "I could help my kids, take care of grandkids."
- "Get married, have a family, have a nice house."
- "I would be debt-free."

RATINGS OF MOTIVATION AND CONFIDENCE

This exercise was introduced as another way to get an idea about how the gambler was feeling about his or her gambling and the possibility of change. We asked people to imagine a ruler with markings from 0 to 10 and asked them two questions:

"If we had a ruler in front of us, and 0 on the ruler was 'not at all motivated to change anything about my gambling,' and 10 on the ruler was 'absolutely motivated to make changes in my gambling'— where would you put yourself right now?"

"If you decided you did want to make changes in your gambling, how confident are you that you could—with 0 being not at all confident and 10 being absolutely confident you could do it if you set your mind to it?"

After each exercise we explored why a particular number had been chosen. If the person rated his or her motivation as a 5, we might ask more questions. If they seemed quite negative and yet chose a 5, we might comment, "Wow, it sounds like, even though you're worried about what changing would be like, you still rate your motivation as a 5." This could be followed with questions such as "Why are you a 5 and not a zero?" or "What would it take for your motivation to move to a 7 or 8? What would have to happen?" Responses ranged from enthusiastic—some even said 12 on the 10-point scale, for example—to extremely doubtful. This was another opportunity for the gamblers to think about whether or not changing gambling was something they were really interested in doing at this time.

DECISION DISCUSSION

At the end of the interview we summarized the discussion and acknowledged that talking about their gambling with a stranger could be very difficult. This was not only intended to continue the practice of affirming the clients, a central MI concept, but also to let them know that we were aware that they had allowed us to share in painful and difficult areas of their lives. We also expressed our appreciation for their willingness to take part in the interview, acknowledging that by doing so they were not only helping with our research but also doing something to care for themselves. Next we asked participants to tell us their thoughts after having gone through the interview. We encountered a wide range of responses to this question. At this point gamblers often expressed ambivalence about change. Some people were quite clear that they wanted to quit or cut down substantially and made statements about fairly specific changes they wanted to make. We reinforced these plans and encouraged further thought and planning about how change could take place. Others were not ready to consider any changes. People who were not ready to change were encouraged to continue to think about the discussion and refer to the workbook if they were interested at a later date. We acknowledged that we had covered a lot of territory in the interview and that the participant was the person who was the best authority on what he or she should be doing (or not doing).

"We've talked about a lot of things today—what do you think about all this?"

- "I feel overwhelmed, it makes me sick."
- "I'd quit if I really thought it was a problem or it started to affect my health."
- "I really have to do something."
- "I would have to stay away from the casino/bar, those friends."
- "I would have to make some different arrangements about money."
- "I would have to start exercising."
- "I have to do it cold turkey."
- "I could make a list of things I want to spend my money on instead of wasting it."
- "It made me think about everything I could lose."
- "I'm not wanting to change right now."

PROBLEMS AND SUGGESTED SOLUTIONS

Generally the MI approach appears to work extremely well with problem gambling and pathological gambling. One potential complication, however, is the extremely high prevalence of comorbid mental health disorders (substance abuse, mood and anxiety, personality) with gambling disorders, which can impact the course and outcome of the gambling problem (Cunningham, 2005; Hodgins, Peden, & Cassidy, 2005; National Gambling Impact Study Commission, 1999; Petry, Stinson, & Grant, 2005). To date, little is known about the implications of comorbidity for gambling treatment. It is not clear whether one or the other disorder should be tackled first or whether treatment should be concurrent (separate interventions) or integrated, or whether client preference should dictate the sequencing. In the absence of evidence-based guidelines, the solution is flexibility on the part of the therapist to move where the client needs to move, which requires a broad base of training and experience. Being able to summon expertise in each of the comorbid disorders is the ideal situation. As the chapters in this book illustrate, the general MI approach can be tailored to the unique characteristics of a diverse range of mental health disorders.

Another complication with gambling disorders is the need to focus on financial issues as part of therapy. Individuals cannot typically pay down huge debt loads quickly and, therefore, must learn to manage them effectively over time. Financial pressures, if not dealt with, can erode motivation and be a risk for relapse (Hodgins & el-Guebaly, 2004). Therapists working with gambling problems must either develop financial counseling expertise or provide concurrent help in this area, even when just offering a brief MI intervention.

RESEARCH

Promoting Self-Recovery in Pathological Gamblers Using Motivational Enhancement

As described above, a randomized clinical trial comparing motivational enhancement plus workbook to a workbook-only condition and a waiting-list control has been completed. Participants were followed for 24 months, and the results showed a significant advantage for the group receiving the motivational intervention. For example, at 3 months, 42% of the motivational group were abstinent and an additional 39% were categorized as improved, compared with 19% and 56% of the workbook-only group (Hodgins et al., 2001). At 24 months, although 37% of the people were abstinent across groups, 54% of the motivational group had improved, compared with 25% of the workbook-only group (Hodgins, Currie, el-Guebaly, & Peden, 2004). These results suggest that the brief telephone motivational intervention is a wise investment of resources in enhancing the likelihood of individual success.

We are currently conducting a study to replicate and extend these findings. In the ongoing study we are comparing a waiting-list group to a workbook-only group, a motivational telephone intervention plus workbook group, and a group that, in addition to the initial motivational telephone call, receives a monthly therapist motivational check-in call for 5 months. The rationale for this latter condition is to determine whether a motivational booster would maintain and improve outcomes over time. In addition, we are interested in understanding the mechanisms of improvement. Does the intervention increase motivation that subsequently affects behavior? Recruitment has been completed (n = 314), and a 12-month follow-up is in progress.

One-Session Motivational Intervention for Problem Gambling

This study involved a randomized clinical trial comparing a motivational intervention with a control interview (Diskin, 2006). We advertised for participants who were concerned about their gambling and who were willing to participate in a study evaluating interview style on subsequent gambling behavior. Participants were not required to be wanting to reduce their gambling but simply to be experiencing some level of concern. The inclusion criteria for the study were intentionally as broad as possible. The only exclusion criteria for participation were that potential participants must have gambled within the preceding 2 months and that they had obtained a score of 3 or greater on the Problem Gambling Severity Index of the Canadian Problem Gambling Index (Ferris, Wynne, & Single, 1998), which is indicative of an "at-risk" level of problem. Participants were randomly assigned to one of two groups. Half the participants were given the motivational interview described above. The other half spent a similar amount of time with an interviewer talking about their gambling and completing various semi-structured personality measures. Two clinicians conducted both the motivational and nonmotivational interviews. All participants were given a copy of the self-help workbook. We followed participants for a 12-month period with follow-up calls at 1, 3, 6, and 12 months.

We intended this to be a fairly stringent test of the effectiveness of MI with problem gamblers. Everyone received a workbook, and everyone spent about 45 minutes to an hour speaking with a clinically trained interviewer. We used a 12-month follow-up period because we wanted to take into account the high rate of natural recovery in this population.

Immediately after the interviews we asked participants to evaluate their experiences of the interview and of their interviewer. The two groups did not differ in their ratings of their interviewer, with both groups rating their interviewers quite highly in terms of empathy, trustworthiness, respect, and understanding. However, the groups did differ in their ratings of the interview they received. Gamblers rated the motivational intervention higher in terms of several variables, including helpfulness, overall satisfaction, and whether problems were worked on effectively.

Since participation in the study did not require that participants intend to quit gambling (or even intend to make any change in their gambling), we decided to use the number of days gambled per month and monthly gambling expenditures as the dependent variables of interest. Both groups were gambling a mean amount of approximately $1,300 Cdn per month in the 2 months preceding the interview, and both groups were gambling about 7 days per month.

For the participants who completed the study, we found that over the 12-month period the gamblers who had received a motivational intervention gambled less often and spent less money gambling than the control group. During the 3 months preceding the final interview the motivational group gambled approximately 2.2 days per month, whereas the control group gambled about 5 days per month. In the final 3-month period preceding the 12-month interview the motivational group also gambled less money on a monthly basis as compared to the attention control group. The motivational intervention participants spent an average of about $340 Cdn gambling per month, but the control group participants spent an average of $912 monthly.

A very interesting and unexpected result was related to level of problem gambling severity. Almost all the gamblers in the study were experiencing significant levels of gambling problems. We had expected that gamblers with comparatively less severe problems would likely find the motivational intervention more helpful than those who were experiencing more severe problems. Instead, we found that, for the people who completed the 12-month follow-up, those with less severe problems improved in a similar fashion whether they received a motivational interview or were in the control condition. Those with more severe problems reduced their gambling significantly if they received a motivational intervention, but they did not do so if they were in the control group.

Over the course of the study gamblers in the comparatively lower-severity group who received a motivational interview spent about $325 per month on gambling, while those in the control group spent about $265 per month (this difference was not statistically significant). It seems that for those whose gambling problems were comparatively less severe the motivational intervention did not have a significant effect over and above receiving the self-help manual and participating in the study. Lower-severity participants in both groups decreased the dollars they spent over 12 months considerably.

However, gamblers in the higher-severity group who received a motivational interview spent about $300 Cdn gambling per month. Those in the control group spent about $1,100 per month. For those in the comparatively more severe group, the motivational intervention was helpful in reducing both dollars and days spent gambling. All of the participants in the study were willing to make some effort to explore their concerns about gambling (enough to make and keep an appointment for an interview). For those with less severe problems, this effort and the availability of the manual may have been enough. For those with more severe problems, participating in the MI made a significant difference. It is unclear at this point which elements of the interview were

246 Motivational Interviewing in the Treatment of Psychological Problems

effective in helping people with severe problems maintain changes in their gambling behavior over the course of 12 months. To the extent that we were able to adhere to the spirit of MI, it may be that the opportunity to explore their ambivalent feelings about gambling in a nonjudgmental atmosphere was helpful in empowering them to decide to make significant changes. New work on exploring the connection between language and process in MI will be helpful in exploring what it is about MI that is effective (Amrhein, Miller, Yahne, Palmer, & Fulcher, 2003).

CONCLUSIONS

The research we have presented above and our clinical experience support the value of MI for problem and pathological gambling. In two studies a motivationally based intervention plus a self-help workbook was clearly associated with better outcomes than a comparison workbook-only condition. In one study the intervention was via telephone, and in the other it was face to face. One study recruited individuals who were seeking to address their gambling problem, albeit without using formal treatment, and the other recruited individuals who were concerned but not necessarily ready to change. Although the evidence is limited to these two studies, the consistency of the results supports their veracity. Brief motivational interventions appear to be a way of extending the options provided by traditional treatment and encouraging reluctant gamblers to initiate the change process.

Further refinement and research are required in a number of areas. Comorbidity rates are high, and the implications of comorbidity for recovery and treatment are unclear. It is possible that, for more complicated clinical presentations, imbedding MI principles in a more intensive treatment intervention is more beneficial than offering brief interventions. Further development of treatment compliance methods using motivational principles is also important, given the high dropout rates reported. Dropping out may be more likely among those with comorbid disorders as well.

MI has the potential to play an important role in the gambling disorder treatment system as it continues to evolve. Treatment for pathological and problem gambling, as compared to other mental health disorders, is still in its infancy. As a result, the system may be more readily influenced by empirical effectiveness and efficacy research than in other areas of mental health.

NOTE

1. The workbooks are available through *www.addiction.ucalgary.ca.*

REFERENCES

American Gaming Association. (2007). *2007 State of the States. The AGA survey of casino entertainment.* Available at *www.americangaming.org/assets/files/aga_ 2007_sos.pdf*

American Psychiatric Association. (2000). *Diagnostic and statistical manual of mental disorders* (4th ed., text rev.). Washington, DC: Author.

Amrhein, P. C., Miller, W. M., Yahne, C. E., Palmer, M., & Fulcher, L. (2003). Client commitment language during motivational interviewing predicts drug use outcomes. *Journal of Consulting and Clinical Psychology, 71,* 862–878.

Bernstein, P. L. (1996). *Against the gods: The remarkable story of risk.* New York: Wiley.

Cunningham, J. A. (2005). Little use of treatment among problem gamblers. *Psychiatric Services, 56,* 1024–1025.

Cunningham-Williams, R. M., & Cottler, L. B. (2001). The epidemiology of pathological gambling. *Seminars in Clinical Neuropsychiatry, 6,* 155–166.

Diskin, K. M. (2006). *Effects of a single session motivational intervention on problem gambling behaviour.* Unpublished doctoral dissertation, University of Calgary, Alberta.

Ferris, J., Wynne, H., & Single, E. (1998). *Measuring problem gambling in Canada: Interim report to the inter-provincial task force on problem gambling.* Toronto: Canadian Interprovincial Task Force on Problem Gambling.

Gerstein, D., Murphy, S., Toce, M., Hoffman, J., Palmer, A., Johnson, R., et al. (1999). *Gambling impact and behavior study: Report of the National Gambling Impact Study Commission.* Washington, DC: National Gambling Impact Study Commission.

Grant, J. E., Kim, S. W., & Potenza, M. N. (2003). Advances in the pharmacological treatment of pathological gambling disorder. *Journal of Gambling Studies, 19,* 85–109.

Heather, N. (2005). Motivational interviewing: Is it all our clients need? *Addiction Research and Theory, 13,* 1–18.

Hodgins, D. C., Currie, S. R., el-Guebaly, N., & Peden, N. (2004). Brief motivational treatment for problem gambling: A 24-month follow-up. *Psychology of Addictive Behaviors, 18,* 293–296.

Hodgins, D. C., Currie, S. R., & el-Guebaly, N. (2001). Motivational enhancement and self-help treatments for problem gambling. *Journal of Consulting and Clinical Psychology, 69,* 50–57.

Hodgins, D. C., & el-Guebaly, N. (2000). Natural and treatment-assisted recovery from gambling problems: A comparison of resolved and active gamblers. *Addiction, 95,* 777–789.

Hodgins, D. C., & el-Guebaly, N. (2004). Retrospective and prospective reports of precipitants to relapse in pathological gambling. *Journal of Consulting and Clinical Psychology, 72,* 72–80.

Hodgins, D. C., & Makarchuk, K. (2002). *Becoming a winner: Defeating problem gambling*. Edmonton: AADAC.

Hodgins, D. C., Mansley, C., & Thygesen, K. (2006). Risk factors for suicide ideation and attempts among pathological gamblers. *American Journal on Addictions, 15*(4), 303–310.

Hodgins, D. C., Peden, N., & Cassidy, E. (2005). The association between co-morbidity and outcome in pathological gambling: A prospective follow-up of recent quitters. *Journal of Gambling Studies, 21,* 255–271.

Hodgins, D. C., & Petry, N. M. (2004). Cognitive and behavioral treatments. In J. E. Grant & M. N. Potenza (Eds.), *Pathological gambling: A clinical guide to treatment*. New York: American Psychiatric Association Press.

Hodgins, D. C., Wynne, H., & Makarchuk, K. (1999). Pathways to recovery from gambling problems: Follow-up from a general population survey. *Journal of Gambling Studies, 15,* 93–104.

Miller, W. R., & Rollnick, S. (1991). *Motivational Interviewing: Preparing people to change addictive behavior.* New York: Guilford Press.

Miller, W. R., & Rollnick, S. (2002). *Motivational Interviewing: Preparing people for change* (2nd ed.). New York: Guilford Press.

Milton, S., Crino, R., Hunt, C., & Prosser, E. (2002). The effect of compliance-improving interventions on the cognitive-behavioral treatment of pathological gambling. *Journal of Gambling Studies, 18,* 207–230.

National Gambling Impact Study Commission. (1999). *National Gambling Impact Study Commission final report*. Washington, DC: Author. Available at *govinfo.library.unt.edu/ngisc/reports*

National Research Council. (1999). *Pathological gambling. A critical review*. Washington, DC: National Academy Press.

Petry, N. M., Stinson, F. S., & Grant, B. F. (2005). Comorbidity of DSM-IV pathological gambling and other psychiatric disorders: Results from the National Epidemiologic Survey on Alcohol and Related Conditions. *Journal of Clinical Psychiatry, 66,* 564–574.

Shaffer, H. J., & Hall, M. N. (2001). Updating and refining prevalence estimates of disordered gambling and behavior in the United States and Canada. *Canadian Journal of Public Health, 92,* 168–172.

Toneatto, T., & Ladouceur, R. (2003). Treatment of pathological gambling: A critical review of the literature. *Psychology of Addictive Behaviors, 17,* 284–292.

Volberg, R. A. (2001). *When the chips are down: Problem gambling in America*. New York: The Century Foundation Press.

Welte, J., Barnes, G., Wieczorek, W., Tidwell, M., & Parker, J. (2004). Alcohol and gambling pathology among U.S. adults: Prevalence, demographic patterns and comorbidity. *Journal of Studies on Alcohol, 62,* 706–712.

CHAPTER 10

Motivational Interviewing for Medication Adherence in Individuals with Schizophrenia

Stanley G. McCracken
Patrick W. Corrigan

Individuals with schizophrenia spectrum disorders[1] (SSD) experience a variety of symptoms that produce significant distress and interfere with social and role functioning. The most widely used approaches for treating individuals with these conditions include the use of antipsychotic medications. A common reason for treatment failure is nonadherence to medications, and the most common form of nonadherence is underuse of these medications (Nose, Barbui, & Tansella, 2003). The results of nonadherence include relapse of psychotic symptoms, rehospitalization, and disruption of functioning at home and work (Dolder, Lacro, Leckband, & Jeste, 2003). While the rate of medication nonadherence among individuals with SSD is quite high, estimated to be from 10 to 80% with a median around 50%, the rate of nonadherence is within the range of other individuals with chronic illnesses requiring complex treatment, for example, insulin-dependent diabetes and hypertension (Dolder et al., 2003; Fenton, Blyler, & Heinssen, 1997; Gray, Wykes, & Gournay, 2002). Motivational interviewing (MI) has been proposed to address substance use problems (Baker et al., 2002; Barrowclough et al., 2001; Graeber, Moyers, Griffith, Guajardo, & Tonigan, 2003; Ziedonis & Trudeau, 1997), goal identification (Corrigan, McCracken, & Holmes, 2001), insight and treatment adherence (Rusch & Corrigan, 2002), and medication adherence (Kemp, Hayward, Applewhaite, Everitt, & David, 1996; Kemp, Kirov, Hayward, Everitt, & David, 1998; O'Donnell et al., 2003) in individuals with SSD. We will review some of the symptoms experienced by individuals with SSD and interventions that have been demonstrated as effective in improving medication adherence in this population. We will end by making a number of recommendations based on the research literature and our own experience in using MI with individuals with SSD.

THE CLINICAL POPULATION AND USUAL TREATMENTS

Individuals with SSD experience symptoms that are a distortion of function, called positive symptoms, and symptoms that are a diminishment of function, called negative symptoms (American Psychiatric Association, 2000). Positive symptoms include the kinds of symptoms that are often the hallmark of psychosis, such as hallucinations, delusions, disordered speech and thinking, and disordered behavior or catatonia. While the negative symptoms, such as alogia, anhedonia, avolition, and blunted affect, are less dramatic than the positive symptoms, they are just as debilitating and may be more refractory to treatment (Diamond, 2002). In addition to positive and negative symptoms, people with SSD also may have cognitive deficits of different kinds. Several cognitive deficits may interfere with the functioning of people with SSD, including attention, memory, and executive functions such as decision making (Spaulding, Reed, Poland, & Storzbach, 1996). These deficits may augment SSD symptoms as well as directly limit social, coping, and other independent skills. A diagnosis of schizophrenia requires that the individual have at least one period in which he or she experiences at least two criterion A symptoms (the positive symptoms listed above and negative symptoms) for 1 month, social or occupational dysfunction, and a total duration of symptoms for at least 6 months (American Psychiatric Association, 2000). Other psychotic disorders differ in the required pattern of criterion A symptoms, duration of the illness, degree of impaired functioning, and the presence of additional symptoms, such as the presence of mood syndrome in schizoaffective disorder (American Psychiatric Association, 2000). Positive, negative, and cognitive symptoms of SSD can interfere with engagement with treatment providers, deciding to participate in treatment once engaged, and adherence to treatment once participation is agreed upon. For example, persecutory and paranoid delusions may produce distrust and fearfulness of family, friends, and treatment providers; withdrawal and the urge to isolate may impede making and keeping appointments; and cognitive impairment can interfere with learning and implementing illness and medication management skills.

The most widely used treatments for SSD are aimed at symptom reduction and include traditional/typical and atypical antipsychotic medications. While these medications are effective in relieving the symptoms of SSD, they have side effects that can be uncomfortable, disfiguring, quality-of-life interfering, and even life-threatening. Furthermore, a number of these medications and the medications used to relieve side effects (such as anticholinergic, anti-Parkinsonian medications) increase cognitive impairment (Corrigan & Penn, 1995). Not surprisingly, side effects are often given as reasons for nonadherence. Since people do not immediately relapse when they decrease or discontinue taking their medications, treatment providers and family members may not be aware of the nonadherence until the individual has relapsed. Many antipsychotic medications are available in forms that can be injected every 2–4 weeks (depot medications), and it was hoped that this mode of administration would lead to improved adherence. Unfortunately, even with the use of depot medications, nonadherence continues to be a significant problem, and the improvement in adherence is likely due to the fact that providers are more aware when the individual does not show up for a shot than when he or she does not take a pill (Diamond, 2002). Similarly, it was hoped that the use of atypical antipsychotic medications, with their reduced incidence of movement-related side effects (such as tardive dyskinesia, Parkinsonian side effects, and akathisia) and their improved ability to relieve negative and mood symptoms, would improve adherence. Nevertheless, nonadherence remains a problem even with the newer medications (Dolder et al., 2003).

The risk of stigma is one important reason why nonadherence to medication occurs (Corrigan, 2004). Stigmas are marks that lead to harm. The mark for people with mental illness is a label: that person A is different and somehow inferior to the majority. Labels occur by association, either an explicit and public statement that "a person is mentally ill" or other associations that lead to discrimination, such as receiving talk therapy or psychotropic mediation. Two forms of discrimination may result from these stigmas: (1) public stigma, the loss of social opportunities when the majority endorses the stigma and acts in a discriminatory manner; and (2) self-stigma, the harm that results from internalizing stigma, challenging one's self-esteem and self-efficacy. Stigma arises in subtle ways as a barrier to adherence. Intervention plans that seek to improve adherence may need to address stigma-related barriers.

In addition to factors related to the illness, the medications used to treat the illness, and the stigma, there are a number of other factors that may lead to nonadherence, including nonmedical (street) drug use; negative individual and family attitudes about medication taking; complex medication regimens, sometimes involving multiple medications taken at different times of the day; lack of insight about the illness; and cultural factors related to the illness and its management (Fenton et al., 1997; Nose et al., 2003; Rusch & Corrigan, 2002). The wide range of variability in estimates of medication adherence results from the use of differing populations and treatment settings, and particularly from differing definitions of adherence and methods used to assess adherence (Fenton et al., 1997; Young, Zonana, & Shepler, 1986). Medication nonadherence includes both errors of omission (e.g., failure to take doses or completely ceasing use of medication) and errors of commission (e.g., taking too much or additional medications) (Blackwell, 1976). For antipsychotic medications nonadherence is primarily underuse of medications.

Research on medication adherence rarely reports the specific pattern of nonadherence. For example, did the individual completely cease taking the medication, take it at the prescribed time but in lesser amounts, or take the prescribed amounts but intermittently? In clinical settings the pattern of nonadherence may provide useful information about the nature of the adherence problem. Figure 10.1 shows four patterns of adherence, each of which represents 50% adherence. The reason behind the nonadherence for each pattern may be quite different. The individual in Row 1 may have run out of money and been unable to refill his prescription, may have experienced aversive side effects, or may have improved and felt he or she did not need to take the medication any more. The individual in Row 2 may not have had money to pay for the prescription, may have experienced increased symptoms, or may have received a visit from his or her case manager. The individual in Row 3 may be experiencing side effects or may be trying to make his or her medication last longer. The individual in Row 4 also may be experiencing side effects, or the reduced dose may be more effective. Not all adherence problems lead to less effective treatment; sometimes people can titrate themselves to a more appropriate dose. Each of these situations is the result of a different adherence issue and would lead to a dif-

Row	Pattern of Adherence							
1	X	X	X	X	0	0	0	0
2	0	0	0	0	X	X	X	X
3	X	0	X	0	X	0	X	0
4	½	½	½	½	½	½	½	½

X = Took pill;   0 = Did not take pill;   ½ = Took half a pill.

FIGURE 10.1. Examples of differing patterns of 50% medication adherence.

ferent intervention, several of which may involve the use of MI methods, beginning with reflective listening to assess and understand the individual's view of the problem.

RATIONALE FOR USING MI FOR INDIVIDUALS WITH SSD

With the increasing number of medications with established efficacy in treating SSD and the serious consequences of relapse, facilitating participation in medication programs is a major priority in the treatment of individuals with SSD. There are three main models or approaches to understanding and promoting adherence. These include models, such as the health belief model, that focus on the individual decision-making process, in which the patient weighs the probable risks and benefits of adhering or not adhering to a course of treatment; models based on the treatment and communication process and the relationship between the provider and the patient; and models that focus on parallel processing on the cognitive level through disease and treatment schemas and on the motivational level through emotional response (Zygmunt, Olfson, Boyer, & Mechanic, 2002). MI has components that address processes central to each of these major approaches to adherence. MI promotes a collaborative relationship between the provider and the individual, encourages the individual to conduct a decisional balance weighing the risks and benefits of change, uses an empathic response to the individual's exploration of his or her emotional and cognitive ambivalence about the illness and treatment, and promotes the individual's self-efficacy regarding change. How these elements are operationalized in working with individuals with SSD is detailed in the remainder of this chapter.

CONDUCTING MI WITH INDIVIDUALS WITH SSD

Process of Change in Individuals with SSD

The transtheoretical or stages of change model describes the process of change that an individual goes through in deciding to make significant changes in behavior (Prochaska, DiClemente, & Norcross, 1992). Table 10.1 lists the six stages of change and characteristics of individuals in each of these stages. Though this model initially was most often used in describing change in individuals with chemical dependence problems, it also has been used to describe the process of development of insight, problem recognition, and medication adherence in individuals with SSD (Corrigan et al., 2001; Rusch & Corrigan, 2002). Since this model has been described in detail elsewhere (e.g., DiClemente & Velasquez, 2002; Prochaska et al., 1992), we will confine our discussion to two important considerations when applying this model to work with individuals with SSD. First, it is important to understand the subgroups of individuals in the precontemplation stage (reluctant, rebellious, resigned, and rationalizing) in order to properly use MI in discussing medication adherence. How each of these subgroups presents in indi-

TABLE 10.1. Stages of Change

Stage of change	Characteristics
Precontemplation	Individual unaware or underaware of the problem; sees no costs to behavior; not even thinking about change.
Contemplation	Individual is ambivalent; sees both costs and benefits to behavior, but costs outweigh benefits; no intention to change at this time.
Preparation	Individual preparing to change; costs outweigh benefits of former behavior; lacks plan for change.
Action	Individual changing through a plan; learning and using skills to change behavior.
Maintenance	Individual consolidating gains; continuing to use and master skills; shift of focus to wellness and lifestyle improvement.
Relapse	Individual experiences a return of problem behavior; may recycle back to early stage.

Note. From DiClemente and Valasquez (2002). Copyright 2002 by The Guilford Press. Adapted by permission.

viduals with SSD will be discussed in detail in a later section. Second, relapse in individuals with SSD should be thought of in two ways. One way is that relapse is recycling through the stages, from action or maintenance back to precontemplation or contemplation. This is how relapse is typically thought of in the transtheoretical model—as a return of the problem behavior or as a failure to adhere to a behavior change plan. A failure to adhere to antipsychotic medications would be considered an example of this view of relapse. The other way that relapse is thought of among individuals with SSD is a return of psychotic and associated symptoms, possibly resulting in rehospitalization. While the most common reason for relapse of the illness is not taking medication, adherence to medication or any other component of treatment does not guarantee that the illness will not return, that is, adhering to a behavior change plan may not necessarily prevent a return of symptoms of the illness. Thus, any discussion of adherence should be conducted with a deep sense of humility and with the recognition that the benefits of treatment may be limited for some individuals.

Basic Principles

The specific elements of MI to address adherence in individuals with SSD are outlined in Table 10.2, but before discussing the specifics we will review the basic principles of MI. MI is best thought of as a way of being with people—emphasizing collaboration, evocation, and autonomy (Miller & Rollnick, 2002). Four basic principles underlie MI: express empathy, develop discrepancy, roll with resistance, and support self-efficacy (Miller & Rollnick, 2002). Expressing empathy and reflective listening are fundamental to MI and are the foundation upon which many clinical skills are built. These skills establish an atmosphere of acceptance and help the individual feel that the counselor is listening. Expressing empathy facilitates engagement with the individual and leads to the development of a collaborative relationship. This acceptance provides a context in which the individual can express concerns about the illness, identify goals, and discuss the advantages and disadvantages of treatment. For example, in an empathic environment an individual can more easily describe the side effects of medication, how these side effects affect his or her life, and how they influence his or her adherence to the medication regimen. By developing discrepancy, the counselor does not try to persuade the individual to accept a diagnosis or a particular treatment but rather elicits the individual's views of how a particular behavior might help achieve or interfere with his or her self-

TABLE 10.2. Elements of MI to Address Adherence in Individuals with SSD

- Using MI to address medication adherence should be conducted with the knowledge that adherence to medication and other components of the treatment program will not necessarily prevent a return of symptoms of SSD or rehospitalization.
- MI should be integrated into all components of the treatment program, used by all members of the team, and used at many different times during the course of treatment.
- The interview context and the individual's clinical condition influence how MI is conducted.
- Motivation should be assessed and not assumed.
- Do not insist on acceptance of the diagnosis.
- Conduct discussions of medication adherence in the context of the individual's goals.

identified goals. For example, a counselor might elicit from the individual ways in which refusing to take medication might influence the likelihood of relapse and thus conflict with his or her goal of getting and keeping a job. This approach also helps overcome cognitive deficits by focusing on familiar problems and personal goals rather than abstract concepts (Rusch & Corrigan, 2002). It also provides a context for empowerment by focusing on the individual's rather than the therapist's goals. Rolling with resistance is a means of avoiding confrontation and the psychological reactance that coercion typically elicits. Ambivalence or reluctance are not opposed but accepted as a natural part of the change process. Rather than arguing over whether the individual has a diagnosis of schizophrenia, the counselor might elicit a discussion of the fear associated with delusions and whether the individual would be interested in taking steps to decrease that fear. Increasing self-efficacy is often one of the more difficult aspects of doing MI with individuals with SSD due to negative symptoms such as anergia and avolition. Providing the individual with specific skills that are clearly connected to identified goals is an important part of increasing self-efficacy.

The Desirability of Using MI in All Components of the Intervention, by All Members of the Treatment Team, and at Different Times during Treatment

MI works well as the foundation of an individualized intervention that includes psychoeducation about the illness and its treatment; family involvement and support; community support, including community-based case management and supportive services targeting work, education, and housing; and concrete behavioral approaches such as skills training, problem solving, and the use of concrete cues for adherence once the individual has determined that medication is to be a part of treatment (Drake & Goldman, 2003). Both the spirit and the strategies of MI are relevant to delivery of all of these interventions. For example, MI is explicitly mentioned as a component of the integrated dual disorder treatment model (Mueser, Noordsy, Drake, & Fox, 2003). MI also is used frequently by staff providing supported employment, supported housing, and assertive community treatment. We have found MI to be an interaction style that can be used to facilitate adherence and behavior change in all elements of psychiatric rehabilitation.

In addition to being able to use MI in delivery of other psychiatric rehabilitation interventions, it is suggested that all members of the team be able to use MI to address medication adherence. Case managers, job coaches, individual counselors, skills trainers, and providers of family psychoeducation often find it necessary to discuss medication adherence with the individual with SSD, even though the psychiatrist has the most direct responsibility for prescribing and monitoring medication. Regardless of the setting, discussions of medication adherence can relate to the specific issue at hand. For example, the psychiatrist or a counselor providing individual therapy may use MI when discussing the role of medication early in treatment, while a case manager or job coach may use MI when discussing medication adherence after the individual has been symptom-free for a long time and is living independently. This example illustrates the idea that, while medication adherence should be addressed early in treatment, staff may need to be prepared to use MI to address adherence throughout work with the individual. For many if not most individuals, the decision to take medication is revisited at many points during the course of treatment. Thus, counselors may find MI useful to address medication adherence at many different times during treatment.

Influence of Interview Context and Individual's Clinical Condition on MI

The context of the interview and the condition of the individual influence how MI is conducted with an individual with SSD. The context of the interview and condition of the individual are often, though not always, highly correlated. That is, interviews with individuals who are still experiencing prominent positive (psychotic) symptoms and are highly distressed and disorganized are often conducted on psychiatric inpatient units, while interviews with individuals who are more stable and whose positive symptoms are absent or attenuated are often conducted in the community. Because of the condition of the individual and the time constraints often placed on counseling sessions, initial MI interviews on psychiatric inpatient units are often brief, focused on establishing a collaborative working relationship, and typically address questions related to "What is happening to me, and why am I here?" The interviewer may need to provide a high degree of structure to the interview—particularly with individuals experiencing high levels of negative symptoms and cognitive impairment—than necessary in interviews with individuals who are less impaired. For example, an individual with alogia (speaking in very brief statements or rarely initiating conversation) may not continue speaking if the interviewer attempts to maintain the exchange by relying on reflective listening. Thus, the interviewer may need to provide prompts or questions more frequently than might be necessary at other times. Similarly, negative symptoms and cognitive impairment often make it hard to discuss general motivational issues, but it may be possible to focus on the consequences of a problem behavior for the individual and his or her goals (Rusch & Corrigan, 2002).

Engaging the Individual

Expressing empathy through the use of reflective listening is key to engaging and communicating acceptance of the individual and to developing a collaborative relationship. It is important that motivation be assessed and never assumed when engaging an individual with SSD. This mindset is helpful not only in working with an individual experiencing a first episode but also is important when working with people who have been in treatment for some time. It is not unusual that an individual with SSD will have experienced providers who have used confrontation, warnings of dire consequences of nonadherence, and even threats of loss of access to personal funds or opportunities for employment as a means of coercing adherence. The individual is likely to have a learning history in which expressing ambivalence, reluctance, and resistance is punished and the verbal expression of motivation is reinforced. Thus, counselors often find it helpful to spend some time at the beginning of treatment exploring and assessing motivation through listening, reflecting, and accepting ambivalence.

As mentioned earlier, it is recommended that the counselor using MI in working with individuals that are symptomatic not insist on acceptance of diagnoses or labels. It is not unusual for an individual admitted to a hospital to deny that he or she has a mental illness and to frame the admission in terms of someone forcing him or her to come to the hospital. Not insisting on acceptance of a diagnosis may be a difficult concept to team members accustomed to basing treatment on diagnosis and who see acceptance of the diagnosis as fundamental to treatment. Note that not forcing a diagnosis on the individual does not mean that psychoeducation about the illness and its care should not be provided. Psychoeducation is an important component of the treatment of SSD, but the person presenting the material should allow participants not to frame their own condition in terms of a specific diagnosis.

Vignette 1: Engaging the Client In the Hospital

Jimmy was a 27-year-old unmarried man living with his mother. He was brought to the emergency room by the police, who were called when his mother became worried about Jimmy's refusal to take medication and about the increasing severity of his paranoia and auditory hallucinations, which were telling him that people were trying to kill him. His diagnosis was schizophrenia, paranoid type. The following exchange took place shortly after admission, and though his symptoms were reduced, he was still suspicious and guarded. He denied hearing voices, but staff suspected that he did hear voices when he was not engaged in an activity of some sort. The goal of this interview was to work on developing a collaborative relationship and to get Jimmy's views about what had happened and why he was in the hospital.

COUNSELOR: Jimmy, today I'd like to understand what happened and why you are here. As you know, I have spoken with your mother, but I want to get your views about this. Is that OK?

JIMMY: Sure, I guess so. I'm not really sick; I'm here because my mom and I got into an argument, and she called the cops.

COUNSELOR: So, you're here because the cops brought you here after your mom called them.

JIMMY: Yeah. They came in and grabbed me, and they put me in the police car.

COUNSELOR: It sounds like you didn't want to come here, that they brought you here against your will. That must have been very frightening. [expressing empathy]

JIMMY: It was, and it made me mad too. People are always making me do stuff that I don't want to do. My mom keeps trying to make me take those pills.

COUNSELOR: You feel pushed into doing things like taking pills. Is that what you were arguing about?

JIMMY: Yeah. That, and some other stuff.

COUNSELOR: Would you be comfortable telling about that? [asking permission]

JIMMY: I don't know; why do you want to know about that?

COUNSELOR: It would be helpful for me to know what happened and to see whether there is anything I can do to help you. Of course, you don't have to talk about anything that you don't want to. That's up to you. [emphasizing personal control]

JIMMY: Well, I guess that might be OK, but I don't want to keep taking these pills. They make me feel like shit.

COUNSELOR: My goal for right now is just to try to understand what was going on. [avoiding argumentation]

JIMMY: OK, but some of it is a little confused. You might think some of it is crazy.

COUNSELOR: It's hard to remember everything . . .

JIMMY: I remember that I was really upset with my mom; I couldn't get her to understand. I was afraid that people were trying to hurt me, but all she would talk about is the damned pills. What do you think of that?

COUNSELOR: That was really scary and frustrating. You couldn't even get your mom to understand what was happening. [expressing empathy]

JIMMY: Yeah. There were voices threatening me, and it was all so confusing. It was really awful, and she just wouldn't get it.

COUNSELOR: Things just kept piling up.

JIMMY: . . . and then the police came. I wouldn't hurt my mom; I've never hurt her or anyone else.

COUNSELOR: All you wanted was to be safe.

JIMMY: Yeah. Why don't they get that?

Note that in this vignette the counselor postponed talking about medications and avoided labels. This interview focuses on the first fundamental principle of MI—expressing empathy. Understanding the client's view of what happened and developing a trusting relationship are the main goals in this interview. Although Jimmy is a bit confused, he does not appear to have serious cognitive impairment. The interviewer was able to use reflective listening and to express empathy much the same way that he would have with a client who did not have SSD.

Identifying Goals

We have found that identifying goals in an individual with SSD is an essential part of later discussions about adherence to antipsychotic medications, since these discussions usually include consideration of how taking the medication will interfere with or promote the attainment of these goals—that is, developing discrepancy between the individual's goals and not taking medication. While some goals may be illness-related—staying out of the hospital or not getting sick—some of the most important and frequently mentioned goals are related to functioning, for example, getting a job, finding someone with whom to have a close relationship, living independently, and being self-reliant. Unfortunately, characteristics of the illness, such as pervasive passivity, may impair the individual's ability to identify goals. Questions about what one would like life to be like in the future may be meaningless. In these situations, the interviewer may need to use a sequence of specific concrete questions about each major domain of functioning, starting with "What is going on now?" For example, the series of questions for how one spends one's time might include:

- "How do you spend your time during the day?" (Some answers might include watching television, attending a day treatment program, or working at a job.)
- "What do you like about what you do?"
- "Are there things that you don't like about what you do?"
- "Is there something that you would rather do?" Or "Is this something that you would like to change?"
- "Is this something that you would like to work on now? Do you want to make this a goal?" (If several goals are mentioned, we try to identify the one's that are most important, such as by asking, "Is this goal very important or just a little important?")

For some individuals their goal might be just getting along without hassles in their current situation. That is, their goal might be something they want to avoid rather than something they want to gain. For example, avoiding conflict with family members, roommates, and caregivers or just being left alone and not bothered may be identified as the individual's major goals. Avoiding going back to jail is, of course, a frequent goal of individuals with criminal justice involvement. Many of these goals (particularly those related to functioning and avoiding hassles) do not require acknowledgment of the existence of an illness. If properly framed, even illness-related goals do not require acknowledgment that one is sick. For example, an individual who has paranoid thoughts may not be willing to acknowledge the paranoia but may be willing to acknowledge feeling fearful or wanting to feel safe. Similarly, an individual may accept the fact that a medication may make him or her feel better and help attain goals without acknowledging a particular diagnosis or even an illness. One of the important contributions of MI to the discussion of medication adherence is recognition of the importance of avoiding arguments over diagnosis and other labels.

Vignette 2: Identifying Goals in an Individual with Significant Cognitive Impairment

Darlene was a 30-year-old woman who lived in a long-term care facility. She was diagnosed with schizophrenia, undifferentiated type, and marijuana dependence disorder. Her positive symptoms (hallucinations and disorganized speech) were well controlled by the medication, but she had a number of negative symptoms and significant cognitive impairment, which was made worse by smoking marijuana. In previous interviews about this issue, she readily acknowledged that smoking pot made her more confused, but her response was "I'd rather be confused and stoned than straight and not confused." The goal of this interview was to identify client goals that can later be used in discussions of medication adherence.

COUNSELOR: Today, I'd like to talk with you about goals that you might have for the future. Would that be OK?

DARLENE: OK. Will this take very long?

COUNSELOR: Only as long as you're willing to talk with me. [emphasizing personal control] Would 20 minutes be all right?

DARLENE: OK.

COUNSELOR: What are your goals for the next 5 years?

DARLENE: (*long pause*) I don't know.

COUNSELOR: So, you don't really have any particular things that you would like to do in the next few years.

DARLENE: (*long pause*) No. I guess not.

COUNSELOR: Would you tell me about where you live?

DARLENE: Well, you know I live at Lakeview Terrace.

COUNSELOR: What do you like about living there?

DARLENE: Not much. The food is OK. I don't have to stay inside all the time.

COUNSELOR: So, there's not much to like about living there?

DARLENE: No.

COUNSELOR: Are there some things you don't like about living there?

DARLENE: I didn't get to pick my roommate, and it's boring. I can't smoke in my room. People won't leave me alone.

COUNSELOR: There's lots you don't like about living there and not much that you do like.

DARLENE: Yeah.

COUNSELOR: Would you like to change where you live?

DARLENE: Yeah.

COUNSELOR: So, you would like to live somewhere where you have more freedom to choose your roommate, to choose what you do, and to not have people bothering you.

DARLENE: Yeah.

COUNSELOR: Is moving someplace else a little important or very important?

DARLENE: I guess it's very important.

COUNSELOR: (*Continues to inquire about another domain of functioning, such as what Darlene does with her time.*)

Note that this individual was not very talkative. There are a number of reasons that a person can be relatively nonverbal. One may be bored, unhappy, or angry about being in the interview, or not sure what to say or how to respond. Alternatively, people with SSD may be nonverbal because of negative and cognitive symptoms such as alogia, passivity, anergia, and confusion. Additionally, as mentioned earlier, people with SSD may not be able to identify future goals without considerable assistance. This interview was much more structured and directive than the first vignette. After reviewing several domains (e.g., how she spends her time, who she associates with, and how much money she has to spend) and possibly identifying goals in some of them, the counselor will try to find out which of these areas is most important to Darlene. This may mean identifying the domains that are currently most dissatisfying to her. Obviously, being dissatisfied doesn't necessarily mean that she will take steps to change her situation. The counselor may need to increase the salience of possible change by arranging for her to talk with someone who has left the facility and is living independently or arranging for her to visit a supported housing program, for example. It may also be useful to teach Darlene some independent living skills, such as cooking, in order to develop self-efficacy and enhance motivation for other goals. The goals that Darlene identifies during this discussion will later be used in discussions of adherence to medication, as in the discussion below. For example, "How will taking your medication help you be able to move into a place where you have more freedom?"

Future medication discussions are conducted in the context of the individual's goals and aspirations. How does taking medication either facilitate or interfere with attaining the individual's goals? Known as cost–benefit or decisional balance discussions, these conversations lead the individual to consider whether the presumed benefits, such as reducing the likelihood or the severity of relapse and reducing symptoms, outweigh the costs of current and potential side effects and the stigma of taking medication. Information relevant to the cost–benefit discussion should be provided, using an MI approach; that is, one should ask permission to provide information rather than forcing information on the individual. For example, the clinician might ask, "Would you like to hear about a medication that is less likely to cause sexual problems?" If the individual recognizes the potential for medication to help achieve her goals, then results of previous cost–benefit discussions can be used to help identify a medication that reduces the most upsetting side effects.

Vignette 3: Conducting a Cost–Benefit Discussion of How Medication Taking Might Facilitate or Interfere with Attaining a Goal

Darrel was a 28-year-old man who had recently moved into his own apartment. Before his first psychotic episode at age 21, he had completed about 2½ years of a business and accounting program at a local college. He was participating in a supported employment program in which he had a job coach, who helped him find and adjust to competitive employment. He had recently been promoted from working in the mailroom to working as a bookkeeper. His current job was more sedentary, and he was having difficulty with drowsiness. He was thinking about discontinuing his medication. His diagnosis was schizophrenia, paranoid type.

COUNSELOR: Darrel, you said that you're thinking about stopping your Risperdal. Tell me about that.

DARREL: Well, when I was in the mailroom the sleepiness wasn't so bad because I was moving around more. I could stay awake.

COUNSELOR: . . . and now that you are sitting in one place you are having more problems with drowsiness.

DARREL: Yeah, last Tuesday my boss came in and found me nodding off. It was really embarrassing; he probably thought I was high or something. I've been doing really well for several months now. I think it's time to stop the Risperdal. I missed a day a couple weeks ago, and I felt fine.

COUNSELOR: Well, would you be willing to talk about this with me? [asking permission]

DARREL: I suppose so, but I won't change my mind.

COUNSELOR: That's up to you. [rolling with resistance by emphasizing personal control] We've worked together long enough for you to know that I'm not going to try to force you to do something you don't want to do. (*Laughs.*) It wouldn't work anyway; you'd just take off and not come back.

DARREL: You got that right.

COUNSELOR: OK. You mentioned that the medication makes you sleepy at work. Are there any other things about the medication that interfere with your goal of keeping a good job?

DARREL: Well, the sleepiness is the main thing, though I have been a little concerned by what I have been hearing about the risk of diabetes with these kinds of medications. I was a little nervous and had a headache when I first started the medication, but that went away and it didn't interfere much with my work in the mailroom. It would interfere with my current job if it came back. Oh, and I gained a little weight, but not that much. That doesn't interfere with work.

COUNSELOR: So, the main problem is being sleepy at work, and you're a little concerned about diabetes, though you haven't really gained much weight.

DARREL: That's right, especially after lunch; I'm really sleepy then. Now, I suppose you want me to list the advantages of the medication. Well, it really helped my thinking when I first started taking it. I couldn't have worked on the books with my thinking so confused, and I wouldn't have been able to work at all with the thoughts of people watching me. But, I don't know if it does anything for me now.

COUNSELOR: OK. On the one hand, the sleepiness makes it hard to stay awake, particularly after lunch. On the other hand, the medication has really helped your thinking. You're less confused, and you don't feel like people are watching you. All that is particularly important now that you are working more with your mind. [summarizing] Are there any other advantages or disadvantages to taking your medication?

DARREL: That's it.

COUNSELOR: Now, let's look at how stopping your medication would either help or interfere with your goal of keeping a good job. [developing discrepancy]

DARREL: Well, the main advantage is that I would be more alert at work. I suppose the disadvantage is that I might get sick again. But, I really feel good now, and I didn't notice anything different the other day when I didn't take my pills.

COUNSELOR: So, the advantage of stopping is that you'd be more alert at work. The disadvantage is that you might relapse, but you aren't so sure about that.

DARREL: Right.

COUNSELOR: Tell me, what has happened in the past? When you stopped taking your meds, did you get sick right away or did it take a while?

DARREL: It didn't happen right away; I mean not immediately. There were different lengths of time. Once it was about a month. Other times it was several months, but I wasn't working then.

COUNSELOR: I'm not sure I understand. Do you think that working would prevent or delay a relapse or that working would make you relapse sooner?

DARREL: I don't know. Most of the time I really like work. I like the people I work with. I like getting paid. I like feeling like I am pulling my own weight. I like it when my supervisor tells me I am doing a good job, and I really liked getting promoted. I do get nervous sometimes and feel stressed.

COUNSELOR: Not just about falling asleep, you mean.

DARREL: No. I mean like when we have deadlines or at the end of the month when I have to put together the attendance reports. I can't make a mistake or someone might not get paid or have the wrong vacation days on his check.

COUNSELOR: So, on the one hand, there are lots of things that you like about work, but there are some stressful things that could be pretty hard to cope with. How do you think this might affect relapse if you were to stop your medication?

DARREL: I don't know. I guess that's a little scary.

COUNSELOR: . . . that you might get sick again and lose your job.

DARREL: Yeah.

COUNSELOR: Is there anything else? I mean . . . are we leaving anything out?

DARREL: Not really.

COUNSELOR: If you, Dr. Glass [Darrel's psychiatrist], and I could figure out a way to deal with the sleepiness, would you be interested in trying this a bit longer? [asking permission to make a recommendation]

DARREL: Maybe. I really don't want to lose this job. It's the best one that I have ever had. I am even thinking about going back and finishing my degree—maybe even becoming a CPA.

COUNSELOR: Then let's do some problem solving to see what other options there are. Let's start by looking at what is going on at night—how long and how well you are sleeping. Then, maybe we can come up with some things that we can discuss with Dr. Glass: what time you take your meds, your risk of diabetes . . . stuff like that. OK?

DARREL: OK.

Note that the counselor rolled with Darrel's resistance and did not warn him of the consequences of stopping his medication, threaten him, or otherwise try to persuade him to take his medication. Obviously, this discussion is based on a long-standing and very good therapeutic relationship. Many clients would not even acknowledge that they were thinking about discontinuing their medication, let alone discuss this before the fact. This conversation is similar to one that occurred earlier in treatment, in that medication taking is discussed in relationship to Darrel's goals. This makes the discussion concrete rather than abstract. It also slips easily into problem solving, once the decision has been made to continue medication for the time being. It should also be noted that there is an implication of a collaborative rather than hierarchical relationship with the psychiatrist. The psychiatrist in this vignette is part of a decision-making complex consisting of the individual, the nonmedical therapist, and the psychiatrist. This sort of relationship is very important in doing MI to promote medication adherence and one of the reasons for everyone on the team to learn and use MI. A hierarchical relationship (I tell you what to do and you do it) has the potential to deteriorate into confrontation, resistance, and refusal. Instead of telling him what to do, the counselor developed (or highlighted) the discrepancy between Darrel's goals—keeping his job and going back to school—and discontinuing his medication.

PROBLEMS AND SUGGESTED SOLUTIONS

A number of problems and solutions related to cognitive impairment and negative symptoms have already been discussed. In this section we will address the presentation and potential solutions to the four Rs of precontemplation in individuals with SSD: reluctant, rebellious, resigned, and rationalizing.

Reluctant participants are those who through lack of knowledge or inertia do not want to consider change (DiClemente & Velasquez, 2002). One of the most common reasons behind the reluctance seen in individuals with SSD is the presence of such negative symptoms as anergia, avolition, and apathy. Inertia also can be the result of medication side effects, such as Parkinsonian side effects, and the drugged feeling associated with antipsychotic medications, particularly the typical medications. Individuals with reluctance secondary to negative symptoms and medication side effects benefit from ongoing support, coaching, and reinforcement. We have found that motivational approaches need to take place quite frequently, even daily with some individuals. Case managers, family members, or job coaches may need to do a quick review of goals and reestablish commitment at the beginning of each day. It is also important to identify a clear sequence of very short-term (i.e., daily) goals that clearly lead to the individual's longer-term goal. This includes consideration of how taking medication fits into accomplishing the goal for the day. Finally, support will need to be available to help the individual avoid discouragement, since many reluctant people with SSD get discouraged easily.

Rebellious persons with SSD, those who are invested in not being told what to do, typically fall into two groups: (1) individuals who no longer believe that they are sick and (2) those who are tired of being told to take medication, participate in rehabilitation, and so on. At times, the appearance of rebellion is actually a good sign and may indicate the development of independence. People in the first group may be high-functioning and often experience a course of illness characterized by repeated psychotic episodes (active phase of the illness) with no symptoms or quite minimal symptoms between episodes. The individual may believe that the illness is completely gone and see no reason to continue taking medication. Some individuals develop a pattern of repeated cycling between an active phase, symptom relief and high functioning, discontinuing medication, and relapse. Often stigma plays a role in this pattern. Whether the rebellion is the result of a belief that the individual is no longer ill or because he or she is tired of being told what to do, we have found that reviewing the costs and benefits of medication and the menu of options available works fairly well. Reviewing past patterns of medication cessation and relapse while acknowledging that the ultimate decision is up to the individual is often helpful. Focusing on the medication-taking behavior as the most immediate decision and looking at this as a decision that is chosen for today also may be beneficial. Finally, consider avoiding discussions about "taking medication for the rest of your life."

The resigned person with SSD has given up on the possibility of change and is overwhelmed by the problem (DiClemente & Velasquez, 2002). This is a characteristic response among individuals who have symptom relapse despite being adherent to medication and other interventions. It is important to *carefully* provide the individual with a more realistic range of expectations for long-term illness management. Unfortunately, some individuals have the expectation, perhaps from their providers, that taking medication will prevent relapse. A more realistic expectation is that medication and other illness management approaches may, if successful, increase the length of time between relapses, decrease the severity of the relapse, and shorten the relapse. A part of instilling hope is conveying the message that just because one medication proves to be ineffective does not mean that another one won't work (Diamond, 2002). In addition to these interventions, the MI counselor may find it useful to review and renew commitment to goals and to reframe the relapse as a setback rather than a failure.

Finally, the rationalizing person appears to have all the answers; sessions with them feel like a debate (DiClemente & Velasquez, 2002). A common type of rationalizing individual with SSD is the individual who believes that what he or she is experiencing is not SSD but something else, for example, a sensitivity to environmental contaminants or foods, a vitamin deficiency, or spiritual distress. Stigma related to mental illness is often a factor in developing these beliefs, since sensitivity to foods and environmental contaminants poses less of a stigma than having a mental illness. These beliefs also may develop as the result of family and cultural beliefs, shame, and guilt. In addition to using empathy and reflective listening, the MI practitioner should take special steps to maintain contact with the individual. It is likely that MI will have to take place over one or more relapses. If the MI counselor is working with an individual with good computer skills, for example, he or she might offer to assist the individual in doing a literature search for information about the alternative in question. There are an increasing number of search engines that are available without subscription (e.g., Google Scholar—at *scholar.google.com*). Information that the counselor gathers through the search may be presented and used in the same way that other data are presented and used in MI; that is, information is offered with permission, and conclusions are elicited and not imposed.

RESEARCH

A number of interventions have been proposed and studied to increase the rate of medication adherence among individuals with SSD (for reviews, see Dolder et al., 2003; Fenton et al., 1997; Gray et al., 2002; Zygmunt et al., 2002). Dolder and colleagues (2003) grouped interventions into three programmatic categories based on whether the approach relied primarily on educational, behavioral, or affective strategies. Educational strategies focus on verbal or written interventions with a knowledge-based emphasis designed to provide information, such as individual or group teaching and audiovisual or written materials. Behavioral strategies focus directly on adherence behaviors by using techniques designed to identify, shape, and reinforce specific behaviors, such as training in medication self-management skills (e.g., using reminders to take medication, self-administering medication, negotiating medication issues with the physician), modeling, contracting, medication packaging, and dose modification. Finally, affective interventions seek to influence adherence through appeals to emotions, social relationships, and social supports, such as family support, counseling, and supportive home visits.

It was found that purely educational interventions are the least successful in improving adherence to antipsychotic medications, while interventions that use a combination of educational, behavioral, and affective approaches are the most successful. Additionally it was found that longer-term interventions and a positive alliance with the provider are also important for success (Dolder et al., 2003). The authors noted such other additional benefits of successful treatment as reduced relapse rates, decreased hospitalization, decreased psychopathology, improved social functioning, increased medication knowledge, and improved insight into the need for treatment—results that further underscore the importance of maintaining antipsychotic medication adherence in individuals with SSD. Zygmunt and colleagues (2002) found similar results in their review of the literature, which included studies conducted in China and Malaysia as well as in the West. Interventions relying solely on psychoeducation were typically ineffective; successful interventions commonly used concrete problem-solving or motivational techniques. Zygmont and colleagues also found that interventions that specifically targeted adherence were more successful than more broadly based interventions. Interestingly, half of the broad-based interventions that were effective in improving adherence involved supportive rehabilitative community-based services, such as assertive community treatment and intensive case management (Zygmunt et al., 2002). Finally, these authors noted that adherence problems often recur and recommended the use of booster sessions.

Most of the work using MI with individuals with SSD has focused on reducing substance use in individuals with co-occurring SSD and substance use disorders (e.g., Barrowclough et al., 2001; Bellack & DiClemente, 1999; Graeber et al., 2003; Ziedonis & Trudeau, 1997). MI alone and as a component of approaches that include other methods such as skills training has been found to be effective in helping individuals with co-occurring conditions increase motivation to address substance use problems.

There have been few controlled randomized studies that have specifically examined the effectiveness of MI in increasing adherence to antipsychotic medication. Kemp and colleagues have based their intervention, called compliance therapy, on principles of motivational interventions (Kemp et al., 1996, 1998). Their intervention consisted of four to six 20- to 60-minute sessions conducted twice a week. The control group received a similar number of sessions (of comparable length) of supportive counseling. In the first two sessions, participants in compliance therapy were invited to review their history of illness and conceptualize the problem. The next two sessions were more specific and were focused on symptoms and the side effects of treatment. The benefits and drawbacks of treatment were discussed; ambivalence was explored; and discrepancy between the individual's actions and beliefs was highlighted. The last two sessions addressed the alleged stigma of medication treatment and the notion that medication is a freely chosen strategy to enhance quality of life. Finally, self-efficacy was encouraged, and the value of staying well was connected to the need for prophylactic treatment (Kemp et al., 1996).

The authors found that the compliance rate among individuals who received compliance therapy was significantly higher than that of the control group. These differences were observed on completion of the intervention and at 3-, 6-, and 18-month follow-up intervals (Kemp et al., 1996, 1998). It should be noted that the Kemp study included individuals with severe affective disorders as well as subjects with psychotic disorders. O'Donnell and colleagues (2003) made a similar comparison of five 30- to 60-minute sessions of compliance therapy (based on the Kemp manual) with nonspecific (supportive) counseling that did not address the issue of medication adherence. They failed to find a difference between compliance therapy and nonspecific counseling at 1 year. Rates of adherence prior to 1 year were not reported. These authors found that baseline adherence, attitudes toward treatment, female gender, and carer involvement in the educational program best predicted adherence rates (O'Donnell et al., 2003). The O'Donnell sample only included individuals with schizophrenia. Both of these tests of compliance therapy evaluated a very brief version of MI administered early in treatment. Given the recommendations of Zygmunt and associates (2002), it may be that an intervention needs to be longer than five to six sessions delivered at the beginning of treatment in order to produce major changes in adherence. Their recommendations fit with our experience in working with individuals with SSD—the commitment to adherence is not made at one point in time but must be renewed repeatedly during the course of treatment. The approach to medication adherence that we have proposed in this chapter has not been tested. Research is clearly needed to see whether integrating MI into all components of the program and used repeatedly throughout treatment promotes adherence to medication and other components of treatment.

CONCLUSIONS

As stated in the introduction, a common reason for failure of treatment of individuals with SSD is nonadherence to medications, and the most common form of nonadherence is underuse of medications (Nose et al., 2003). As pharmacological treatments for SSD improve, the importance of adherence to these medications grows accordingly. A number of adherence-promoting interventions have been proposed, tested, and demonstrated to have varying degrees of effectiveness in improving medication taking. Both research and clinical experience suggest that interventions to promote adherence to antipsychotic medication in individuals with SSD should be based on a strong therapeutic alliance, should take a long-term perspective specifically targeting nonadherence, and should use concrete problem-solving and motivational techniques (e.g., Dolder et al., 2003; Zygmunt et al., 2002).

There are a number of characteristics of MI that suggest that it is useful in promoting adherence in individuals with SMI, among the most significant of which is its emphasis on collaboration, evocation, and autonomy (Miller & Rollnick, 2002). This client-centered style provides a context for empowerment and recovery—far different from the coercive style often seen in programs that serve individuals with SSD. The model proposed in this chapter specifically targets adherence to antipsychotic medications, is long-term, and is recommended to be integrated with other psychiatric rehabilitation interventions. We have suggested that MI interventions targeting adherence should occur in a number of contexts, including supported employment, community-based case management, family support, and dual disorders treatment. This is because discussions of medication occur frequently and with a wide range of providers. The basics of our approach differ little from traditional MI, though we have made a number of suggestions for modifications to address problems that often occur in individuals with SSD. The most significant modifications are in response to illness-related factors such as the presence of negative symptoms, cognitive impairment, and medication side effects. MI may hold promise as a method for enhancing adherence and treatment delivery with individuals with SSD, with improvements in symptom control and quality of life. We look forward to empirical evaluation of these methods in future research work with this important population.

NOTE

1. The literature cited, particularly treatment literature, primarily includes in its samples individuals with a diagnosis of schizophrenia, though most studies also include individuals with other psychotic disorders such as schizoaffective disorder, schizophreniform disorder, psychotic disorder not otherwise specified, and occasionally mood disorders with psychotic features. Since there are more similarities than differences among these conditions, we also will include individuals with other psychotic disorders in our discussion. We will refer to the disorders as a group—schizophrenia spectrum disorders (SSD)—unless the distinction is important, and then we will refer to a specific diagnosis. Few studies reviewed for this chapter included individuals with mood disorders. While we believe that the approach described in this chapter is appropriate for individuals with bipolar and major depressive disorders, space limitations prevent us from addressing some specific modifications necessary when working with people with severe depression and manic symptoms, such as grandiosity and racing thoughts. Thus, we focus our recommendations specifically on individuals with psychotic disorders.

REFERENCES

American Psychiatric Association. (2000). *Diagnostic and statistical manual of mental disorders* (4th ed., text rev.). Washington, DC: Author.

Baker, A. I., Lewin, T., Reichler, H., Clancy, R., Carr, V., Garrett, R., et al. (2002). Motivational interviewing among psychiatric in-patients with substance use disorders. *Acta Psychiatrica Scandinavica, 106*, 233–240.

Barrowclough, C., Haddock, G., Tarrier, N., Lewis, S. W., Moring, J., O'Brien, R., et al. (2001). Randomized controlled trial of motivational interviewing, cognitive behavior therapy, and family intervention for patients with comorbid schizophrenia and substance use disorders. *American Journal of Psychiatry, 158*, 1706–1713.

Bellack, A. S., & DiClemente, C. C. (1999). Treating substance abuse among patients with schizophrenia. *Psychiatric Services, 50*, 75–80.

Blackwell, B. (1976). Treatment adherence. *British Journal of Psychiatry, 129*, 513–531.

Corrigan, P. W. (2004). How stigma interferes with mental health care. *American Psychologist, 59*, 614–625.

Corrigan, P. W., McCracken, S. G., & Holmes, E. P. (2001). Motivational interviews as goal assessment for persons with psychiatric disability. *Community Mental Health Journal, 37*, 113–122.

Corrigan, P. W., & Penn, D. L. (1995). The effects of antipsychotic and antiparkinsonian medication on psychosocial skill learning. *Clinical Psychology: Science and Practice, 2*, 251–262.

Diamond, R. J. (2002). *Instant psychopharmacology* (2nd ed.). New York: Norton.

DiClemente, C. C., & Velasquez, M. M. (2002). Motivational interviewing and the stages of change. In W. R. Miller & S. Rollnick, *Motivational interviewing: Preparing people for change* (2nd ed., pp. 201–216). New York: Guilford Press.

Dolder, C. R., Lacro, J. P., Leckband, S., & Jeste, D. V. (2003). Interventions to improve antipsychotic medication adherence: Review of recent literature. *Journal of Clinical Psychopharmacology, 23*, 389–399.

Drake, R. E., & Goldman, H. H. (Eds.). (2003). *Evidence-based practices in mental health care* (compendium of articles from *Psychiatric Services*). Arlington, VA: American Psychiatric Press.

Fenton, W. S., Blyler, C. R., & Heinssen, R. K. (1997). Determinants of medication compliance in schizophrenia: Empirical and clinical findings. *Schizophrenia Bulletin, 23*, 637–651.

Graeber, D. A., Moyers, T. B., Griffith, G., Guajardo, E., & Tonigan, S. (2003). Addiction services: A pilot study comparing motivational interviewing and an educational intervention in patients with schizophrenia and alcohol use disorders. *Community Mental Health Journal, 39*, 189–202.

Gray, R., Wykes, T., & Gournay, K. (2002). From compliance to concordance: A review of the literature on interventions to enhance compliance with antipsychotic medication. *Journal of Psychiatric and Mental Health Nursing, 9*, 277–284.

Kemp, R., Hayward, P., Applewhaite, G., Everitt, B., & David, A. (1996). Compliance therapy in psychotic patients: Randomised controlled trial. *British Medical Journal, 312*, 345–349.

Kemp, R., Kirov, G., Everitt, B., Hayward, P., & David, A. (1998). Randomized controlled trial of compliance therapy. 18-month follow-up. *British Journal of Psychiatry, 172*, 413–419.

Miller, W. R., & Rollnick, S. (2002). *Motivational interviewing: Preparing people for change* (2nd ed.). New York: Guilford Press.

Mueser, K. T., Noordsy, D. L., Drake, R. E., & Fox, L. (2003). *Integrated treatment for dual disorders: A guide to effective practice*. New York: Guilford Press.

Nose, M., Barbui, C., & Tansella, M. (2003). How often do patients with psychosis fail to adhere to treatment programmes:? A systematic review. *Psychological Medicine, 33*, 1149–1160.

O'Donnell, C., Donohoe, G., Sharkey, L., Owens, N., Migone, M., Harries, R., et al. (2003). Compliance therapy—a randomized controlled trial in schizophrenia. *British Medical Journal, 327*, 834–837.

Prochaska, J. O., DiClemente, C. C., & Norcross, J. C. (1992). In search of how people change: Applications to addictive behaviors. *American Psychologist, 47*, 1102–1114.

Rusch, N., & Corrigan, P. W. (2002). Motivational interviewing to improve insight and treatment adherence in schizophrenia. *Psychiatric Rehabilitation Journal, 26*, 23–32.

Spaulding, W. D., Reed, D., Poland, J., & Storzbach, D. M. (1996). Cognitive deficits in psychotic disorders. In P. W. Corrigan & S. C. Yudofsky (Eds.), *Cognitive rehabilitation for neuropsychiatric disorders* (pp. 129–166). Washington, DC: American Psychiatric Press.

Young, J. L., Zonana, H. V., & Shepler, L. (1986). Medication noncompliance in schizophrenia: Codification and update. *Bulletin of the American Academy of Psychiatry and the Law, 14*, 105–122.

Ziedonis, D. M., & Trudeau, K. (1997). Motivation to quit using substances among individuals with schizophrenia: Imlications for a motivation-based treatment model. *Schizophrenia Bulletin, 23*, 229–338.

Zweben, A., & Zuckoff, A. (2002). Motivational interviewing and treatment adherence. In W. R. Miller & S. Rollnick, *Motivational interviewing: Preparing people for change* (2nd ed., pp. 299–319). New York: Guilford Press.

Zygmunt, A., Olfson, M., Boyer, C. A., & Mechanic, D. (2002). Interventions to improve medication adherence in schizophrenia. *American Journal of Psychiatry, 159*, 1653–1664.

CHAPTER 11

Motivational Interviewing with Dually Diagnosed Patients

Steve Martino
Theresa B. Moyers

Motivational interviewing (MI; Miller & Rollnick, 2002) is a highly recommended component of a comprehensive treatment approach for patients who suffer from co-occurring severe mental illness such as schizophrenia or schizoaffective disorder and alcohol or drug use disorders (Carey, 1996; Drake et al., 2001; Minkoff, 2001). Yet, how would a practitioner proceed to use MI with psychotically ill substance-abusing patients? Is a direct application of MI appropriate without alteration, or must one modify the practice of MI to accommodate the clinical challenges presented by these dually diagnosed patients?

Like others (Bellack & DiClemente, 1999; Carey, Purnine, Maisto, & Carey, 2001; Handmaker, Packard, & Conforti, 2002; Martino, Carroll, Kostas, Perkins, & Rounsaville, 2002), we take the position that some modification of MI practice is necessary to address the complex needs of dually diagnosed patients. This chapter describes recommended modifications to MI when working with patients impaired by psychotic functioning. We first detail the unique clinical issues presented by patients impaired by psychosis. Next, we present recommended modifications to MI through case vignettes and discuss situations where skill-building, supportive, and crisis interventions are more appropriate than MI. We conclude the chapter with a summary of how MI has been applied in dual diagnosis treatment and the related research, and future directions needed to advance these and other dual diagnosis MI applications.

CLINICAL POPULATION AND USUAL TREATMENTS

Psychotic disordered dually diagnosed patients commonly present to treatment with several unique clinical issues that affect their motivation for behavior change. These issues include (1) the need for integrated psychiatric and substance abuse treatment, (2) cognitive impairments, (3) positive psychotic symptoms, (4) negative psychotic symptoms, and (5) acute symptoms requiring intervention.

Need for Integrated Treatment

Psychotically ill dually diagnosed patients have a serious mental illness that interacts with their alcohol and illicit drug use. These interactions may involve substance use that (1) lessens negative psychotic symptoms, (2) reduces discomfort caused by positive psychotic symptoms, (3) facilitates social interactions, and (4) masks burgeoning psychotic symptoms as solely substance-induced. Helping patients improve their functioning requires understanding how their dual problem areas affect each other and treating these problems at the same time (Drake, McLaughlin, Pepper, & Minkoff, 1991). An integrated and comprehensive treatment also extends the targets of behavior change to other areas deemed essential to dual diagnosis recovery. In particular, antipsychotic medication adherence is a critical treatment target that addresses the impaired brain structures and neural mechanisms involved in psychosis (Harrison, 1999). In addition, dually diagnosed patients' numerous treatment needs (e.g., medical/dental, vocational, financial, housing) often involve them in many sectors of the service system. Adopting strategies to foster patient engagement and retention in integrated treatment is important.

Cognitive Impairment

Dually diagnosed patients also may have significant cognitive impairments. On average, patients with schizophrenia score about one standard deviation unit lower on cognitive performance measures than the average group of healthy comparison patients (Heinrichs, 2004). Across studies, patients with schizophrenia show deficits in word generation, abstract reasoning and mental flexibility, attention and concentration, verbal learning, and working memory. Chronic alcohol and drug abuse likely worsens these areas by further independently contributing to poorer cognitive performance (e.g., inefficiencies in problem solving, abstraction, visual-spatial abilities, perceptual-motor functioning, mental flexibility, speed of information processing, and learning and memory) (Bolla, Brown, Eldreth, Tate, & Cadet, 2002; Lawton-Craddock, Nixon, & Tivis, 2003; Nixon & Phillips, 1999; Parsons, 1998). Modifying treatments to accommodate dually diagnosed patients' cognitive impairments is a significant clinical challenge.

Positive Psychotic Symptoms

Most idiosyncratic to psychotic patients are positive psychotic symptoms. Typical positive symptoms include delusions, hallucinations, disordered thinking, and unusual or bizarre behaviors (e.g., disorganized speech such as circumstantiality or tangentiality). If these symptoms become severe enough, patients may require psychiatric hospitalization, crisis intervention, and/or medication intervention. However, many patients with schizophrenia function with episodic or chronic positive symptoms that do not reach dramatic levels of expression but challenge the ability of clinicians to accurately understand and enhance the motivation of their patients.

Negative Psychotic Symptoms

Equally characteristic of schizophrenia is the presence of negative psychotic symptoms. Negative psychotic symptoms involve the restriction or absence of thoughts, feelings, and behaviors that most people experience. Typical negative symptoms include feeling emotionally flat, having slowed thinking and speech production, diminished motivation, energy, and pleasure, and being socially isolated. These impairments may make it difficult for patients to engage in an interview or to respond with much spontaneity and fluency. Instead of recognizing how these patients may have difficulty ascertaining and describing their experiences, clinicians may mistakenly presume these patients are unmotivated for change. Negative symptoms are quite common among schizophrenic patients and constitute the most enduring symptoms of psychotic illness. Addressing them in treatment is another central challenge for clinicians.

Acute Symptoms Requiring Intervention

At times dually diagnosed patients may have insufficient psychiatric stability to attend to the content of an interview and remain reality-based. They also have higher rates of suicidality and homicidality than substance-abusing patients without co-occurring psychiatric conditions (Drake, Osher, & Wallach, 1989; Lyons & McGovern, 1989; Turner & Tsuang, 1990). Clinicians working with these patients must have the capacity to accurately assess mental status and risk to safeguard dually diagnosed patients and provide them with the most appropriate treatments (e.g., crisis intervention, hospitalization).

RATIONALE FOR USING MI WITH DUALLY DIAGNOSED PATIENTS

While there has been extensive consideration of clinical issues in dual diagnosis patients (see Drake et al., 2001; Managed Care Initiative Panel on Co-Occurring Disorders, 1998), less attention has been paid to developing strategies to motivate these patients for behavioral change. Typically, MI is noted as a recommended evidence-based practice to use with this population (Bellack & DiClemente, 1999; Carey, 1996; Drake et al., 2001; Osher & Kofoed, 1989). The combination of the MI style for eliciting motivation for change and emphasis on harm reduction is seen as an attractive alternative to more confrontational and abstinence-oriented addiction treatment approaches that are not as effective with drug and alcohol problems and might even exacerbate psychotic symptoms (Carey, 1996).

Yet, there have been relatively few attempts to modify and evaluate MI for dually diagnosed patients. Recently, several clinical investigators have begun to describe and test their initial efforts to specifically apply MI to dually diagnosed patients (Carey et al., 2001; Graeber, Moyer, Griffith, Guajardo, & Tonigan, 2003; Handmaker et al., 2002; Martino et al., 2002; Van Horn & Bux, 2001). While these applications have been implemented at different clinical levels of care (e.g., outpatient, ambulatory) and modalities (individual, group) and with varying degrees of independence from other treatment services (add-on to integrated treatment, stand-alone intervention), the investigators all highlight how they have applied MI to address critical dual diagnosis clinical issues. In the remainder of this chapter, we will describe and synthesize these modifications of MI and use clinical examples to illustrate their use.

CLINICAL APPLICATION OF MI
WITH DUALLY DIAGNOSED PATIENTS

We organize our discussion of how to apply MI with dually diagnosed patients according to the challenges these patients' clinical issues pose to MI practice. Namely, we discuss (1) accommodating multiple interacting behavior targets, (2) accommodating cognitive impairments, (3) addressing positive psychotic symptoms, (4) managing negative psychotic symptoms, and (5) knowing when MI is appropriate. Table 11.1 summarizes recommended modifications to MI in each of these areas. Because we believe it is best to learn how to swim in the shallow part of the pool with a capable instructor rather than to be thrown into the deep end without support, we strongly recommend that those interested in applying MI in dual diagnosis treatment already have training, experience, and credentials for working with this patient population and, similarly, have developed their MI skills in less challenging clinical waters.

Accommodating Multiple Interacting Behavior Targets

The addition of psychiatric problems to the traditional alcohol and illicit drug use targets of MI complicates clinicians' efforts to enhance dually diagnosed patients' motivation for change. Clinicians must attend to the patients' motivations for addressing their substance abuse and psychiatric problems and understand their interactions. For example, a patient who has developed endocarditis may want to stop using heroin for health reasons. However, the patient may continue to use it to reduce the intensity of derogatory auditory hallucinations. Another patient may use cocaine to temporarily feel euphoric instead of emotionally flat despite later having financial hardships from purchasing cocaine. Other patients who feel stigmatized because of their psychotic illness may use drugs to fit in with their age peers and not attend dual diagnosis treatment programs to avoid viewing themselves as psychiatric patients. Clinicians must understand these interacting motivations to effectively treat dual diagnosis patients.

Many MI techniques are amenable to addressing these interactions. Use of such open-ended questions or statements as "What effect does your drinking have on your voices?" or "Tell me about what happens to you psychiatrically when you smoke crack" elicit discussion about the relationship between substance use and psychotic symptoms. Likewise,

TABLE 11.1. Clinical Issues, Challenges to MI, and Recommended Modifications

Clinical issues	Challenges to MI	Recommended modifications
1. Need for integrated psychiatric and substance abuse treatment that also targets related important behavioral domains.	MI needs to accommodate a larger range of interacting behavioral targets that mutually may affect the patients' motivation to change any one behavioral area. Clinicians must recognize, reinforce, and elicit change talk regarding other target behaviors.	a. Attend to motivations for using substances, addressing psychosis, and how these motivations interact. b. Use open-ended and evocative questions that elicit discussion of psychiatric concerns and their interactions with substance use. c. Target medication and treatment program adherence in addition to substance use. d. Extend strategies such as decisional balance activities and personalized feedback to encompass medication and treatment adherence areas.
2. Multiple aspects of cognition are impaired, including attention, working memory, encoding acquisition, word generation and verbal fluency, and executive ability problems such as abstract reasoning and mental flexibility.	Patients may have difficulty with self-reflection, cognitively tracking what the clinician asks or says, appraising the consequences of problem behaviors, and holding in balance combined and competing motivations for change.	a. Question, reflect, and summarize in clear and concise terms. b. Liberally use successive reflections and summaries. c. Use concrete and engaging materials and methods for eliciting change talk.
3. Positive psychotic symptoms such as delusions, hallucinations, related bizarre behaviors, and disorganized speech may be present.	Psychotically organized expressions and behaviors during the session complicate the reflective listening process when patients talk in ways that may be confusing, digressive, or bizarre. Patients may worsen symptomatically if the clinician reflects emotionally charged material or prolongs the patients' contemplation of ambivalent states.	a. Paraphrase often to maintain reality-based and organized patient–clinician dialogue. b. Use metaphor or simile to make sense of patients' seemingly bizarre statements and gestures. c. Use caution in exploring despairing patient statements and negative life events or expressed emotions. d. Succinctly summarize ambivalence and quickly employ strategies to elicit change talk to resolve the ambivalence in favor of change.

(continued)

TABLE 11.1. (continued)

Clinical issues	Challenges to MI	Recommended modifications
4. Negative psychotic symptoms such as thought blocking, social isolation, decreased emotional expression, impoverished thinking, processing speed, and speech, and diminished volition and drive may be present.	Patients may appear disinterested or disengaged in the session and have difficulty participating in it. Their motivation to not use substances may be diminished by the baseline phenomenology that remains in the absence of substance use. They may not see participation in treatment programs, social or vocational rehabilitation efforts, or self-help groups as desirable.	a. Paraphrase often to stimulate patient discussion. b. Give patients sufficient time to respond to questions and reflections. c. Affirm patients' participation in the session. d. Use personalized and structured feedback, including assessment instruments and other prompts, to facilitate participation.
5. Multiple dual diagnosis problems may require other types of interventions. Psychotic symptom severity may worsen. Acute suicidality and homicidality are likely to occur among dually diagnosed patients more than with primary substance-abusing patients.	Patients may require interventions that are not MI or that remove the patients' freedom of choice and personal autonomy, depending on their symptom severity and global functioning.	a. Flexibly shift to skill-building and supportive interventions to address complex and multiple dual diagnosis problems. b. Develop capacity and professional support to handle crisis situations. c. Determine when patients are too psychotic to benefit from MI.

evocative questions such as "What problems does marijuana cause you mentally?" or "Instead of drinking or drugging, what have you done in the past that has helped you feel less paranoid?" may draw out change talk relevant to the intersection of both problem areas. In addition, decisional balance activities and personalized feedback activities can address psychiatric-related behaviors in addition to substance-related ones. Both Handmaker and colleagues (2002) and Martino and colleagues (2002) suggest examining the costs and benefits of dual diagnosis treatment program adherence and nonadherence with patients. Martino and colleagues used a color-coded bar chart comparing recent (past 30 days) Addiction Severity Index (ASI; McLellan et al., 1992) ratings with the corresponding subjective patient ratings on functional areas tapped by the instrument. During the feedback portion of the interview, clinicians and patients examined the rating similarities and differences and how substance use affects the patients' functioning, particularly in the psychiatric domain. In a similar manner, these investigators used the Positive and Negative Syndrome Scale (PANSS; Kay, Fizbein, & Opler, 1987) to provide patients with specific information about the patients' psychotic symptoms and used this information to talk about how substance use and positive and negative symptoms affected each other.

As implied, the target behaviors for motivational enhancement need to expand to behaviors essential for recovery from psychotic disorders, and clinicians must recognize, reinforce, and elicit patient change talk in these areas. Specifically, motivation for treatment adherence to prescribed pharmacotherapy and dual diagnosis services is critical (Handmaker et al., 2002; Martino et al., 2002). Nonadherence in these areas has been associated with poorer substance use and psychiatric patient outcomes (Drake et al., 1991; Owens, Fischer, Booth, & Cuffel, 1996) where failure to adhere to treatment removes patients from the active therapeutic agents that presumably may help them be more successful in recovery (Zweben & Zuckoff, 2002). Pharmacotherapies that attempt to treat the neurobiological substrates of schizophrenia are essential, particularly with the advent of atypical antipsychotic agents that have fewer side effects, more efficacy for treating negative psychotic symptoms, and the potential to reduce cravings that prompt illicit drug use (Brady & Malcolm, 2004; Owens et al., 1996). When working with dually diagnosed patients using MI, clinicians inquire how patients view taking medications and attend to obstacles (e.g., uncomfortable side effects, limited effectiveness, complicated regimens, costs) that may impede adherence. With the expanding range and availability of pharmacotherapeutic options and the growing number of guidelines to improve the neuroleptic care of dually diagnosed patients, increased hope and optimism about the benefits of antipsychotic medications may be warranted and create new opportunities for practitioners and patients to collaborate on viable medication strategies that increase the likelihood of adherence (Mellman et al., 2001).

Patient engagement and retention in integrated dual diagnosis services also is necessary for successful long-term recovery from severe and persistent psychotic and substance use disorders (Drake, Mercer-McFadden, Mueser, McHugo, & Bond, 1998). These program services provide patients with essential supports for obtaining housing, accessing employment and medical services, developing non-substance-using social networks and stronger family connections, and improving social coping skills. The capacity of clinicians to continuously promote patients' involvement in this type of comprehensive integrated system of care to develop patient stability and functional improvement is critical (Drake et al., 2001). In this regard, MI used within dual diagnosis treatment may require more than a brief intervention of one to four sessions, as it is typically practiced. Rather, it is better construed as a clinical tool that clinicians use when the patients' shifting levels of motivation across multiple behavior change areas and phases of treatment become an impediment to progress (Martino et al., 2002). Once the patient is actively working toward a treatment goal, the use of MI is likely to be unnecessary, although the clinician may still wish to place emphasis on the collaborative spirit of this method.

Handmaker and colleagues (2002) describe an outpatient stage-matched integrated dual diagnosis treatment model that adopts this type of long-term perspective of keeping patients involved in treatment appropriate to their level of motivation. Patients attend a variety of groups to address different stages of readiness for different problem areas over time. Thus, a patient may stop using illicit drugs and attend a group designed to practice drug relapse prevention skills, but he or she may continue to drink excessively on occasion and have ambivalence about entering into a supportive housing program. The patient would attend a "talk about change" group to address the patient's mixed motivations for changing these latter areas. If the patient decides to change behavior that he or she had previously resisted, then the patient moves to action planning and practice groups for this new behavioral target (e.g., developing interviewing skills for a housing program). If the patient's motivation wavers, the patient may move back to a group that is more suitable for the patient's level of motivation. In this manner, the patient continues to participate in targeted treatment appropriate to his or her evolving level of motivation across behavior change areas.

Accommodating Cognitive Impairments

Cognitive impairments may complicate the MI process by making it more difficult for patients to self-reflect, cognitively track what clinicians ask or say, appraise the consequences of problem behaviors, and hold in balance combined and competing motivations for change. If such processing problems are evident, modifying MI to accommodate these impairments is needed to make the highly reflective approach appropriate for use with the dually diagnosed patient population. Several recommendations have emerged in the literature.

Of foremost importance is the need for simplicity and clarity throughout the interview. Open-ended questions should be stated in clear and concise terms rather than compounding or overcomplicating them with multiple requests for elaboration within the same query. For example, the question "How did your last hospitalization occur and what did your use of substances, medications, or any other issues have to do with it?" burdens the patient with parsing apart multiple questions, holding them in memory, and responding in a sequenced manner— clearly a challenge for someone impaired by psychosis. Instead, the clinician should avoid these types of questions and simplify them by inquiring about smaller chunks of information in a straightforward manner, for example:

> "Tell me about what you think are the main reasons for your being hospitalized."

Additionally, liberal use of successive and clearly stated reflections and summaries during an interview helps patients attend to, remember, and logically organize the conversation. The clinical vignette below illustrates the utility of successive reflective and summary statements with a man struggling with schizoaffective disorder and cocaine dependence and interviewed on an inpatient unit after he had been hospitalized for 5 days.

PATIENT: I'm depressed, man. I couldn't keep going on. The voices didn't let up. ..

CLINICIAN: The voices didn't let up, and you became more and more depressed. You felt like giving up.

PATIENT: It's hard living on the street. I'm not staying in the shelter. It's not safe in there. (*pause*) Drugs.

CLINICIAN: In addition to hearing voices, you haven't felt safe in the shelter, where drugs are all around you. You've been doing the best you can to survive on the street.

PATIENT: (*Tears up.*) My girlfriend is in jail. She makes me go out and get drugs for her. She yells and screams at me until I do it. The voices get so bad. When she went to jail, I had nowhere to stay. I'm not going back to a shelter.

CLINICIAN: So, you haven't had a safe place to live for some time. When you were staying with your girlfriend, she was using and pushed you to get drugs for her. After she went to jail, you lost your housing. You tried staying in a shelter, but people around you were using and you felt unsafe. Without a safe place to live and hearing voices that got so bad, you became more and more depressed.

PATIENT: Yeah. I smoked crack because I couldn't take it anymore. I thought I might try to kill myself. (*Tears up.*) I didn't have any more money.

CLINICIAN: You were completely spent.

PATIENT: Nothing was working. Then I lost my medications. So, I went to the emergency room.

CLINICIAN: You were looking for some way to feel better. Crack didn't help. Living on the streets didn't help. Losing your medications didn't help. Being around people who use—like your girlfriend or people in the shelter—didn't help. The voices and depression became unbearable. At first, you thought taking your life would be a way out. Instead, you decided to go to the emergency room. I'm glad you did.

PATIENT: I don't want to die. I have a son.

The clinician continues in this fashion and clarifies that the patient's mother is raising his son and that the patient wants to be more involved in his son's life and obtain work to help his mother financially. The clinician evokes the ways in which smoking crack makes his voices and depression worse in the end, contributes to his losing his medications, and doesn't help him achieve his employment and parenting goals.

Several alterations to direct methods for eliciting change talk often are helpful to accommodate cognitive impairments. Strategies such as exploring a decisional balance, clarifying goals and values, and providing objective feedback may need to be simplified and delivered in more structured and engaging ways. Regarding the decisional balance, patients with schizophrenia may have difficulties seeing the relationship between their use and subsequent negative consequences. They also may have difficulty reflecting very long on the costs and benefits of changing versus not changing behavior. Bellack and DiClemente (1999) suggest identifying only one or two specific negative consequences that strongly impact the patient and then focusing on these significant drawbacks in motivating the patient to reduce or quit substance use. Martino and colleagues (2002) report that many patients with psychotic disorders find completing a 2 × 2 matrix (e.g., costs and benefits of substance use vs. quitting) confusing. They recommend simplifying the task by focusing only on the positive and negative consequences of changing behavior. Alternatively, Carey and colleagues (2001) have patients discuss the reasons for not changing and the reasons for changing instead of specifically differentiating the pros and cons within these two categories. Handmaker and colleagues (2002) concretize this approach further by stacking blocks for both sets of reasons and then talking with patients about which side has more. They also have recorded reasons to stop using substances on color-coded cards (red for stop) that patients carry with them and then review whenever they feel an urge to use.

Modifying strategies for developing discrepancy may be useful. Carey and colleagues (2001) recommend using a conceptually simple and highly structured "personal strivings" list to help patients articulate what they would like to achieve in the future. Clinicians and patients complete a worksheet that asks patients to identify up to three goals that they would like to accomplish. For each identified goal, the worksheet contains a prompt that asks the patients how cutting down or quitting substance use would affect their goal attainment. If patients have difficulty generating personal goals, clinicians prompt patients to consider possible goals related to dual diagnosis recovery (e.g., symptom improvement, accessing employment programs). Moreover, clinicians ask patients to consider how adhering to treatment (medications, formal programs, case management services) would affect goal attainment. Graeber and colleagues (2003) utilized the Personal Values Card Sort (Miller, C'de Baca, Matthews, & Wilbourne, 2001). However, they modified it to reflect more concrete achievements relevant to patients with schizophrenia (e.g., "autonomy" was adapted to "have control of my own money") and then used these simplified identified values as the foundation for discrepancy development. An updated version of this modified card sort (Moyers & Martino, 2006) is available on the University of New Mexico Center on Alcoholism, Substance Abuse, and Addictions website (*casaa.unm.edu*).

While providing personalized feedback is not unique to MI, this strategy most often is included in MI interventions (Burke, Arkowitz, & Menchola, 2003), and many practitioners have described ways in which they have adapted it to accommodate dually diagnosed patients' cognitive impairments. In general, it is a useful strategy for engaging patients in self-reflection about their substance use and their experience of their psychotic disorders when they have not generated this material on their own (Carey et al., 2001). Use of visual aids (graphs, charts), simplifying the presentation of material into small units of information, and using engaging formats to keep patients focused on what is presented commonly are recommended. For example, use of thermometer-like scales to prompt discussions about levels of commitment to cutting down or quitting substance use may help patients talk about their level of motivation and what might raise or strengthen their commitment to change (Carey et al., 2001). Use of color-coded pie or bar charts may help patients better understand their pattern of use relative to population norms instead of describing percentiles to them (Carey et al., 2001). Preparing pamphlets that organize the presentation of feedback also may be helpful for patients to consider important dual diagnosis recovery issues (Martino et al., 2002). Finally, simplifying technical terms into patient-friendly language that captures their experiences enhances the feedback process. Martino and colleagues (2002) found that when using the PANSS global positive and negative psychotic symptom scale scores in a patient feedback activity many patients become confused by the term "positive" symptoms, in that it suggested something beneficial about being psychotic. One patient cleverly suggested that we refer to positive symptoms as "hot symptoms" (i.e., symptoms that make patients feel like they are boiling inside) and negative symptoms as "cold symptoms" (symptoms that make patients feel like they are frozen inside). Thereafter, we presented the information in bar-chart form and color-coded the "hot" symptom bar red and the "cold" symptom bar blue, and found that patients responded well to this visual image. This modified feedback technique generated more patient discussion and elaboration than the original format.

Addressing Positive Psychotic Symptoms

Positive psychotic symptoms such as auditory hallucinations, delusions, and disorganized thinking challenge the ability of clinicians to accurate understand and reflect what patients say. While these symptoms sometimes make the patients' statements very difficult to understand, we have found that patients may continue to convey useful intended meaning even when positive psychotic symptoms color what they have said.

Our central recommendations for addressing positive psychotic symptoms in MI revolve around the use of reflective listening. In particular, the capacity of clinicians to reflect the majority of the time using paraphrases (or complex reflections) has been highlighted as an important preliminary proficiency standard (Miller & Mount, 2001; Moyers, Martin, Catley, Harris, & Ahluwalia, 2003). This skill becomes even more essential when working with dually diagnosed patients who may say things that at first may seem illogical or unusual, at best. Without the clinicians' active efforts to bring order and reasoning to the conversation, confusion for both parties will occur and patients may become symptomatically worse.

In dual diagnosis MI, therefore, reflective listening functions both to express the clinician's empathy and to serve the additional function of keeping the patient–clinician dialogue reality-based and logically organized when patients speak in marginally coherent ways. We have found that liberal use of paraphrasing—perhaps even more than in MI for patients unimpaired by psychosis—is necessary. Several examples illustrate this process. In the first example, a male patient with chronic paranoid schizophrenia and a past history of alcohol and marijuana abuse is participating in an intake evaluation for an intensive outpatient program. After the clinician provides an opening statement describing how the intake will proceed, the clinician begins the interview with a patient-centered open-ended question designed to elicit the reasons the patient has sought program services. The patient's suspiciousness is prominent.

CLINICIAN: Tell me about what's led you to seek treatment in our program.

PATIENT: I'm not seeking treatment. Treatment is seeking me.

CLINICIAN: It's not that you want to come here for treatment. Treatment is being forced on you.

PATIENT: My housing counselor and my therapist are after me. Partners in crime, that's what they are.

CLINICIAN: They've recommended that you come here and it seems like an injustice to you. You don't want to be here.

PATIENT: What right do they have to tell me I have to come here just because they think I'm drinking?

CLINICIAN: You feel falsely accused of drinking, and even if you did drink, it's none of their business.

PATIENT: I did drink, but not much. They are making way too much out of it. My counselor went into my room without asking and has been following me around the house. He found an empty beer bottle in my room and said I had to come here for an evaluation. I don't need help for my drinking. It's a free country. I should be able to buy what I want.

CLINICIAN: You don't want to be forced into treatment for drinking. Maybe other things are of concern to you. You want the freedom to choose what you will work on in treatment, that is, if you decide to invest in treatment for yourself.

PATIENT: Yeah, I get angry. I don't trust other people—sometimes for good reason. I might want to work on that, but I only had one beer. I don't think he or my therapist should make so much over it. That really pisses me off.

CLINICIAN: You don't think you have a problem with drinking. You sometimes get angry for good reason, like over this situation. To your credit, you recognize that sometimes you might get pissed off at people when they really didn't mean any harm. Sounds like that is more of what you might want to work on. Their focus on your drinking isn't helping you address your main concern.

In this example, the patient has some awareness about his inaccurate suspiciousness. Use of reflection with paranoid patients is appropriate when the patient's delusions are not fixed. However, if a patient rigidly adheres to delusional beliefs and become increasingly paranoid when the clinician reflects these beliefs, continued reflection of the paranoid delusions would be inappropriate. Such intervention might foster more paranoid ideation. Under those circumstances, we would recommend that the clinician simply acknowledge the patient's beliefs and shift the focus to other areas where motivational enhancement opportunities might exist.

Using deeper levels of reflection involving paraphrases that incorporate metaphor or simile are also helpful in anchoring the patients' statements in reality while promoting empathic listening. In this example, a 19-year-old student on an extended medical leave from college is talking with his clinician during an outpatient session. He had used hallucinogens and MDMA (ecstasy) at college numerous times. He barely passed his courses during his first semester, uncharacteristic of his usual academic proficiency. He told his parents that he had difficulty in adjusting to college life initially and that he would improve his grades during the second semester. He nonetheless seemed more withdrawn during winter break and made little effort to initiate contact with high school friends. At the beginning of his second semester, he stopped attending classes and began to demonstrate increasingly bizarre behavior. After a brief hospitalization and initiation of pharmacotherapy, he took a medical leave, returned to live with his parents, and began to attend individual therapy. He continued to demonstrate overly abstract speech and episodically behave in unusual ways. In the session, the clinician and patient are talking about his use of LSD and ecstasy and the impact it has had on his functioning.

CLINICIAN: What have been the negative effects of using these drugs?

PATIENT: It's been a mind-blowing experience of septic proportions.

CLINICIAN: You feel that drugs have fouled up your mind.

PATIENT: You know I can't see college on my horizon right now.

CLINICIAN: Your mind is not working the way it used to, in part due to the drugs, and it's hard to see going back to college right now.

PATIENT: I can't concentrate very well, and it's hard to remember things. Will I be convicted when others have not?

CLINICIAN: You wonder why this has happened to you. Others have used drugs, stopped, feel fine later, and continue to function. You aren't sure how things will end up.

PATIENT: (*Gets up out of his chair, walks to the office door, opens and slams it, and then stands in the middle of the room looking confused.*)

CLINICIAN: You're not sure if the door has been shut for you to return to college. You want to do what you can to open it, but you are not sure what you can do.

PATIENT: (*Looks at the clinician.*) What can I do? (*Sits down.*)

At this point the clinician provides feedback about neuroleptic medication, drug abstinence, therapy, and minimizing stressful circumstances that might exceed his current coping capacities.

Another common MI technique for deepening reflections is to paraphrase emotional states or feelings the patients express. Psychotic patients, however, often have difficulty coping with depressed and anxious feelings. Intensely negative affect may lead to cognitive disorganization, delusional thinking, increased hallucinations, or even hostility among aggressively prone and paranoid patients. Thus, clinicians minimize excessive focus on despairing patient statements and negative life events that are likely to evoke negative emotional states. They also avoid exploring distressing feelings when such deeply attendant reflective listening may be disorganizing for patients. When reflection of feeling occurs, clinicians typically repeat or rephrase what the patient has expressed directly. In the last example the clinician reflects the patient's concern about his ability to return to college and then provides solicited feedback to manage the patient's anxiety rather than to explore the patient's fear that he might not fully recover psychiatrically or achieve important life goals.

Similarly, because dually diagnosed patients often have difficulty weighing competing or discrepant motivations, they may experience excessive emotional discomfort and agitation when considering the normal ambivalence in changing their maladaptive behaviors. Prolongation of this experience during the interview may prompt or exacerbate their psychiatric symptoms (e.g., disordered thinking, paranoia) and decrease their ability to benefit from MI. In dual diagnosis MI, we recommend that clinicians carefully attend to the patients' discomfort when reflecting patient ambivalence and use a lower threshold of discomfort as an indicator to concentrate more on one side of the ambivalence or the other. At this juncture, rather than repeatedly reflecting or amplifying the patients' ambivalence as a primary strategy for the patients to resolve it, as is commonly practiced in MI, in dual diagnosis MI clinicians move more quickly toward succinctly summarizing the patients' ambivalence and using strategies to elicit change talk to resolve the ambivalence in favor of change. In the example below, a patient describes his ambivalence about attempting a new medication. The counselor chooses not to reflect his intense ambivalence but to move toward a resolution in a directive manner.

PATIENT: I know I ought to do it, but I've tried so many of them. I don't like feeling like a guinea pig. For this one, they have to test my blood once a month, too. Like I'm not here enough as it is. But one of my friends has been on it for 6 months, and he looks pretty good. He even got his own apartment. I wish I could get my own apartment.

CLINICIAN: There is something in you that has hope for this particular medication.

PATIENT: Yeah. But I don't like needles.

CLINICIAN: You're even thinking you could get your own place. That would be something. It might even be worth it for the blood tests.

PATIENT: It would be worth it if I could get my own place.

CLINICIAN: There's a big payoff if this medicine could work as well for you as for your friend.

PATIENT: I wish it could work like that for me.

CLINICIAN: Yep, there's that hope I was talking about.

Managing Negative Psychotic Symptoms

Negative psychotic symptoms present several challenges to MI. Patients may have little internal drive to manage their dual disorders or sustain motivation in the absence of reinforcing supports (Bellack & DiClemente, 1999). They also may talk little in sessions and take more time to respond to the clinician. Thus, the notion of the patient talking more during a session than the clinician as an indicator of clinician MI proficiency and client collaboration (Moyers et al., 2003) should be discarded when working with patients significantly impaired by negative symptoms. With patients who have a predominantly positive psychotic symptom picture, MI functions to structure and sometimes constrain the conversation. With patients impaired by negative symptoms, the challenge is to stimulate discussion and generate material that may facilitate motivational enhancement (Carey et al., 2001).

To accomplish this task, MI clinicians may have to talk as much or more than patients by frequently paraphrasing what the patients have implied in their limited communications, by providing patients with sufficient time to consider and respond to the reflections, by affirming their participation when it might otherwise go unnoticed, and by using structured tasks within each session. In the dialogue below, a clinician is interviewing her patient, who has diagnoses of chronic undifferentiated schizophrenia and cocaine abuse. The patient has a history of repeatedly stopping his antipsychotic medications 4–6 weeks after discharge from inpatient hospitalizations. Recently, he had been prescribed Olanzapine (Zyprexa) to better treat his enduring negative symptoms and to reduce the side effect profile that he had reported prompted his medication nonadherence in the past. He has adhered to the Zyprexa for an unprecedented 8 weeks. During the past week, however, he was not home on two occasions when his visiting nurse came to check on his medication adherence. The nurse called the clinician, who then scheduled an appointment to talk about what had happened.

CLINICIAN: I appreciate you coming in to see me today. The fact that you're here tells me you're willing to talk about how things are going with Zyprexa.

PATIENT: (*Gazes at the floor.*) Yeah.

CLINICIAN: How are things going with Zyprexa?

PATIENT: (*Is silent for a few seconds and then speaks with little animation.*) OK.

CLINICIAN: (*Pause—considers whether the patient's flatness is purely symptomatic or implies ambivalence about taking Zyprexa.*) In some ways, Zyprexa works OK, and in some ways it's not OK.

PATIENT: It's better. (*silence*)

CLINICIAN: How is Zyprexa better for you than other medication?

PATIENT: I *think* better. My body works better. (*silence*)

CLINICIAN: Better.

PATIENT: I can sit still and watch TV longer and talk in the group [adjunctive group therapy] more.

CLINICIAN: So taking Zyprexa has helped your mind and body work better. You've noticed your attention and concentration have improved, and you can talk to others more than you had been. Zyprexa also helps you feel physically more comfortable. For these reasons, and maybe others, you've continued to take Zyprexa longer than you've taken other medications. I give you lots of credit for your effort and your ability to know what medications work for you.

PATIENT: (*long silent pause*) I know what works best for me.

CLINICIAN: And by taking Zyprexa for 8 weeks, you're letting me, your psychiatrist, and your nurse know that Zyprexa works for you. On the other hand, you weren't around twice when your nurse came to visit you. She says she doesn't know if you took your medication, and she was concerned about you.

PATIENT: (*pause*) I was around. (*pause*) I just didn't answer the door.

CLINICIAN: You were home. You just didn't want to see her.

PATIENT: I don't need her to always check to see if I take my medication.

CLINICIAN: You've decided to take the Zyprexa. At this point, you don't feel you need her checking up on you every day. There may be other things she might be able to help you with when she visits, but you don't like constantly being monitored about your meds.

PATIENT: Yeah. (*pause*) I took Zyprexa on the days she didn't see me.

The interview continues with the patient speaking about how he had been "raped by syringes" (forcibly medicated during inpatient treatments) in the past, graphically communicating his aversion to authoritative medication management strategies. The clinician deftly identifies the importance of the patient's having more autonomy over his medication regimen to promote continued antipsychotic medication adherence at this critical juncture. The session continues with the clinician and patient discussing preferable medication adherence options and how the visiting nurse might be most helpful (e.g., titrating visits, less medication monitoring during visits).

Sometimes careful and active reflective listening or use of evocative questions will be insufficient in drawing out discussion among patients impaired by negative symptoms. Patients may have difficulty generating material and need more active prompting than is customary in a traditional delivery of MI. As with cognitive impairments, the use of structured feedback that is straightforward, visual, and engaging to elicit discussion about the patients' substance use and psychiatric symptoms may be useful for stimulating motivational enhancement discussions with patients impaired by negative symptoms. Carey and colleagues (2001) also recommends using assessment instruments like the decisional balance scale (King & DiClemente, 1993) and the Alcohol and Drug Consequence Questionnaire (Cunningham, Sobell, Gavin, Sobell, & Breslin, 1997) to help patients identify reasons to use or not use substances. Similarly, they prompt patients with lists of goals to generate and discuss the patients' personal goals, and then they inquire about how substance use and treatment nonadherence may conflict with goal attainment.

Knowing When MI Is Appropriate

The complex and multiple counseling challenges dually diagnosed patients present to clinicians cannot be addressed solely with MI. Other dual diagnosis treatment interventions (e.g., case management, social skills training and relapse prevention, vocational rehabilitation, family counseling) are needed to teach patients recovery skills and provide them with supportive services that will help them make behavioral changes and sustain these changes over time (Bellack & DiClemente, 1999). While clinicians may continue to employ the underlying empathic and collaborative MI counseling style in the patient's overall treatment or formally use MI as needed to systematically resolve recurring or new motivational dilemmas, skilled clinicians flexibly shift between targeted motivational, skill-building, supportive, and crisis interventions to address the patients' dual diagnosis treatment needs. For example, dually diagnosed patients who have become motivated for changing their substance use may find prolonged exploration of their motivations redundant and unproductive. Instead, focusing on the development of dual diagnosis relapse prevention skills and recovery supports is more appropriate (Ziedonis & Trudeau, 1997). Clinicians should not use MI when acute exacerbations of the patients' psychiatric symptoms seriously impair the patients' capacity to make informed decisions, function autonomously, or maintain their own or other people's safety. In these situations, the clinicians' medical-legal responsibilities usurp their patients' freedom of choice, and clinicians may employ coercive force (call police, write emergency evaluation requests) to make patients do what they feel are in the patients' best interests (e.g., involuntary hospitalization) even when the patient disagrees. MI is inappropriate under these circumstances (Miller & Rollnick, 2002). Because grave symptomatic deterioration and crisis situations are more prevalent with dually diagnosed patients than with substance-abusing patients without co-occurring conditions (Drake et al., 1989; Lyons & McGovern, 1989; Turner & Tsuang, 1990), clinicians conducting dual diagnosis MI must be capable of performing mental status and risk assessments proficiently and know how to handle patients when they become seriously impaired.

What is less clear, however, is the threshold of psychotic functioning above which a patient cannot make use of MI. In other words, at what point does a patient become too psychotic to benefit from MI when he or she has not yet reached levels of grave disability? We believe the answer to this question lies in the patient's responses. After a period of clinician–patient dialogue, clinicians determine the degree of the patient's positive and negative psychotic symptoms and general cognitive functioning. Excluding cases in which significant symptom resolution or serious exacerbation has occurred and the appropriateness or inappropriateness of MI is obvious, clinicians often are interviewing patients who have a mixed presentation of positive and negative symptoms and/ or cognitive impairments. As the clinicians employ MI strategies, they pay careful attention to how patients respond and adjust their use of MI accordingly (Miller & Moyers, 2007). If a patient responds, for example, to reflections by becoming more disorganized, then the clinician might consider using a more highly structured intervention instead. They may better serve their patients through case management, problem-solving, social rehabilitation, and medication interventions. When patients achieve greater psychiatric stability and cognitive clarity, MI may re-enter the therapeutic picture. On the other hand, if in response to clinician interventions patients consistently become less symptomatic, more organized and logical in speech, and demonstrate capacity to recall and consider the discussion, we deem MI appropriate to use with dually diagnosed patients. In appropriate situations, then, MI effectively functions to evoke reality-based and related patient perceptions that can then be incorporated into the motivational enhancement process. Thus, in dual diagnosis MI, clinicians gauge how to proceed in the interview by listening to the balance of patient change talk and resistance and by monitoring how psychiatrically symptomatic the patients are. Clinicians will follow the patients' lead only if it literally makes sense to do so.

RESEARCH

Three different applications of MI for dually diagnosed patients have been described and studied in the literature: (1) referral engagement, (2) standard treatment supplement, and (3) stand-alone intervention. We briefly describe these applications and then discuss future research directions.

Referral Engagement

MI has been used to help patients transition from inpatient to outpatient settings. Swanson, Pantalon, and Cohen (1999) used a two-session interview to motivate psychiatric patients, 77% of whom had substance-related disorders, to follow up with an initial outpatient appointment. They randomly assigned patients to MI or standard discharge planning. The two-session MI more than doubled the rate of treatment engagement (42 vs. 16%) among dually diagnosed patients. Most recently, in a randomized controlled trial of 78 outpatients with schizophrenia or schizoaffective disorder and tobacco dependence, Steinberg, Zeidonis, Krejci, and Brandon (2004) determined that a significantly greater proportion of participants receiving a one-session MI contacted a tobacco dependence treatment provider and attended the first counseling session by 1-month follow-up, as compared with those receiving standard psychoeducational counseling or advice only.

Standard Treatment Supplement

MI also has been used to supplement standard integrated dual diagnosis treatment (i.e., combined treatment of substance use and psychiatric problems with intensive case management and rehabilitation supports). Martino, Carroll, O'Malley, and Rounsaville (2000) randomly assigned 23 subjects with mood, psychotic, and substance use disorders to receive a one-session preadmission MI or a standard psychiatric intake as a prelude to entering a dual diagnosis partial hospital program. Use of this brief intervention resulted in improved rates of program attendance and involvement. However, differences in rates of substance relapse and medication noncompliance were not significant. Likewise, Carey and colleagues (2001) described a four-session MI for dually diagnosed patients to supplement ongoing mental health treatment in an outpatient setting. In this model, MI was administered to patients with low readiness to change, as indicated by current use, and/or low levels of engagement in substance abuse treatment. To date, they have not published study results detailing the efficacy of this approach.

Stand-Alone Intervention

MI has been used as a stand-alone psychosocial treatment for motivating patients to change their substance use patterns. In a randomized controlled pilot study, Graeber and colleagues (2003) showed that 36 non-treatment-seeking veterans who had comorbid schizophrenia and alcohol dependence significantly reduced their number of drinking days and daily alcohol consumption when they received a three-session dual diagnosis MI instead of an equivalently long psychoeducational intervention.

Future Research Directions

The preliminary efforts to incorporate MI into dual diagnosis practice are encouraging. While methodological improvement in future studies are needed (larger sample sizes, therapist MI fidelity checks, more than one or two therapists, and longer follow-up periods), many promising additional opportunities exist to advance our understanding of the application of MI to dually diagnosed patients. For example, the potential effectiveness of more extensive MI interventions delivered over several stages within longer-term dual diagnosis treatment programs (e.g., Bellack & DiClemente, 1999; Carey et al., 2001; Handmaker et al., 2002) should be tested. Moreover, the efficacy of MI delivered in a group format, the most common way of providing counseling interventions within mental health and addiction treatment services, is an unexplored area of clinical research importance (Handmaker et al., 2002).

Future studies also might include more homogeneous groups of dually diagnosed patients with specific combinations of psychiatric and substance use disorders. As in the current MI outcome literature, MI might work best with psychotically ill patients who primarily abuse or are dependent on alcohol. To date, the only MI study that has demonstrated significant effects on substance use outcomes for dually diagnosed patients included schizophrenic and alcohol-dependent outpatients where the patients' drinking was the target of intervention (Graeber et al., 2003). How effective MI is for treating drug-abusing and -dependent psychotically ill patients is unknown and may differ, depending on the patients' type of primary drug problem. Likewise, the effectiveness of MI may vary with the severity of the patients' psychotic symptoms and social deficits. Finally, clinicians' dual diagnosis MI skills, such as the frequent use of complex reflections, may be a particularly important factor that affects treatment outcome. The modifications we have described in many ways embody standards of highly proficient MI performance and advanced stages of learning MI (Miller & Moyers, 2007). It may be that MI makes its impact with dually diagnosed patients only when clinicians perform it at the highest skill levels to accommodate the marked symptom and social impairments posed by psychotic illness. The relationship of clinician MI adherence and competence to dual diagnosis treatment outcomes needs future examination.

CONCLUSIONS

MI is a key treatment component within a comprehensive integrated dual diagnosis service system. Extending the application of MI to populations for which it was not designed has made it necessary to modify the approach to accommodate the unique cognitive, symptomatic, and clinical challenges that dually diagnosed patients bring to treatment. We believe that recommendations to use crisp open-ended questions and reflections, successive organizing summaries, frequent paraphrasing, metaphor to elucidate meaning in seemingly odd statements or gestures, and simple, concrete, and engaging materials and methods maximize the effectiveness of dual diagnosis MI and make good sense for MI practice in general. Given these patients' complex treatment needs, including essential pharmacotherapies, crisis management, and other psychosocial interventions, clinicians must also be able to flexibly stage and switch treatment approaches as clinical circumstances dictate. These skills may require clinicians to perform MI at the highest levels of proficiency for the approach to work well with dually diagnosed patients. Nonetheless, ventures into the motivational underpinnings of psychotically ill substance-abusing patients will become confusing at times, and both clinicians and patients may not know what to say or how to proceed to bring about desired behavioral changes. One patient aptly captured this dilemma by posing the following question to her clinician after she had returned to a program following a recent relapse into cocaine use. She inquired, "When you are born in a soundless environment, and you go to a noisy one, can you hear what the other people hear?" In dual diagnosis MI, clinicians and patients may have to listen harder.

REFERENCES

Bellack, A. S., & DiClemente, C. C. (1999). Treating substance abuse among patients with schizophrenia. *Psychiatric Services, 50*, 75–80.

Bolla, K. I., Brown, K., Eldreth, D., Tate, D., & Cadet, J. L. (2002). Dose-related neurocognitive effects of marijuana use. *Neurology, 59*, 1337–1343.

Brady, K. T., & Malcolm, R. J. (2004). Substance use disorders and co-occurring axis I psychiatric disorders. In M. G. Gallanter & H.D. Kleber (Eds.), *Textbook of substance abuse treatment* (3rd ed.). Washington, DC: American Psychiatric Publishing.

Burke, B. L., Arkowitz, H., & Menchola, M. (2003). The efficacy motivational interviewing: A meta-analysis of controlled trials. *Journal of Consulting and Clinical Psychology, 71*, 843–861.

Carey, K. B. (1996). Substance use reduction in the context of outpatient psychiatric treatment: A collaborative, motivational, harm reduction approach. *Community Mental Health Journal, 32*, 291–306.

Carey, K. B., Purnine, D. M., Maisto, S. A., & Carey, M. P. (2001). Enhancing readiness-to-change substance abuse in persons with schizophrenia. *Behavior Modification, 25*, 331–384.

Cunningham, J. A., Sobell, L. C., Gavin, D. R., Sobell, M. B., & Breslin, F. C. (1997). Assessing motivation for change: Preliminary development and evaluation of a scale measuring the costs and benefits of changing alcohol and drug use. *Psychology of Addictive Behaviors, 11*, 107–114.

Drake, R. E., Essock, S. M., Shaner, A., Carey, K. B., Minkoff, K., Kola, L., et al. (2001). Implementing dual diagnosis services for clients with severe mental illness. *Psychiatric Services, 52*, 469–476.

Drake, R. E., McLaughlin, P., Pepper, B., & Minkoff, K. (1991). Dual diagnosis of major mental illness and substance disorder: An overview. *New Directions for Mental Health Services, 50*, 3–12.

Drake, R. E., Mercer-McFadden, C., Mueser, K. T., McHugo, G. J., & Bond, G. R. (1998). Review of integrated mental health and substance abuse treatment for patients with dual disorders. *Schizophrenia Bulletin, 24*, 589–608.

Drake, R. E., Osher, F. C., & Wallach, M. A. (1989). Alcohol use and abuse in schizo-phrenia: A prospective community study. *Journal of Nervous and Mental Disease,* *177,* 408–414.

Graeber, D. A., Moyers, T. B., Griffith, G., Guajardo, E., & Tonigan, S. (2003). A pilot study comparing motivational interviewing and an educational intervention in patients with schizophrenia and alcohol use disorders. *Community Mental Health Journal, 39,* 189–202.

Handmaker, N., Packard, M., & Conforti, K. (2002). Motivational interviewing in the treatment of dual disorders. In W. R. Miller & S. Rollnick, *Motivational interviewing: Preparing people for change* (2nd ed.). New York: Guilford Press.

Harrison, P. J. (1999). The neuropathology of schizophrenia: A critical review of the data and their interpretation. *Brain, 122,* 593–624.

Heinrichs, R. W. (2004). Meta-analysis and the science of schizophrenia: Variant evi-dence or evidence of variants? *Neuroscience and Biobehavioral Reviews, 28,* 379–394.

Kay, S. R., Fizbein, A., & Opler, L. A. (1987). The Positive and Negative Syndrome Scale (PANSS) for schizophrenia. *Schizophrenia Bulletin, 13,* 261–276.

King, T. K., & DiClemente, C. C. (1993). *A decisional balance measure for assessing and predicting drinking behavior.* Poster presented at the annual meeting of the Asso-ciation for the Advancement of Behavior Therapy, Atlanta, GA.

Lawton-Craddock, A., Nixon, S. J., & Tivis, R. (2003). Cognitive efficiency in stimu-lant abusers with and without alcohol dependence. *Alcoholism Clinical and Experimental Research, 27,* 457–464.

Lyons, J. S., & McGovern, M. P. (1989). Use of mental health services by dually diag-nosed patients. *Hospital and Community Psychiatry, 40,* 1067–1069.

Managed Care Initiative Panel on Co-Occurring Disorders. (1998). *Co-occurring psy-chiatric and substance disorders in managed care systems: Standards of care, practice guidelines, workforce competencies, and training curricula.* Rockville, MD: Center for Mental Health Services.

Martino, S., Carroll, K., Kostas, D., Perkins, J., & Rounsaville, B. (2002). Dual diagno-sis motivational interviewing: A modification of motivational interviewing for substance-abusing patients with psychotic disorders. *Journal of Substance Abuse Treatment, 23,* 297–308.

Martino, S., Carroll, K. M., O'Malley, S. S., & Rounsaville, B. J. (2000). Motivational interviewing with psychiatrically ill substance abusing patients. *American Jour-nal on Addictions, 9,* 88–91.

McLellan, T. A., Kushner, H., Metzger, D., Peters, R., Smith, I., Grissom, G., et al. (1992). The 5th edition of the Addiction Severity Index. *Journal of Substance Abuse Treatment, 9,* 199–213.

Mellman, T. A., Miller, A. L., Weissman, E. M., Crismon, M. L., Essock, S. M., & Marder, S. R. (2001). Evidence-based pharmacologic treatment for people with severe mental illness: A focus on guidelines and algorithms. *Psychiatric Services, 52,* 619–625.

Miller, W. R., C'de Baca, J., Matthews, D. B., & Wilbourne, P. L. (2001). Personal values card sort. Available at *www.casaa.unm.edu*

Miller, W. R., & Mount, K. A. (2001). A small study of training in motivational interviewing: Does one workshop change clinician and client behavior? *Behavioral and Cognitive Psychotherapy, 29,* 457–471.

Miller, W. R., & Moyers, T. (2007). Eight stages in learning motivational interviewing. *Journal of Teaching in the Addictions, 5,* 3–17.

Miller, W. R., & Rollnick, S. (2002). *Motivational Interviewing: Preparing people for change* (2nd ed.). New York: Guilford Press.

Minkoff, K. (2001). Developing standards of care for individuals with co-occurring psychiatric and substance use disorders. *Psychiatric Services, 52,* 597–599.

Moyers, T., Martin, T., Catley, D., Harris, K. J., & Ahluwalia, J. S. (2003). Assessing the integrity of motivational interviewing interventions: Reliability of the motivational interviewing skills code. *Behavioural and Cognitive Psychotherapy, 31,* 177–184.

Moyers, T., & Martino, S. (2006). *Personal values card sort for dually diagnosed patients.* Available at *www.casaa.unm.edu*

Nixon, S. J., & Phillips, J. A. (1999). Neurocognitive deficits and recovery in chronic alcohol abuse. *CNS Spectrums, 4,* 95–110.

Osher, F. C., & Kofoed, L. L. (1989). Treatment of patients with psychiatric and psychoactive substance abuse disorders. *Hospital and Community Psychiatry, 40,* 1025–1030.

Owens, R. R., Fischer, E. P., Booth, B. M., & Cuffel, B. J. (1996). Medication noncompliance and substance abuse among patients with schizophrenia. *Psychiatric Services, 47,* 853–858.

Parsons, O. A. (1998). Neurocognitive deficits in alcoholics and social drinkers: A continuum? *Alcoholism Clinical and Experimental Research, 22,* 954–961.

Steinberg, M. L., Zeidonis, D. M., Krejci, J. A., & Brandon, T. H. (2004). Motivational interviewing with personalized feedback: A brief intervention for motivating smokers with schizophrenia to seek treatment for tobacco dependence. *Journal of Consulting and Clinical Psychology, 72,* 723–728.

Swanson, A. J., Pantalon, M. V., & Cohen, K. R. (1999). Motivational interviewing and treatment adherence among psychiatrically and dually diagnosed patients. *Journal of Nervous and Mental Disease, 187,* 630–635.

Turner, W. M., & Tsuang, M. T. (1990). Impact of substance abuse on the course and outcome of schizophrenia. *Schizophrenia Bulletin, 16,* 87–95.

Van Horn, H. A., & Bux, D. A. (2001). A pilot test of motivational interviewing groups for dually diagnosed inpatients. *Journal of Substance Abuse Treatment, 20,* 191–195.

Ziedonis, D. M., & Trudeau, K. (1997). Motivation to quit using substances among individuals with schizophrenia: Implications for a motivation-based treatment model. *Schizophrenia Bulletin, 23,* 229–238.

Zweben, A., & Zuckoff, A. (2002). Motivational interviewing and treatment adherence. In W. R. Miller & S. Rollnick, *Motivational interviewing: Preparing people for change* (2nd ed., pp. 299–319). New York: Guilford Press.

CHAPTER 12

Motivational Interviewing in the Correctional System

An Attempt to Implement Motivational Interviewing in Criminal Justice

Carl Åke Farbring
Wendy R. Johnson

PRISON POPULATIONS AND USUAL TREATMENTS

Prisons, with the obvious exception of lifelong incarceration, have demonstrated serious shortcomings in stopping offenders from reoffending (Lipsey, 1992; Wooldredge, 1988). Offenders who have been imprisoned have been shown to have recidivism rates approximately 7% higher than offenders who have been supervised in communities (Smith, Goggin, & Gendreau, 2002). Results from a variety of rehabilitation programs have been poor (Lipsey & Wilson, 1998). Some even increase recidivism (Petrosino, Turpin-Petrosino, & Buehler, 2002). "Scared Straight," one such program, takes at-risk youths into jails and prisons to be confronted by hardened criminals, typically inmates serving long or even life sentences. These inmates confront them graphically with the realities of prison life and the downside of crime. Shock incarceration, typically referred to as "boot camp," was created in response to prison overcrowding and designed for younger nonviolent offenders on their first offense. The common elements among boot camps include their strict military atmosphere, intensive physical activity, and goal of future crime deterrence, although they vary widely in their other components (MacKenzie & Hebert, 1996). A meta-analysis of research on boot camps (Kider, MacKenzie, & Wilson, 2003) indicates that this politically popular method increases recidivism instead of reducing it. Many other programs show no beneficial effects at all on such outcomes as recidivism.

The Implementation of "What Works"

In recent years governments in many countries have funded strategies to reduce recidivism associated with drug use in adjudicated populations. These programs are often grouped under the "what works" banner, implying that such programs are based on research evidence for their efficacy. The term "what works" is actually a backlash against the phrase "nothing works," which was popularized by a 1974 article reporting on the dismal outcomes of rehabilitation programs (Martinson, 1974). Interestingly, Martinson himself rejected his original opinion just 5 years later in an often overlooked article (Martinson, 1979).

Cullen and Gendreau (1988) find five guiding principles that increase the effectiveness of correctional treatment, regardless of the program. These are authority, anticriminal modeling, problem solving, use of community resources, and quality interpersonal relationships. The first, authority, refers to the clarity and predictability of rules and expectations. Anticriminal modeling must be demonstrated by all workers coming into contact with the offenders. Anticriminal behaviors and expressions by offenders must be reinforced. Problem-solving efforts include actively engaging the offender in resolving those issues that prevent him from engaging in a prosocial lifestyle. Community resources include any element in the offender's nonincarcerated environment that may facilitate a prosocial lifestyle. This may include family ties, employment opportunities, spiritual resources, and recreational opportunities. Finally, the humanistic counseling values of warmth, genuineness, empathy, and active listening must be present in all interactions with the offender. These five principles are the cornerstones underlying the delivery of effective correctional treatments.

The most commonly encountered rehabilitation programs within correctional treatment systems include cognitive behavioral programs and therapeutic communities. Cognitive behavioral approaches have long been the gold standard in correctional treatment. Based on the premise that changing thinking changes behavior, most criminal justice programs address criminal thinking and cognitive restructuring in some fashion. Cognitive behavioral and social learning treatments have showed substantially larger effect sizes in reducing recidivism as compared to nonbehavioral approaches (Dowden & Andrews, 2000; Lipton, Pearson, Cleland, & Yee, 2002).

Therapeutic communities (TCs) are residential programs with highly structured environments. Residents of a TC work together to run the community, with the help of professional staff (Lipton, 2001). Important elements of a TC include social modeling, cognitive restructuring, problem-solving skills, and accountability for one's actions. Treatment within a TC may include group and individual counseling, 12-step facilitation, didactic education, and residential job duties (Anglin & Hser, 1990). TCs have consistently been found to be effective at reducing recidivism and drug use among adjudicated populations (Anglin & Hser, 1990; Butzin, Martin, & Inciardi, 2002; Pearson & Lipton, 1999; Wexler, DeLeon, Thomas, Kressel, & Peters, 1999). The most successful long-term intervention ever made in a Swedish prison has been a TC where relapse in experimental groups was between 14 and 21% lower ($p < .005$) as compared to controls during a follow-up period of 2–5 years (Farbring, 2000).

"What works" programs generally target deficits in cognitive skills but also more specifically target offending behavior, aggression, drug dependency, domestic violence, and sexual offending. The overall results of the "what works" implementation have been mixed. The Home Office in the United Kingdom has reported reductions of 4.5 and 3.6% in juvenile recidivism in 2001 and 2002, respectively (Home Office, 2004). These figures are small but by no means unimportant. The comparable report regarding adults shows a 1.8% reduction within 2 years for offenders released from custody or community sentences in the first quarter of 2001, compared to the same period in 2000. The latest report on a 2002 cohort group shows a small but nonsignificant improvement over the 2000 results (Home Office Statistical Bulletin, 2005).

Sweden, and to an increasing degree other Scandinavian and European countries, have emulated the U.K. implementation of "what works" programs in many details, but with fewer funds. The total number of inmates completing evidence-based programs in Sweden has increased by a third from 2003 to 2004, to a total of 1,569. The motivational program described in this chapter represents 73% of that increase.

RATIONALE FOR USING MOTIVATIONAL
INTERVIEWING IN PRISON

Corrections-based treatment is frequently directive, confrontational, and restrictive. Offenders are typically mandated to enter treatment, and unwillingness to do so is punished with loss of privileges. Once in treatment, offenders are confronted with their thinking errors and history of poor life choices in order to convince them to change. Unfortunately, when people experience external demands to change, their resistance increases. Because motivational interviewing (MI; Miller & Rollnick, 2002) avoids confrontation, resistance is diminished and internal motivation may have a chance to grow. MI holds much promise for transferring external motivation for change to internal motivation (Mann, Ginsburg, & Weekes, 2002).

Another good reason to believe MI would be helpful in engaging criminals in treatment is that it steers clear of labeling and judgment. Offenders, like alcoholics, have long been on the receiving end of negative labels, value judgments, and stigma. MI may reduce the experience of stigma associated with being in prison or being convicted of a crime. Furthermore, it has been demonstrated that MI works especially well with persons high in anger (Allen et al., 1997), suggesting its usefulness with correctional populations.

Because MI is appropriate for people in the precontemplative and contemplative stages of change (Prochaska & DiClemente, 1982), it may help offenders utilize other programming more effectively. Most correctional rehabilitative programs begin with the implicit assumption that the offender is ready to change. Much effort is then made to teach a variety of prosocial life skills. However, these efforts may be wasted if the individual either does not want to change or has not resolved his or her ambivalence about changing. Like people addicted to drugs, offenders have ambivalence about making changes in their lives. Although extremely risky, engaging in crime can be exciting and financially rewarding, at least in the short run. Criminal networks may provide a person with a sense of community and belonging, especially when more conventional social opportunities are closed. Through MI, offenders can explore the pros and cons of making changes and work to resolve their ambivalence about criminal behavior.

Substance abuse and involvement with the criminal justice system go hand in hand. Some 60–80% of prison and jail inmates either are under the influence of substances (including alcohol) at the time of their arrest, committed the offense to support a drug habit, or were charged with an alcohol- or drug-related crime (Belenko & Peugh, 1998). This high rate of co-occurring substance abuse and incarceration is not merely a result of criminalizing drug possession: people under the influence have a higher likelihood of committing a crime. Over 50% of violent crime, 60–80% of child abuse and neglect, 50–70% of property crimes, and 75% of drug manufacturing or distributing involve drug use by the offender (Belenko & Peugh, 1998; National Institute of Justice, 1999). Because MI has been successful in helping people change substance-abusing behaviors, it stands to reason that criminal behaviors associated with such addictions may change as well.

On the whole, there is scant research on MI in corrections and consequently no evidence to support the efficacy of MI in prisons in reducing drug use or recidivism. There is, however, reason to believe that the same mechanisms that work with alcoholics and drug users also would apply to drug-using offenders and might be particularly appropriate for helping criminally involved individuals make prosocial changes.

CLINICAL APPLICATIONS OF MI IN CORRECTIONS

Program Description

In 2003 an MI intervention was introduced within the Swedish prison system. A brochure was circulated inviting inmates to participate in the program by talking about themselves confidentially with a counselor. The brochure assured clients there were no right or wrong answers, nothing would be forced upon them, and that the program was designed to help counselors understand how inmates were thinking about their future. Today, word of mouth from other inmates accounts for most of the referrals to the program, and there is even a waiting list. The number of clients completing the program has swelled from 175 in 2003 to 1,011 in 2006, making MI the most extensively delivered intervention in the Swedish correctional system.

The manual, titled *Beteende–Samtal–Förändring* (BSF, translated as *Behavior–Interviewing–Change*; Farbring & Berge, 2003), describes a semistructured five-session MI intervention focusing on drug use and criminal behavior. The five sessions are in sequence with the Prochaska and DiClemente (1982) stages-of-change model. A standardized taxonomy for change talk is presented, based on the Amrhein (2000) coding manual.

Prior to the actual intervention, the counselor meets with the client to introduce the concept of change and the transtheoretical model, and asks the client to complete the self-report motivational scales: the Stages of Change Readiness and Treatment Eagerness Scale (SOCRATES; Miller & Tonigan, 1996) and/or the University of Rhode Island Change Assessment (URICA; McConnaughy, Prochaska, & Velicer, 1983). The client is assured of confidentiality. The client is also encouraged to choose a graphical position indicating his or her stage of change regarding a self-selected problem (see Figure 12.1; Prochaska & DiClemente, 1982). The position is measured by degrees from zero and is used to compare with his or her chosen position after the fifth session of the MI program. The client is given a workbook containing all the exercises from the intervention.

The first session consists of providing feedback to the client based on the introductory meeting. Topics addressed include how change might appear for the client, how his or her friends have made changes, and the like. The client is encouraged to examine different stages of change in relation to different problem areas.

During session 2, the counselor and client explore the positive and the negative aspects of maintaining a specific behavior. The explicit

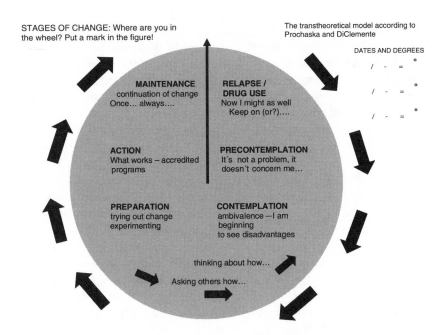

FIGURE 12.1. Stages-of-change model. Clients are encouraged to decide their position before and after the program. The long vertical arrow represents 0 degrees.

purpose is to encourage the client to see the positive side of change and to elicit change talk. In the "force field" exercise in this session, the client is encouraged to assign emotional weights to arguments for and against the status quo. Here, the counselor deliberately avoids reflecting on arguments for status quo and elicits too many of those with the intention to try to stay the course toward change. Other exercises include rating scales of importance, confidence, priorities, and inner or external motivation about making a change. In this exercise clients are encouraged to place 10 1-kilo weights on either of the two sides, depicting internal or external (e.g., pressure from family) motivation for change. These exercises are also repeated as posttests.

The third session introduces the topic of values and the Values Card Sort exercise (Miller, C'de Baca, Matthews, & Wilbourne, 2001). The client is encouraged to write down his or her most important values in the workbook and to explore the discrepancies between these values and personal current behavior in order to elicit change talk. An exercise from this session, the "motor of change," focuses on the emotional side of differences between the status quo and change alternatives. This exercise taps into emotions—without which the motor of change is not likely to start. "John, when you were stealing from your parents to buy heroin, how did that affect your relationship with your loved ones? What did they say, and how did you feel about that?" As many have said before, there would not be any smokers in the world if rational understanding alone were enough to engender behavior change.

The fourth session refers to the balance exercise in the second meeting about internal or external motivation and picks up on what clients mentioned as instrumental in external motivation. The client works with two exercises: a social network map and a cognitive restructuring of negative remarks from family members about his or her lifestyle. The client's network is a primary cause of relapse (Andrews & Bonta, 2003). Most clients in corrections need to make changes in relationships in order to eliminate or decrease antisocial associations.

The fifth session elicits the personal strengths and qualities of the client. Previous mistakes may have eroded self-efficacy. The client is taught to reframe what he or she has considered to be failures. The exercise involves the client's writing down all the qualities and resources that he or she possesses. The fifth meeting must end on a positive note with respect to change talk (Amrhein, Miller, Yahne, Palmer, & Fulcher, 2003). Therefore, there is an option between creating a short-term change plan and a crystal ball exercise in which the client is invited to imagine the future. If the client is unwilling to make a concrete plan, change might be more acceptable in hypothetical form: "Well, I know you don't feel like it right now, but *if* you were to take steps toward change, what would be most suitable for you?" (Farbring, 2003). "What if" planning may pave the way for new cognitive structuring. The meeting ends by completing posttests and an evaluation form. Finally, the client is asked if he or she is interested in a follow-up session in a few months.

Training and Treatment Fidelity

There are arguments for and against using standardized manuals to ensure that the therapy protocol is being followed (Hettema, Steele, & Miller, 2005; Project MATCH Research Group, 1997). Porporino and Fabiano (2002) point out that motivational work must be integrated into behavioral and cognitive programs to avoid the risk that clients feel alienated from the agenda for change. A preliminary evaluation of the Swedish drug treatment program in corrections by the Brottsförebyggande Rådet (Swedish National Council for Crime Prevention, 2005) concluded that there were no immediate signs of positive results following the massive MI education initiative in the penal system. In fact, none of the clients in special motivational housing units was aware that he or she had participated in motivational sessions. The launch of the BSF manualized program was based on this lack of results from the training and the need for *in vivo* practice to enhance skills. A manual was deemed essential to monitor program implementation and treatment adherence while respecting client autonomy and collaboration.

Training and Supervising Therapists

In Sweden, a program was funded from 2001 through 2003 to instruct the trainers and to train virtually all the staff members in prisons and probation units in MI. In March 2003, all prison program counselors completed 3 days of training in MI with additional training in the BSF manual. Given prior research experience (Miller, Yahne, Moyers, Martinez, & Pirritano, 2004), it was also necessary to develop a plan for ongoing supervision and monitoring of the newly trained therapists.

Integrated into the last part of the BSF manual is the content-related integrity instrument 1-PASS by Resnicow (2002), slightly modified with the author's permission to meet the needs of the correctional service. A module that monitors the counselor's ability to elicit change talk and a dimension called compass direction have been added, and the interpretation of some other modules has been extended to include more skills in the program. The purpose of using the 1-PASS is to enhance therapist skills by observing and evaluating the skills that have been used in sequence with the sessions of the program. Even though the integrity instrument for monitoring and scoring skills was integrated into the manual, monitoring and supervision was explicitly voluntary during the first year, until more familiarity with the manual was attained. In order not to create resistance against monitoring, it was deemed important to keep it nonthreatening at the outset. This MI-consistent method seemed to be well received and served to reduce anxiety.

An organization of prison supervisors trained in MI and the BSF program was created in 2005 to monitor, give feedback, and certify counselors. Counselors meet with supervisors in geographical regions every 5 weeks. They listen to a tape brought by a member of the "peer review team" and use the 1-PASS form (Resnicow, 2002) to monitor and render constructive feedback. Counselors also meet privately with their supervisor in order to be certified, which is an official recognition featured on the correctional website. After certification, counselors continue to participate in the peer review groups and enhance learning by helping others. To remain certified, a new training tape must be approved by the supervisor every year. These procedures make it clear that adequate implementation, monitoring, and feedback are of crucial importance in ensuring that MI is taking place correctly.

MI on the Organizational Level

A research project aiming primarily at reducing stress and anxiety among prison staff members is being implemented in concert with the research on the inmates. It is derived from MI and contains three simple styles of communication people typically use in everyday conversations in varying blends: telling (instructing), listening, and guiding. Steve Rollnick has developed a short intervention based on these three styles in collaboration with the Swedish Criminal Justice (Farbring). This involves a Web-based interactive program designed for prison officers, but which can easily be adapted to suit staffers in other settings as well. Staff personnel in prisons, mental hospitals, youth institutions, and the like often face difficult situations in which levels of frustration are high. Härenstam (1989) concluded that the levels of stress among staff members in prisons were two to three times higher than in similar professions in Sweden and represented a danger to their health. The hypothesis of the current research is that better communication skills on the part of the officers will reduce their stress. Consequently, stress levels for inmates in those institutions should be lower, and the resulting climate should be more conducive to change. Staff members of seven different prisons have been randomly assigned either to receive training in enhancing communication skills or to a control condition. Every training participant receives a CD and a manual. The CD contains scenarios in which actors illustrate situations where different blends of listening, instructing, and guiding should be applied, in part in an interactive mode. Pre- and posttest measurements will assess the effects on certain psychological and physiological dimensions, such as stress cortisol and other medical tests. Preliminary results (May 2007) show reductions of stress reactions following the intervention.

CLINICAL ILLUSTRATIONS

The following are excerpts from manualized sessions with prison inmates.

A is about age 30. He talks slowly, and there are many reflective pauses during the interview. He has indicated there is a 60% chance he will continue to commit crimes.

INTERVIEWER: So, there is a 60% chance that you will relapse in crime. Why not more—why not 70% or 80%?

A: I am thinking about my family . . .

INTERVIEWER: You have a lot of love for your family . . .

A: Yes, there is so much love.

INTERVIEWER: What can your family do to help you?

A: Only by being there. When I see my sisters and my brothers . . . it's going to be a big difference. That's enough for me to quit. I want to be together with my family alot.

INTERVIEWER: It sounds as if you've made up your mind that you can do it. That's the kind of person you are.

A: Yes, I am that kind of person—that's who I am.

INTERVIEWER: It seems as if you can resist the pressure from others here on the ward to carry on with drugs and crime.

A: There are weak people here, but I'm strong.

INTERVIEWER: You seem to be the kind of person who can manage on your own. Nothing can stop you if you make up your mind. [reflective listening and affirmation; attributing positive characteristics to the client]

A: Yes, it's very difficult to stop me.

B is a 50-year-old client from Stockholm who has used many different drugs since he was a teenager, including heroin, amphetamines, and cannabis. Children and parenthood are topics that can serve, when relevant, to increase emotionally rooted discrepancy. The interviewer first skillfully renders feedback on the SOCRATES (Miller & Tonigan, 1996), then raises the issue of family.

INTERVIEWER: It's clear that you score very high on ambivalence. This is very good; it means that you're the kind of person who reflects a lot about change and also you understand what it means. [affirmation and positive feedback]

B: Yes, I'm not a criminal in general—only when I'm using drugs. Maybe it's because I worked before; I know what it's like.

A bit further into the interview they are discussing that B is older than most drug users and he doesn't know if he will live for 10 more years if he continues to use drugs.

INTERVIEWER: So, what's left for you to do in your life? How is your relationship with your children?

B: I have to build their confidence in me again. I'm not the father I want to be.

INTERVIEWER: They feel sad about that.

B: Yes, I'm sad, too. I cry when we say goodbye, when I leave them. Once, on a train, I was crying for hours, and another time when I was leaving them I drove my car slowly because I wanted to miss the connecting flight.

INTERVIEWER: These are strong feelings.

B: I've let them down; I know they love me even though I am a drug user.

C estimates that he has made only modest progress in the stages-of-change model (from 262 to 280–285 degrees) due to his participation in the BSF program. He believes it was a good thing for him to be sentenced to imprisonment. This is a reminder for policymakers that it is a good investment to use the time in prison to enhance motivation to change for clients and to offer easily accessible treatment alternatives.

INTERVIEWER: How did you start to think about change—how did you come this far in your thinking?

C: It's because I ended up here. That's when I started to think, "I don't want to come here again." [external motivation that has helped to develop internal motivation]

INTERVIEWER: So if you had not ended up here . . .

C: I would have continued my criminal life.

Seeing his own strengths is difficult for C, since he is so accustomed to hearing about his problems and character deficits. In the fifth meeting he struggles with describing his positive attributes ("easier to tell what I am bad at . . ."), and the counselor comes up with a good idea.

INTERVIEWER: What made you a successful criminal? You managed to sell a lot of drugs.

C: I am a good businessman. I am good at planning and I don't waste my money.

INTERVIEWER: Those are good personal resources, aren't they. You could use them in whatever goal you want to attain.

C: That's right. I am also flexible; I know to set the right price for different people.

INTERVIEWER: It sounds as if you are intelligent in socializing with people.

C: Yes, I don't judge people, and I am also very hard-working.

INTERVIEWER: Those are excellent qualities. How could you use them differently?

C: I guess the best would be if I could have my own coffee shop in Amsterdam . . . (*still ambivalent, but later*) I want to go to a treatment house, it all starts there.

SOME CONSIDERATIONS REGARDING
MI IN CORRECTIONS

Genuine Empathy

Working in criminal justice with a legally prescribed agenda to "help" clients to change always seems to raise the issue of manipulation versus genuine empathy. In an ideal world, counselors will always help clients on the basis of unconditional and genuine empathy, but sometimes this view is challenged by the demands of prison and probation. It is not uncommon for counselors to lack sincere hope for the client or to think the client is undeserving of sympathy. If genuine empathy is not there, should the counselor give up on the client and concentrate on others, or try to do the best he or she can do with each one? An example may help illustrate this issue.

I (Carl Farbring) was heading a therapeutic community in a prison. In a counseling session with an 18-year-old client, I said something to the effect that one cannot always bluntly tell people the truth, because it may cause trouble. Later I was warned by other clients that this client was now threatening me, because I had questioned his father's value of telling the truth in all situations. I was a bit worried because the client had a violent record, and I considered expelling him from the community for breaking the contract not to threaten with violence. I decided to let him stay, invited his father to the prison, and we discussed the matter together and reached an understanding. From that moment on, I spent a lot of time with this client and tried to guide him through his stay in the prison. However, I never felt quite comfortable during our conversations, and I honestly did not have much hope for him.

More than 10 years later I made a presentation. Afterward, I was approached by a social worker who asked me if I remembered the client. When I said that I did, the social worker said that the client had been doing well now for about 10 years and was working successfully at a job. When the client discovered from the social worker that I would be at this conference, he asked the social worker to convey this message to me: "Tell him that I would never have made it without his support and his faith in me."

Even when empathy or hope is hard to find, the counselor must dig deeply into him- or herself and understand that clients depend on it.

Reflective Listening

The art of reflective listening involves more than technical skills. Clients in criminal justice often bear grudges against society and the people who have penalized them. As a counselor, one has to sweep one's ego aside to recognize change talk in the face of resistance and hostility. Clients often present two divergent themes in conversation: embedded in their anger and frustration at the system may be hints at values and goals that are important to them. It can be a real challenge for a counselor to detect and reflect these without invalidating the negative emotions. However, to reflect only the frustrated, angry statements may serve to increase frustration and anger. The counselor must recognize and reflect the client's resistance, but then focus on hints at problem recognition and change talk.

Reflective listening may have other hazards too. If, in reflecting what the client has said, one paraphrases it in purely professional or psychological language, there is a risk that it will be experienced by the client as a roadblock. What might be an excellent affirmation with a highly verbal client could be seen as alienating for another. Sometimes it is better to accept the client's own words about a feeling or experience instead of attempting to paraphrase it. Simple reflections seem to work best with clients in criminal justice, and continuing-the-paragraph reflections are an excellent tool when they are phrased in common language.

Motivational Work as a Risk for Backlash

An MI program that increases hope and the desire to change runs the risk of creating frustration when the possibility of fulfilling these hopes is undermined by the corrections system. As a result, clients may give up hope about change. Correctional clients face serious challenges when they are released from confinement. Housing, employment, dysfunctional peer networks and families, and mental health problems are all issues that are difficult to resolve. Increased motivation to change must be met with real opportunities to do so. If not, there may be a serious backlash against the program.

RESEARCH

The Karolinska Institute in Stockholm is performing research on the effects of the BSF intervention. Clients are randomized into three groups. Group 1 receives five BSF manualized semistructured sessions and a workbook. Group 2 receives the same intervention as group 1, but the counselors also receive monitoring and feedback about MI using the 1-

PASS. Group 3 receives "planned ordinary conversations" and a treatment plan. These conversations could contain MI, because all staff members have been trained in the method, but the BSF manual is not used. A protocol has been developed to guide these sessions. Outcome is measured by recidivism, drug use, application to other treatment programs, and retention in treatment.

While the results of the randomized trial are not yet available, the difference between pre- and posttests from the BSF program from 2004 and 2005 have been analyzed (see Table 12.1). On Socrates 8D (designed to measure attitudes toward drug use) changes are in the expected direction on both the problem recognition (2004: $p < .02$, $n = 155$; in total, 2004–2005: $p < .07$, $n = 271$) and taking steps dimensions (2004: $p < .005$; in total, 2004–2005: $p < .0001$, $n = 271$), with no significant changes on the ambivalence dimension. On Socrates 8A (designed to measure attitudes toward alcohol consumption) there are significant changes on the ambivalence (2004–2005; $p < .005$, $n = 81$) and taking steps dimensions ($p < .05$, $n = 81$). On the URICA the same pattern emerges: on the precontemplation dimension the difference goes in the expected direction but does not reach significance ($p < .08$), there is a positive change in the contemplation dimension (2004: $p < .005$, $n = 83$; in total, 2004–2005: $p < .06$, $n = 175$), and changes on the action dimension reach significance ($p < .001$, $n = 175$). From pre- to posttests on scales measuring desire, perceived self-efficacy, perceived priority of actual change compared to other important things in clients' lives, and internal versus external motivation, all differences are significant and in the predicted direction (2004: $p < .0001$, $n = 190$; in total, 2004–2005: $p < .0001$, $n = 332$).

The client's estimated position in the stages-of-change model is clearly more positive after the fifth meeting compared to pretest ($p < .0001$, $n = 286$) and also after the sixth (optional) meeting, which occurs at various time intervals, compared to the fifth ($p < .0001$, $n = 44$).

After the fifth session, counselors are asked to estimate change and answer the questions that appear in Table 12.2. Similarly, clients are asked to assess their thoughts about change, which are reported in Table 12.3.

TABLE 12.1. Changes on the Socrates 8D and A from Pre- to Posttest for the 2004–2005 Population

Measure	Problem recognition	Taking steps	Ambivalence	n
Socrates 8D	0.58 ($p < .07$)	1.53 ($p < .0001$)	−0.27 (n.s.)	271
Socrates 8A	0.28 (n.s.)	1.22 ($p < .05$)	−1.40 ($p < .005$)	81

TABLE 12.2. Counselors' Views on Client Progress, 2004–2005 Population

Question	% yes	% no	% no answer	n
• Does the client intend to enter further treatment?	55.76	32.73	11.51	443
• Does the client want follow-up sessions in BSF?	45.80	32.20	22.20	441
• Have you noticed improvement in collaboration?	54.20	38.55	7.26	441
• Have you noticed improvement in desire to change?	78.68	16.33	4.99	441

CONCLUSIONS

The rate of recidivism in criminal populations is very high and must be reduced. Usually, the focus in prison and probation is on rules and security, and staff members have often been recruited with these expectations in mind. Sometimes these goals are at odds with evidence-based attempts at rehabilitation. Prison-based therapeutic communities and the "what works" initiative have begun to influence correctional work, but many things remain to be improved to accomplish substantial reductions in recidivism. Too many prisons around the world are, in fact, direct contributors to relapse in crime and drug use.

The increasing focus of the Swedish criminal justice system on decreasing crime by reducing drug use has led to an interest in implementing MI. Judging from feedback and from listening to tapes, clients

TABLE 12.3. Clients' Estimates of the Program's Effects on their Thoughts about Change, 2004–2005 Population

Statement	Absolutely not	Maybe	Yes, to some degree	Yes, very much	No answer	n
I am thinking more about change now than I did before the program	0	9.28%	32.99%	43.30%	14.43%	97
I have already started to make some changes	0	4.17%	35.42%	46.88%	13.54%	97

are willing and eager to talk about themselves within their own frame of reference. This represents considerable and humane progress in criminal justice. Judging from the quality of these tapes, counselors not only enjoy doing MI, but they have achieved considerable skill in practicing it.

MI has achieved a positive reputation in the Swedish correctional service as an evidence-based method for talking to clients. It is well recognized outside the network of counselors who are directly involved in therapy with inmates. Although it is less than 3 years old, the BSF programmatic adaptation of MI is already the most widely used program in Swedish criminal justice. It is used both as a stand-alone intervention in probation and in prison for inmates with short sentences but also as an overture to lengthier treatment interventions. The data from the randomized trials will be analyzed during 2007–2008.

MI has already made a considerable contribution in helping clients to consider change alternatives in Swedish prisons and probation programs. It may also improve the atmosphere of the environment, particularly in prisons, which in turn may produce a climate more optimal for change. Not only does MI offer staff members a more effective way to work with inmates, it also holds promise for creating a healthier workplace with fewer feelings of frustration and stress. The fact that it has already changed the treatment culture in prison is in itself something of a cultural revolution.

REFERENCES

Allen, J., Anton, R. F., Babor, T. F., Carbonari, J., Carrol, K. M., Connors, G. J., et al. (1997). Project MATCH secondary a priori hypotheses. *Addiction, 92,* 1671–1698.

Amrhein, P. C. (2000). *A training manual for coding client commitment language, version 1.0.* Albuquerque: Center on Alcohol, Substance Abuse, and Addictions, University of New Mexico.

Amrhein, P. C., Miller, W. R., Yahne, C., Palmer, M., & Fulcher, L. (2003). Client commitment language during motivational interviewing predicts behavior outcomes. *Journal of Consulting and Clinical Psychology, 71,* 862–878.

Andrews, D. A., & Bonta, J. (2003). *The psychology of criminal conduct* (3rd ed.). Cincinnati, OH: Anderson Publishing.

Anglin, M. D., & Hser, Y. (1990). Treatment of drug abuse. In M. Tonry & J. Q. Wilson (Eds.), *Drugs and crime* (pp. 393–460). Chicago: University of Chicago Press.

Belenko, S., & Peugh, J. (1998). *Behind bars: Substance abuse and America's prison population.* New York: National Center on Addiction and Substance Abuse at Columbia University.

Brottsförebyggande Rådet (Swedish National Council for Crime Prevention). (2005). *Evaluation of the program against drugs in corrections during the years 2002–2004.* Stockholm: Author.

Butzin, C. A., Martin, S. S., & Inciardi, J. A. (2002). Evaluating component effects of a prison-based treatment continuum. *Journal of Substance Abuse Treatment, 22,* 63–69.

Cullen, F., & Gendreau, P. (1988). The effectiveness of correctional rehabilitation: Reconsidering the "nothing works" debate. In L. Goodstein & D. L. MacKenzie (Eds.), *The American prison: Issues in research policy* (pp. 23–44). New York: Plenum Press.

Dowden, C., & Andrews, D. A. (2000). Effective correctional treatment and violent reoffending: A meta-analysis. *Canadian Journal of Criminology, 42,* 449–469.

Farbring, C. Å. (2000). The drug treatment programme at Österåker Prison: Experience from a therapeutic community during the years 1978–1998. *American Jails, 14,* 85–96.

Farbring, C. Å. (2003). "IF"—a way of broaching the subject without creating resistance. *MINUET, 10,* 4.

Farbring, C. Å., & Berge, P. (2003). *BSF Beteende–Samtal–Förändring: Fem samtal om förändring. Manual och arbetshäfte.* [Behavior–Interviewing–Change: Five interviews about change: Manual and workbook]. Stockholm: Kriminalvårdsstyrelsen.

Härenstam, A. (1989). *Prison personnel—working conditions, stress and health: A study of 2000 prison employees in Sweden.* Doctoral dissertation, National Institute of Psychosocial Factors and Health, Department of Stress Research, Karolinska Institute, Stockholm.

Hettema, J., Steele, J., & Miller, W. R. (2005). A meta-analysis of research on motivational interviewing treatment effectiveness (MARMITE). *Annual Review of Clinical Psychology, 1,* 91–111.

Home Office. (2004). News and Updates, December 2, 2004. Available at *www.probation.homeoffice.gov.uk/output/page 268.asp*

Home Office Statistical Bulletin. (2005, May 25). *Re-offending of adults: Results from the 2002 cohort.* Available at *www.homeoffice.gov.uk/rds/pdfs05/hosb2505.pdf*

Kider, S., MacKenzie, D. L., & Wilson, D. B. (2003). *Effects of correctional boot camps on offending: A Campbell collaborative systematic review.* Newbury Park, CA: Sage.

Lipsey, M. W. (1992). The effect of treatment on juvenile delinquents: Results from meta-analysis. In F. Lösel, T. Bliesener, & D. Bender (Eds.), *Psychology and law: International perspectives* (pp. 131–143). Oxford, UK: Walter de Gruyter.

Lipsey, M. W., & Wilson, D. B. (1998). Effective intervention for serious juvenile offenders: A synthesis of research. In R. Loeber & D. Farrington (Eds.), *Serious and violent juvenile offenders: Risk factors and successful interventions* (pp. 313–345). Thousand Oaks, CA: Sage.

Lipton, D.S. (2001). Therapeutic community treatment programming in corrections. In C. R. Hollin (Ed.), *Handbook of offender assessment and treatment* (pp. 155–175). Chichester, UK: Wiley.

Lipton, D. S., Pearson, F. S., Cleland, C. M., & Yee, D. (2002). The effectiveness of cognitive behavioural treatment methods on offender recidivism. In J. McGuire

(Ed.), *Offender rehabilitation and treatment: Effective programmes and policies to reduce re-offending* (pp. 79–112). Chichester, UK: Wiley.

Mackenzie, D. L., & Hebert, E. E. (Eds.). (1996). *Correctional boot camps: A tough intermediate sanction.* Washington, DC: National Institute of Justice.

Mann, R. E., Ginsburg, J. I. D., & Weekes, J. R. (2002). Motivational interviewing with offenders. In M. McMurran (Ed.), *Motivating offenders to change. A guide to enhancing engagement in therapy* (pp. 87–102). Chichester, UK: Wiley.

Martinson, R. (1974). What works?: Questions and answers about prison reform. *Public Interest, 35,* 22–54.

Martinson, R. (1979). New findings, new views: A note of caution regarding sentencing reform. *Hofstra Law Review, 7,* 243–258.

McConnaughy, E., Prochaska, J. O., & Velicer, W. F. (1983). Stages of change in psychotherapy: Measurement and sample profiles. *Psychotherapy: Theory, Research and Practice, 20,* 368–375.

Miller, W. R., C'de Baca, J., Matthews, D., & Wilbourne, P. (2001). *Personal Values Card Sort.* Retrieved July 4, 2005, from the University of New Mexico, Center on Alcoholism, Substance Abuse and Addiction Website, *casaa.unm.edu/inst/personal valuescardsort.pdf.*

Miller, W. R., & Rollnick, S. (2002). *Motivational interviewing: Preparing people for change* (2nd ed.). New York: Guilford Press.

Miller, W. R., & Tonigan, J. S. (1996). Assessing drinkers' motivation for change: The Stages of Change Readiness and Treatment Eagerness Scale (SOCRATES). *Psychology of Addictive Behaviors, 10,* 81–89.

Miller, W. R., Yahne, C. E., Moyers, T. B., Martinez, J., & Pirritano, M. (2004). A randomized trial of methods to help clinicians learn motivational interviewing. *Journal of Clinical and Consulting Psychology, 72,* 1050–1062.

National Institute of Justice. (1999). *Annual report on drug use among adult and juvenile arrestees.* Washington, DC: U.S. Department of Justice.

Pearson, F. S., & Lipton, D. S. (1999). A meta-analytic review of the effectiveness of corrections-based treatment for drug abuse. *Prison Journal, 79,* 384–410.

Petrosino, A., Turpin-Petrosino, C., & Buehler, J. (2002). Scared Straight and other juvenile awareness programs for preventing juvenile delinquency. *Annals of the American Academy of Political and Social Science, 589*(1), 41–62.

Porporino, F., & Fabiano, E. (2002). New Reintegration Program for Resettlement Pathfinders/Pre-Course Brochure. Ottawa, ON, Canada: T³ Associates.

Prochaska, J. O., & DiClemente, C. C. (1982). Transtheoretical therapy: Toward a more integrative model of change. *Psychotherapy: Theory, Research, and Practice, 19,* 276–288.

Project MATCH Research Group. (1997). Matching alcoholism treatments to client heterogeneity: Project MATCH posttreatment drinking outcomes. *Journal of Studies on Alcohol, 58,* 7–29.

Resnicow, K. (2002). *1-PASS coding system for motivational interviewing: Introduction and scoring.* Unpublished rating scale.

Smith, P., Goggin, C., & Gendreau, P. (2002). *The effects of prison sentences and intermediate sanctions on recidivism: General effects and individual differences.* Ottawa, ON, Canada: Solicitor General of Canada.

Wexler, H. K., DeLeon, G., Thomas, G., Kressel, D., & Peters, J. (1999). The Amity prison TC evaluation: Reincarceration outcomes. *Criminal Justice and Behavior,* 26, 147–167.

Wooldredge, J. (1988). Differentiating the effects of juvenile court sentences on eliminating recidivism. *Journal of Research in Crime and Delinquency,* 25, 264–300.

Motivational Interviewing in the Treatment of Psychological Problems

Conclusions and Future Directions

Hal Arkowitz
William R. Miller
Henny A. Westra
Stephen Rollnick

Motivational interviewing (MI) is a firmly established treatment for substance use disorders (Hettema, Steele, & Miller, 2005) and health-related problems (Rollnick, Miller, & Butler, in press). It has a solid research base to support its efficacy and is widely used in many different settings and countries. The time seems ripe to examine the extension of MI to other clinical problems. The chapters in this book represent significant beginnings of the application of MI and related procedures to mental health problems and populations not previously treated with MI. We hope that this work will serve as a catalyst for mental health practitioners and researchers to explore the utility of MI for the full range of psychological disorders. The chapters in this book represent the use of MI and related procedures with a variety of mental health problems and populations to facilitate treatment engagement and outcome.

- Westra and Dozois employed a four-session MI pretreatment to enhance the effects of subsequent CBT for anxiety disorders.
- Murphy employed an MI-related program to facilitate problem identification, motivation to change, and treatment engagement for combat veterans with PTSD.
- Tolin and Maltby used a multifaceted four-session intervention drawing from MI and other approaches to help facilitate treatment engagement of clients with obessive–compulsive disorder who refused to participate in exposure therapy.
- Zuckoff, Swartz, and Grote used an MI-related engagement session for depressed women who were not seeking therapy but who were in need of it.
- Arkowitz and Burke employed MI as an integrative framework for the treatment of depression into which other treatments such as cognitive-behavioral therapy (CBT) can be incorporated.
- Zerler used an MI-related approach with suicidal clients to evaluate suicide risk and facilitate subsequent treatment engagement.
- Treasure and Schmidt combined certain aspects of MI with a cognitive-interpersonal therapy approach for clients with eating disorders.
- Hodgins and Diskin developed a one-session MI-related intervention to increase the likelihood that problem gamblers would enter treatment and to enhance the efficacy of treatment.
- McCracken and Corrigan used MI to increase medication adherence for clients with schizophrenic spectrum disorders.
- Martino and Moyers developed an MI-related intervention to increase the motivation of psychotic clients to adhere to prescribed drug treatments.
- Farbring and Johnson described a country-wide application of MI in the Swedish correctional system that includes an individual five-session MI treatment to reduce drug use and recidivism as well as a program to train all prison and probation staff members in MI.

In these chapters, the authors used MI in a variety of ways. Some employed MI as described by Miller and Rollnick (1991) either as a pretreatment or a methodology employed throughout the course of the entire treatment (e.g., Westra & Dozois; Arkowitz & Burke; Zerler; Hodgins & Diskin; McCracken & Corrigan; and Farbring & Johnson). The others used selected components of MI or added other components to it. However, when only some elements of MI are employed (e.g., reflective listening) without the other elements of MI, or when MI is intermixed with other procedures, we consider the intervention to be MI-related but not "pure" MI. The latter includes the MI spirit (collaboration, evocation, autonomy), principles (express empathy, develop discrepancy, roll with resistance, and support self-efficacy) and methods, the most important of which is to elicit and differentially reinforce change and commitment talk to help resolve ambivalence, increase motivation to change, and promote behavior change. While we wish to be clear on what MI is and what an MI-related intervention is, we also wish to encourage the use of *any* methods that help clients.

The data presented by the authors suggest that MI and MI-related procedures have positively influenced the way treatment is conducted, resulting in the enhancement of treatment engagement and outcomes. The clinical applications of these procedures vary considerably in their degree of research support. Some chapters describe clinical proposals that can pave the way for research. Others present either pilot data or initial studies evaluating their approaches. Overall, the preliminary results seem very promising, though clearly much remains to be investigated and learned.

WHY HAS MI DIFFUSED SO RAPIDLY?

Among the many things yet to be understood with regard to MI is why it has diffused so rapidly. Since the publication of the first book on MI (Miller & Rollnick, 1991), the number of publications in the area has been doubling every 3 years, and there are now over 160 randomized clinical trials in print. Adoptions have spread rapidly through the addiction field, where MI was first employed, then into healthcare and health promotion, and most recently into correctional systems. The editors of this book are aware of numerous grant applications, papers in press, and research in progress examining applications of MI and MI-related approaches to a wide variety of clinical problems and populations. This volume represents yet another set of applications of MI as part of treatment in the service of mental health.

One source of its appeal is that MI directly addresses motivational problems that have long vexed the helping professions and that have received insufficient attention in the psychotherapy literature. Often clients were blamed for being "unmotivated," "noncompliant," "resistant," and for "not following through" with what their caregivers prescribed.

In the addiction treatment field this went as far as refusing to treat people with life-threatening conditions until they were sufficiently "ready." The helper's heart knows that there is something wrong with this picture. One contribution of MI has been a change in thinking, a realization that enhancing motivation for change is an important part of the therapist's job. Rather than waiting for sufficient suffering to render the person "ready" for treatment, or dismissing clients because they are "resistant to treatment," it is possible to evoke motivation for change. That makes it possible to treat a broader range of people and to do so earlier than might otherwise occur. This is a point of view that is sorely needed in the field of mental health. It also makes it possible to increase treatment engagement of those who need but are not receiving treatment, those who refuse certain treatments, and those already in treatment.

The MI approach also involves a shift in perspective to the therapist's being more evocative of motivation rather than trying to install it in another person, like software into hardware. MI is predicated on the idea that motivations for change are already there, and it is a matter of calling them forth rather than creating them. When people are suffering, the problem is not usually a lack of motivation for, but rather ambivalence about, change. They want it and yet they don't want it. MI is about resolving that ambivalence in the direction of change.

Many therapies seem to assume that just because a client shows up for a therapy session he or she is motivated, is willing to engage in the therapy, and lacks ambivalence about being in therapy or changing. This assumption is challenged by the resistance, modest adherence, and high dropout rates that are so often encountered in psychotherapy outcome studies as well as in community mental health centers and private practice. MI makes no such assumption. In MI, the client's motivation, engagement, and ambivalence are central and attended to not only in the initial stages but throughout the entire course of therapy.

The practice of MI offers a pleasant relief for clinicians from the alternative of "wrestling" with clients about change. It is quite a burden, and a significant source of professional frustration, to perceive that it's up to you as therapist to make your clients change. In this scenario, you are the champion of change and must overcome the dragons that guard the person's status quo. This is a very difficult battle to win. MI reframes the helper's work from wrestling to dancing. Working with client motivation is no longer a power struggle or contest of wills, but instead a collaborative endeavor.

Another reason for the rapid and continuing dissemination of MI and its expansion to other fields is that it often achieves at least modest success in relatively few sessions (Burke, Arkowitz, & Menchola, 2003; Hettema et al., 2005). Burke and colleagues (2003) found that the average number of MI sessions that clients received in the studies they reviewed was two, and the maximum was four. These brief treatments yielded substantial therapeutic effects. In Project Match (Project Match Group, 1997, 1998), four sessions of an MI-related procedure (motivational enhancement therapy) did as well as 12 sessions of other well-established therapies (CBT and 12-step approaches). However, a comparison of MI with four sessions of these other approaches would be needed to determine if indeed MI works faster. The majority of MI interventions discussed in this book were also rather brief, ranging from one to four sessions. The question of whether there is a "dose effect" for MI such that longer treatments will yield even larger effects is an intriguing one. There is evidence, at least, that a single session of MI is less effective than two or more sessions (Rubak, Sandbaek, Lauritzen, & Christensen, 2005).

The rapid dissemination of a complex treatment method also brings problems. Diffusion can result in a diffuse product. Clinicians invariably adapt the method to their own style, practices, and model of human nature. Adaptation is a natural part of the diffusion process (Rogers, 2003). Questions then arise as to what adaptations are feasible without losing the essence or efficacy of the core method.

Furthermore, practitioners often learn a new practice informally on their own, perhaps through reading or learning about it from colleagues, and misunderstandings can abound. We have witnessed clinicians practicing and trainers teaching "motivational interviewing" that was far from the spirit and method of MI as we understand it. If what they do is respectful of people in distress and is effective, in one sense it doesn't matter whether it's MI. Calling an approach something that it's not, however, can create confusion for people who want to learn it and for interpreting research on the treatment.

Related to the foregoing point are findings from clinical research that there is substantial variability in the effectiveness of MI across clinicians and settings. Even within a highly controlled clinical trial, clients' outcomes vary widely, depending on the clinician who delivers MI (Project Match Research Group, 1998). In addressing a particular problem, MI seems to work in some trials and not others, and its efficacy can even vary by site within a multisite trial (Carroll et al., 2006). This is not unique to, but is certainly characteristic of, MI in studies to date. This raises the question of what accounts for these differences in effectiveness among clinicians and sites. Answers to this question may help us to understand the nature of the effective ingredients of MI.

A further appeal of MI has emerged from recent research. One might expect that a brief intervention would be differentially effective for clients who have less severe problems. Research published to date, however, has yielded little evidence that this is so, and some studies suggest the opposite—that response to MI is greater with increased problem severity (e.g., Handmaker, Miller, & Manicke, 1999; McCambridge & Strang, 2004). Larger between-group effect sizes have been observed for MI with more severely (Bien, Miller, & Boroughs, 1993; Brown & Miller, 1993) than with less severely alcohol-dependent populations (Miller, Benefield, & Tonigan, 1993).

WHAT IS ESSENTIAL TO THE EFFICACY OF MI?

Every psychotherapy contains superstitious elements, components that are believed to be important but are, in fact, optional, inert, or perhaps even obstacles. The challenge is to separate the beliefs of progenitors and practitioners from the realities of clinical outcomes. This is best done not by armchair debate or individual case experience but rather through scientific methods that are designed specifically to test hypotheses and control for human biases. What components or processes of a psychotherapy are truly the "active ingredients" in facilitating change?

In this regard, clinical science is at a relatively young stage in understanding how and why psychotherapies work. Beyond studies to support the efficacy of specific methods for particular problems, attention has been given to hypothesized "common factors" or "common processes," specifiable principles that may promote change across a wide range of therapies (e.g., Arkowitz, 1997, 2002). Among the many common factors that have been proposed, the therapy relationship (Lambert & Barley, 2002) and empathy (Bohart, Elliott, Greenberg, & Watson, 2002) have received the most attention and have been shown to have substantial effects on the outcome of therapy, regardless of the type of therapy employed.

As with other psychotherapies, research is just beginning to clarify how and why MI exerts the effects that have been observed in clinical trials. This chapter is therefore not a mandate but a progress report.

Is It MI Yet?

Some years ago in a television commercial, a child watching as the parent stirred a cooking pot asked eagerly, "Is it soup yet?" We have faced a

similar challenge in training clinicians through successive approximations to the clinical method of MI. The same issue arises as we are asked
to provide fidelity checks for MI interventions being offered in clinical
trials. Practitioners do their best to practice what we preach, and the
question becomes "Is it MI yet?"

It is perhaps easier to recognize what is *not* MI. Painful early experience taught us that clinicians could adopt specific techniques from MI
but entirely miss the essence of the method, from our perspective. They
had the words but not the music. They were emitting MI-consistent responses, and yet it was not MI. In a study of training, Miller and Mount
(2001) found that after a workshop clinicians had incorporated a few
MI-consistent behaviors (such as reflective listening) into their existing
stew of practice habits, but the change was too small to make any real
difference to their clients.

The Spirit of MI

These experiences helped clarify what we believe to be the heart of
MI, the music or "spirit" of this method (Rollnick & Miller, 1995).
The specific treatment methods of MI emanate from and are offered in
service of this underlying spirit. Miller and Rollnick (2002) have described three characteristic elements of the spirit of MI that guide its
practice.

First, the MI spirit involves a *collaborative* client-centered approach. It is a way of working with and not "on" a fellow human being.
The relationship between the interviewer (clinician) and interviewee
(client) emphasizes partnership, what Buber called an I–thou relationship rather than an expert–subject (I–it) discourse (Buber, 1971; Buber,
Rogers, Anderson, & Cissna, 1997). We have likened it to sitting side
by side on a sofa, looking together at a picture album of the person's life.
The person turns the pages and tells the story, while the listener asks a
few gentle questions and seeks to understand the other's life experience.
The client-centered counseling style of Carl Rogers is closely akin to MI
and forms a strong foundation for its practice.

Second, the MI spirit is *evocative* in nature. It does not start from a
deficit model—that the person lacks crucial things that the counselor
can provide: insight, wisdom, knowledge, skills, and such. MI does not
communicate "I have what you need" but rather "You have what you
need." Motivation is not installed, but rather it is evoked from the client's own perspectives and values. To be sure, the counselor may provide expertise when invited by the client, but MI begins with respect for

and interest in the client's own values and perspectives. After all, it is the client's own reasons for change, and not the counselor's, that are likely to be the most persuasive.

Third, the MI spirit recognizes and honors the client's *autonomy*. Self-determination, the ability to choose how one will see and be, is one thing that can never be taken away from a human being, even by the most extreme privations (Frankl, 1963). In this sense, one can never "motivate" another person. No matter how much one may insist that "You can't let clients decide," or tell them what they "must" or "cannot" do, choice remains in the client's hands. Accepting and acknowledging this fact is part of the spirit of MI, and paradoxically it can open the door for change to happen.

These three characteristics of the MI spirit in turn clarify what MI is not. It is not about an expert telling people what they should or must do. It is not about "getting in the face" of clients to "make them see" a reality that is different from their own. MI is not about installing things that the person lacks, or tricking people into doing what they don't want to do. It is not "confrontational" in the usual sense of that term, although MI is all about helping people to explore possibly difficult and painful realities and come face-to-face with their choices.

This "spirit" of MI is not amorphous. Observers listening to counseling tapes can reliably rate its presence (Moyers, Martin, Catley, Harris, & Ahluwalia, 2003), and better client outcomes are predicted by these global ratings, above and beyond the practice of MI-specific behaviors (Moyers, Miller, & Hendrickson, 2005).

Therapist attitudes are of crucial importance in guiding the practice of MI. However, it is the directive component of MI that distinguishes it from client-centered therapy. MI is directive in the sense that it specifically attempts to help the client increase personal motivation to change, resolve ambivalence about change, and increase change talk. Use of the MI spirit without the directive components is not MI and is more similar to Rogers's client-centered therapy. In MI, change talk is consciously evoked by a variety of methods, such as asking particular open-ended questions, the answers to which involve the client's own desire, ability, reasons, and need for change. This is done with an empathic and supportive style, interested in and respectful of the client's own perceptions and experience. The client's personal motivations for change are reflected, affirmed, and collected in summaries. This is a departure from the usual inner experience of ambivalence, which is to think of a reason for change, then to think of a reason not to change, and then to stop thinking about it. MI keeps the process moving, with a goal of resolving ambivalence in the direction of therapeutic change. The specific techniques described in MI are used in service of this guiding axiom.

WHY DOES MI WORK?: THREE HYPOTHESES

Studying what components of MI are crucial to its efficacy points to a more fundamental question—of why this approach works at all. As MI has evolved, various hypotheses have emerged to explain its impact. Interestingly, they lead to somewhat different prescriptions about how MI should be practiced. All assume the presence of the MI spirit.

The first of these posits that people literally talk themselves into change. To the extent that people voice change talk, they tend to move in the direction of actual behavior change. Conversely, to the extent that clients argue against change, they are likely to continue on as before. There is evidence that certain aspects of in-session change talk do predict subsequent behavior change (e.g., abstinence from drugs) (Amrhein, Miller, Yahne, Palmer, & Fulcher, 2003) and that change is inversely related to the amount of resistance voiced during an MI session (Miller et al., 1993). From this it follows that the counselor should seek to differentially evoke and reinforce change talk, and also counsel in a way that minimizes resistance and client arguments against change. This was the original premise of MI (Miller, 1983), also reflected in Miller and Rollnick's (1991, 2002) books on the subject. This might be termed a *directive* hypothesis of MI, emphasizing the importance of differentially eliciting change talk.

A second account of how MI works might be called a *relational* hypothesis. In this perspective, the idea of selectively eliciting and reinforcing change talk is a nonessential aspect, and MI works primarily H-because of the underlying humanistic spirit in which the counselor provides the accepting and affirming client-centered atmosphere described by Carl Rogers (Rogers, 1980; Truax & Carkhuff, 1967). It is this quality of a counseling relationship that is therapeutic, and clients naturally move in the direction of positive change when counselors provide this facilitative atmosphere. This is essentially the underlying theory of nondirective client-centered counseling (Rogers, 1959). Research on the efficacy of client-centered therapy is consistent with this view (e.g., Elliott, Greenberg, & Lietaer, 2004).

The third explanation of MI could be called a *conflict resolution* hypothesis. In this view, it is important for the counselor to thoroughly explore *both* sides of the client's ambivalence: reasons to change and reasons to stay the same. This differs from the first (directive) theory in asserting that it is essential for the client to voice and explore counterchange motivations: the good things about the status quo and the downsides of change. In this perspective, counseling would be incomplete (and ineffective) if it failed to evoke from the client these counterchange as well as prochange arguments. The assumption is that when clients explore *both* sides of their dilemma in an empathic and accepting atmosphere, they naturally tend to resolve their ambivalence. In this sense a conflict resolution hypothesis overlaps with the relational hypothesis but departs from a purely client-centered perspective in the intentional and strategic evocation of both sides of the ambivalence.

Why would exploring both sides of ambivalence bring about change? An assumption here is that the person is immobilized by an active conflict between competing motivations, and it is the working through of this conflict that is crucial. This view has been elaborated by Engle and Arkowitz (2006) and draws heavily on work by Greenberg and his associates (e.g., Greenberg, Rice, & Elliott, 1993) and the early work of Dollard and Miller (1950) on approach–avoidance conflicts. Resolution of the conflict occurs when the two opposing sides become less antagonistic to and more integrated with each other (Clarke & Greenberg, 1986).

These causal hypotheses do lead to conflicting and testable predictions about the relationship between MI process and outcome. Perhaps the clearest point of divergence lies in the importance of having clients voice the disadvantages of change and the motivations for status quo. Intentional evoking of counterchange arguments is generally contraindicated within the directive hypothesis of MI, is foundational in the conflict resolution hypothesis, and is irrelevant within the relational hypothesis.

There is research evidence that relational components such as empathy promote behavior change (Bohart et al., 2002; Burns & Nolen-Hoeksma, 1992; Miller & Baca, 1983; Miller, Taylor, & West, 1980; Valle, 1981). There is also some indication that the directive component of MI adds efficacy beyond that accounted for by relational components (Lincourt, Kuettel, & Bombardier, 2002). The conflict resolution hypothesis remains to be operationalized and tested with regard to MI.

The chapters of this book reflect these varying perspectives on how MI works. Several place emphasis on the relational MI spirit. Several emphasize decisional conflict, advocating the strategic evocation of both prochange and counterchange arguments. Still others reflect a directive and strategic view of MI. It is possible that each of these hypothesized mechanisms contributes overall variance or accounts for change in a subgroup of clients receiving MI.

COMBINING MI AND COGNITIVE-BEHAVIORAL THERAPY

Given the prominence and effectiveness of cognitive-behavioral therapy (CBT) for a wide range of clinical problems, it is worthwhile to consider how MI might be integrated or combined with CBT. Such a combination or integration has much to recommend it. Most work in CBT assumes that the person is motivated to change and usually starts with work in the action stage. With very few exceptions (e.g., Leahy, 2002), CBT does not specifically address issues of motivation, resistance, or ambivalence. Perhaps by the addition of MI to CBT to address these issues, more clients will remain in CBT and cooperate with the tasks of therapy, leading to potentially better outcomes.

One of the clearest ways that MI and CBT may be combined is to use MI as a pretreatment to CBT. The work of Westra and Dozois (Chapter 2, this volume) points to the potential of an MI pretreatment to enhance client engagement and treatment efficacy of subsequent CBT for anxiety disorders. Connors, Walitzer, and Dermen (2002) similarly found positive effects for an MI pretreatment for alcoholism followed by a multifaceted treatment that included many aspects of CBT. They also found that the MI pretreatment was more effective than another pretreatment (a role induction interview) that had been shown to be effective in earlier studies. The amount of MI pretreatment can be tailored to the client's degree of readiness to engage in CBT. For example, Amrhein and colleagues (2003) found that two-thirds of clients responded well to one session of MI, but the remaining third showed reversal of gains when pressed to complete the process in a single session.

MI can be used not only as a pretreatment for CBT but also throughout the course of CBT as necessary. Problems related to low motivation and resistance can arise at any point in therapy. When such problems do arise during the course of CBT, the therapist may switch to MI for part of a session or for one or more sessions as necessary to resolve the resistance and increase the motivation to change.

Such an integrated psychotherapy was developed for the COMBINE study, a multisite trial of treatments for alcohol dependence. The Combined Behavioral Intervention began with motivational enhancement therapy and then proceeded to a menu of CBT modules delivered within the overall clinical style of motivational interviewing (Miller, 2004). Trial results showed that patients receiving this psychotherapy or a medication (naltrexone) or both had significantly better outcomes than those receiving placebo medication without psychotherapy (Anton et al., 2006).

Much of what is written about CBT speaks to the content of specific techniques. However, there is little written and much to learn about the *style* of conducting CBT. That is, much of the focus in the CBT literature is on *what* to do rather than *how* to do it. There is surprisingly little in the CBT literature on how to cultivate and maintain a positive and collaborative working relationship throughout therapy. It may be that the MI spirit can form a relational context for CBT that may enhance the outcome of treatment. However, it should be emphasized that the MI spirit is not unique to MI and, in itself, is not MI. Thus, using the MI spirit to conduct CBT is not really an integration of the two approaches. That would occur only when the principles and methods as well as the spirit of MI were employed. Using MI as a pretreatment as well as episodically throughout CBT as needed, and conducting CBT in the MI spirit, may hold promise for increasing engagement and outcomes in CBT and perhaps even other therapies.

It may be that such a style is particularly important with reluctant and ambivalent clients. Here, preserving autonomy, evoking the client's ideas about what might help or how you can help, and eliciting feedback may prove to be particularly critical to engaging such clients in treatment. As just one illustration, clients are often highly ambivalent about doing exposure therapy. Here, high doses of empathy and validation, developing discrepancy, and rolling with resistance may be crucial to navigating these impasses (see Tolin & Maltby, Chapter 4, this volume).

Much more remains to be discovered about how the manner of conducting CBT contributes to good (and poor) outcomes. Process research in CBT would be particularly important in explicating the principles of relationship that facilitate engagement with CBT. One study found that the therapist quality of empathy strongly predicted drinking outcomes in cognitive-behavioral treatment for alcohol problems (Miller et al., 1980). Marcus, Westra, Angus, and Stala (2007) studied clients' experiences of CBT who were in treatment for generalized anxiety disorder (GAD). They found that good-outcome clients consistently described the therapist as a "guide" in the service of achieving their goals and explicitly contrasted this with an expected, more authoritarian, directive style. One client remarked, "She [the therapist] was a teacher but not a director," Another noted that "I thought it [therapy] would be more opinion-based, but it was more about me than her." Rollnick and colleagues (in press) have described this guiding style of MI as intermediate between a directing-authoritarian style and a following-passive style. While future research needs to determine the causal direction of these findings, such results suggest that adopting an MI spirit in conducting CBT may hold promise in contributing to more positive engagement and better outcomes.

MEASUREMENT AND MECHANISMS IN MI

An important problem in MI research to date has been the frequent lack of clear specification of the treatment being delivered and tested (Burke et al., 2003). It is not sufficient to defer to a manual or describe the intended intervention. Even with careful training and supervision of practitioners, the implementation of MI can be highly variable. Documentation of what was actually delivered is thus essential. The gold standard for doing so is routine recording of MI sessions and systematic coding of sessions. Several coding systems have been developed for this purpose (Lane et al., 2005; Madson & Campbell, 2006; Madson, Campbell, Barrett, Brondino, & Melchert, 2005; Miller & Mount, 2001; Moyers et al., 2003; Moyers, Martin, Manuel, Hendrickson, & Miller, 2005). Such coding also permits informative analyses of the relationships between treatment processes and outcomes (Moyers, Miller, et al., 2005).

Despite the presence of good coding systems for MI sessions, more work needs to be done to measure the specific constructs of ambivalence and motivation. Measurement of these constructs is important for both clinical and research purposes. At the clinical level, reliable and valid measures of motivation and ambivalence can direct our work. To the extent that motivation is low and ambivalence is high, one would need to do more MI work to change the client's status on these measures. If motivation is high and ambivalence low, it's time to move into the action stage of treatment. Miller and Rollnick (2001) suggest various client behaviors that can be used as informal indices of these constructs. However, reliable and valid measures could be even more effective in guiding the clinician. Furthermore, having such measures could allow researchers to study more closely why MI works and to shed additional light on a theory of MI. Does MI indeed increase motivation and reduce ambivalence, and are such effects mediators of change? Right now, research has demonstrated that MI produces significant behavior change, but comparatively little is known about specifically why and how it works.

One promising lead for the measurement of motivation is change talk, particularly that which reflects a *commitment* to change (Amrhein et al., 2003). When such talk has been coded during therapy sessions, it has been found to significantly predict behavior change. Another promising lead is a self-report measure of motivation, including intrinsic motivation, developed by Pelletier, Tuson, and Haddad (1997) and based on Deci and Ryan's (1985) self-determination theory.

At present, there are no adequate measures of ambivalence. Engle and Arkowitz (2006) did a thorough search of the literature and found a number of measures of resistance, none of which were particularly strong, but no measures of ambivalence. Clearly, this is an area where further instrument development is needed.

REMAINING QUESTIONS

There are many other questions and issues relating to MI that need to be addressed. We have listed some of the main ones that have occurred to us below. The list is by no means exhaustive. In fact, it is typically the case in research that answering one question raises many more, so this list is just a beginning to stimulate the thinking of researchers and practitioners about MI.

• How effective is MI for problems other than substance abuse and health-related problems?" The work of the contributors to this book suggest that it may be highly applicable to many other problems, but rigorous randomized controlled trials for these and other problems are needed to answer this question. It may be that MI is more effective for some problems than others. Certain clinical problems, like anorexia, are known to be associated with high levels of resistance. Is MI better for such problems than those which may be less associated with resistance?

• How effective are different ways of using MI?" The chapters in this book demonstrate the remarkable flexibility of the MI approach. It has been used as a pretreatment and a complete treatment. It has also been used in combination with other treatment methods and could be used in a "shifting" manner in which the therapist conducting a different type of therapy shifts into MI when problems relating to resistance arise. Finally, it may be that MI can serve as an integrative framework into which other therapy methods could be incorporated. These different uses of MI need to be further developed and evaluated in controlled research with different people and problems.

• What is the comparative efficacy of MI?" More controlled studies are needed comparing the outcome of MI to outcomes of other established treatments such as CBT and for different people and problems. Furthermore, the comparative efficacy of MI on attrition rates, cooperation with the tasks of therapy, effects on associated problems, and maintenance of change also need to be evaluated.

• Is MI more effective than Rogers's client-centered therapy?" This question relates to the directive aspects of MI. How much, if anything, do they add to client-centered therapy, on which much of MI is based?

• Is MI more effective for some people than others?" Are there certain types of people who do better with MI than others? For example, some results from Project MATCH suggested that anger predicted positive outcomes for MI. This finding needs to be replicated. In addition, other individual differences (e.g., reactance, expectations for change) need to be examined as well to determine how personal characteristics might interact with treatment to influence outcome.

• What characteristics of the therapist are associated with high effectiveness in the use of MI?" Many studies have shown that therapists high in empathy are more effective in CBT and other therapies than those low in empathy. Is this true for MI? What other therapist characteristics may enhance the effects of MI?

• How effective is MI for different populations?" Is MI differentially effective for different age groups? Would children, adolescents, and the elderly do as well with MI as the adult age groups that have been the subjects in most MI studies? How effective is MI for different ethnic groups, inpatient populations, and for people with cognitive deficits?

• How effective is MI employed in couples, family, and group therapy formats?" What impact would it have on the outcome of MI if the focus were not on one but multiple interviewees who are in an intimate system?

• Would longer MI treatment lead to better treatment outcomes?" It's remarkable that MI has achieved the success that it has when it is typically used for relatively few (one to four) sessions. Would more sessions of MI produce better outcomes?

• What is the role of problem-related normative feedback in MI?" Many MI studies in the area of alcohol and substance abuse have included a feedback component in which the client is told where his or her problem ranks in severity as compared to others. Such feedback is not an integral part of the MI approach and yet is widely used. Does such feedback enhance the effectiveness of MI for alcohol and substance abuse? Is there a role for such feedback in such other problems as anxiety, mood, or eating disorders?

- What is the best way to train people in MI?" Recent studies (e.g., Miller & Mount, 2001; Miller, Yahne, Moyers, Martinez, & Pirritano, 2004) have found that the widely used format of introductory workshops to teach MI has only a minimal impact on participants' subsequent practice. Research is needed to evaluate new training formats and methods so that the trainees incorporate MI into their clinical practice consistently in the future.

CONCLUSIONS

We hope this book will stimulate innovations and extensions in the use of MI. The chapters in this book represent creative and flexible uses of MI and its application to clinical problems beyond substance abuse and health-related problems. While most of the chapters present only pilot data, these data generally point in a positive direction. We hope to see reports of the studies that emerge from this pilot data appearing in the literature in the near future.

While the extensive research in substance abuse and health has answered many questions and raised many others, more research and clinical innovation in the use of MI for other disorders and populations is needed as well, along with evaluations of the different uses and forms of MI. If this book serves as a catalyst for such research and practice, then we will have accomplished our goals.

REFERENCES

Amrhein, P. C., Miller, W. R., Yahne, C., Knupsky, A., & Hochstein, D. (2004). Strength of client commitment language improves with therapist training in motivational interviewing. *Alcoholism: Clinical and Experimental Research, 28,* 74A.

Amrhein, P. C., Miller, W. R., Yahne, C. E., Palmer, M., & Fulcher, L. (2003). Client commitment language during motivational interviewing predicts drug use outcomes. *Journal of Consulting and Clinical Psychology, 71,* 862–878.

Anton, R. F., O'Malley, S. S., Ciraulo, D. A., Cisler, R. A., Couper, D., Donovan, D. M., et al. (2006). Combined pharmacotherapies and behavioral interventions for alcohol dependence: The COMBINE study: A randomized controlled trial. *Journal of the American Medical Association, 295,* 2003–2017.

Arkowitz, H. (1997). Integrative theories of change. In S. Messer & P. Wachtel (Eds.), *Theories of psychotherapy: Origins and evolution* (pp. 227–288). Washington, DC: American Psychological Association Press.

Arkowitz, H. (2002). An integrative approach to psychotherapy based on common processes of change. In J. Lebow (Ed.), *Comprehensive handbook of psychotherapy: Vol. 4. Integrative and eclectic therapies* (pp. 317–337). New York: Wiley.

Bien, T. H., Miller, W. R., & Boroughs, J. M. (1993). Motivational interviewing with alcohol outpatients. *Behavioural and Cognitive Psychotherapy, 21,* 347–356.

Bohart, A. S., Elliott, R., Greenberg, L. S., & Watson, J. C. (2002). Empathy. In J. C. Norcross (Ed.), *Psychotherapy relationships that work: Therapist contributions and responsiveness to patients.* New York: Oxford University Press.

Brown, J. M., & Miller, W. R. (1993). Impact of motivational interviewing on participation and outcome in residential alcoholism treatment. *Psychology of Addictive Behaviors, 7,* 211–218.

Buber, M. (1971). *I and thou.* New York: Free Press.

Buber, M., Rogers, C. R., Anderson, R., & Cissna, K. N. (1997). *The Martin Buber–Carl Rogers dialogue: A new transcript with commentary.* Albany: State University of New York Press.

Burke, B. L., Arkowitz, H., & Menchola, M. (2003). The efficacy of motivational interviewing: A meta-analysis of controlled clinical trials. *Journal of Consulting and Clinical Psychology, 71,* 843–861.

Burns, D., & Nolen-Hoeksma, S. (1992). Therapeutic empathy and recovery from depression: A structural equation model. *Journal of Consulting and Clinical Psychology, 92,* 441–449.

Carroll, K. M., Ball, S. A., Nich, C., Martino, S., Frankforter, T. L., Farentinos, C., et al. (2006). Motivational interviewing to improve treatment engagement and outcome in individuals seeking treatment for substance abuse: A multisite effectiveness study. *Drug and Alcohol Dependence, 81,* 301–312.

Clarke, K. M., & Greenberg, L. S. (1986). Differential effects of the Gestalt two-chair intervention and problem solving in resolving decisional conflict. *Journal of Counseling Psychology 33,* 11–15.

Connors, G. J., Walitzer, K. S., Dermen, K. H. (2002). Preparing clients for alcoholism treatment: Effects on treatment participation and outcomes. *Consulting and Clinical Psychology, 70,* 1161–1169.

Deci, E. L., & Ryan, R. M. (1985). *Intrinsic motivation and self-determination in human behavior.* New York: Plenum Press.

Dollard, J., & Miller, N. E. (1950). *Personality and psychotherapy: An analysis in terms of learning, thinking, and culture.* New York: McGraw-Hill.

Elliott, R., Greenberg, L. S., & Lietaer, G. (2004). Research on experiential psychotherapies. In C. R. Snyder & R. E. Ingram (Eds.), *Handbook of psychological change: Psychotherapy processes and practices for the 21st century* (pp. 493–539). New York: Wiley.

Engle, D. E., & Arkowitz, H. (2006). *Ambivalence in psychotherapy: Facilitating readiness to change.* New York: Guilford Press.

Frankl, V. E. (1963). *Man's search for meaning.* Boston: Beacon Press.

Greenberg, L. S., Rice, L. N., & Elliott, R. (1993). *Facilitating emotional change: The moment-by-moment process*. New York: Guilford Press.

Handmaker, N. S., Miller, W. R., & Manicke, M. (1999). Findings of a pilot study of motivational interviewing with pregnant drinkers. *Journal of Studies on Alcohol, 60*, 285–287.

Hettema, J., Steele, J., & Miller, W. R. (2005). Motivational interviewing. *Annual Review of Clinical Psychology, 1*, 91–111.

Lambert, M., & Barley, D. E. (2002). Research summary on the therapeutic relationship and psychotherapy. In J. Norcross (Ed.), *Psychotherapy relationships that work* (pp. 17–36). New York: Oxford University Press.

Lane, C., Huws-Thomas, M., Hood, K., Rollnick, S., Edwards, K., & Robling, M. (2005). Measuring adaptations of motivational interviewing: The development and validation of the behavior change counseling index (BECCI). *Patient Education and Counseling, 56*, 166–173.

Leahy, R. L. (2002). *Overcoming resistance in cognitive therapy*. New York: Guilford Press.

Lincourt, P., Kuettel, T. J., & Bombardier, C. H. (2002). Motivational interviewing in a group setting with mandated clients: A pilot study. *Addictive Behaviors, 27*, 381–391.

Madson, M. B., & Campbell, T. C. (2006). Measures of fidelity in motivational enhancement: A systematic review. *Journal of Substance Abuse Treatment, 31*, 67–73.

Madson, M. B., Campbell, T. C., Barrett, D. E., Brondino, M. J., & Melchert, T. P. (2005). Development of the Motivational Interviewing Supervision and Training Scale. *Psychology of Addictive Behaviors, 19*, 303–310.

Marcus, M., Westra, H. A., Angus, L., & Stala, D. (2007, June). *Client experiences of cognitive behavioural therapy for generalized anxiety disorder: A qualitative analysis*. Paper presented at the annual meeting of the Society for Psychotherapy Research, Madison, WI.

McCambridge, J., & Strang, J. (2004). The efficacy of single-session motivational interviewing in reducing drug consumption and perceptions of drug-related risk and harm among young people: Results from a multi-site cluster randomized trial. *Addiction, 99*, 39–52.

Miller, W. R. (1983). Motivational interviewing with problem drinkers. *Behavioural Psychotherapy, 11*, 147–172.

Miller, W. R. (Ed.). (2004). *Combined Behavioral Intervention manual: A clinical research guide for therapists treating people with alcohol abuse and dependence* (COMBINE Monograph Series, Vol. 1; DHHS No. 04-5288). Bethesda, MD: National Institute on Alcohol Abuse and Alcoholism.

Miller, W. R., & Baca, L. M. (1983). Two-year follow-up of bibliotherapy and therapist-directed controlled drinking training for problem drinkers. *Behavior Therapy, 14*, 441–448.

Miller, W. R., Benefield, R. G., & Tonigan, J. S. (1993). Enhancing motivation for change in problem drinking: A controlled comparison of two therapist styles. *Journal of Consulting and Clinical Psychology, 61*, 455–461.

Miller, W. R., & Mount, K. A. (2001). A small study of training in motivational interviewing: Does one workshop change clinician and client behavior? *Behavioural and Cognitive Psychotherapy, 29*, 457–471.

Miller, W. R., & Rollnick, S. (1991). *Motivational interviewing: Preparing people to change addictive behavior.* New York: Guilford Press.

Miller, W. R., & Rollnick, S. (2002). *Motivational interviewing: Preparing people for change* (2nd ed.). New York: Guilford Press.

Miller, W. R., Taylor, C. A., & West, J. C. (1980). Focused versus broad spectrum behavior therapy for problem drinkers. *Journal of Consulting and Clinical Psychology, 48,* 590–601.

Miller, W. R., Yahne, C. E., Moyers, T. B., Martinez, J., & Pirritano, M. (2004). A randomized trial of methods to help clinicians learn motivational interviewing. *Journal of Consulting and Clinical Psychology, 72,* 1050–1062.

Moyers, T. B., Martin, T., Catley, D., Harris, K. J., & Ahluwalia, J. S. (2003). Assessing the integrity of motivational interventions: Reliability of the Motivational Interviewing Skills Code. *Behavioural and Cognitive Psychotherapy, 31,* 177–184.

Moyers, T. B., Martin, T., Manuel, J. K., Hendrickson, S. M. L., & Miller, W. R. (2005). Assessing competence in the use of motivational interviewing. *Journal of Substance Abuse Treatment, 28,* 19–26.

Moyers, T. B., Miller, W. R., & Hendrickson, S. M. L. (2005). How does motivational interviewing work?: Therapist interpersonal skill predicts client involvement within motivational interviewing sessions. *Journal of Consulting and Clinical Psychology, 73,* 590–598.

Pelletier, L. G., Tuson, K. M., & Haddad, N. K. (1997). Client Motivation for Therapy Scale: A measure of intrinsic motivation, extrinsic motivation, and amotivation for therapy. *Journal of Personality Assessment, 68,* 414–435.

Project Match Research Group. (1997). Matching alcoholism treatments to client heterogeneity: Project Match post-treatment drinking outcomes. *Journal of Studies on Alcohol, 58,* 7–29.

Project Match Research Group. (1998). Therapist effects in three treatments for alcohol problems. *Psychotherapy Research, 8,* 455–474.

Rogers, C. R. (1959). A theory of therapy, personality, and interpersonal relationships as developed in the client-centered framework. In S. Koch (Ed.), *Psychology: The study of a science: Vol. 3. Formulations of the person and the social contexts* (pp. 184–256). New York: McGraw-Hill.

Rogers, C. R. (1980). *A way of being.* Boston: Houghton Mifflin.

Rogers, E. M. (2003). *Diffusion of innovations* (5th ed.). New York: Free Press.

Rollnick, S., & Miller, W. R. (1995). What is motivational interviewing? *Behavioural and Cognitive Psychotherapy, 23,* 325–334.

Rollnick, S., Miller, W. R., & Butler, C. C. (in press). *Motivational interviewing in health care: Helping patients to change behavior.* New York: Guilford Press.

Rubak, S., Sandbaek, A., Lauritzen, T., & Christensen, B. (2005). Motivational interviewing: A systematic review and meta-analysis. *British Journal of General Practice, 55,* 305–312.

Truax, C. B., & Carkhuff, R. R. (1967). *Toward effective counseling and psychotherapy.* Chicago: Aldine.

Valle, S. K. (1981). Interpersonal functioning of alcoholism counselors and treatment outcome. *Journal of Studies on Alcohol, 42,* 783–790.

Index

Page numbers followed by *n* indicate note; *t* indicate table.